Minimally Invasive Therapy
of the Liver and Biliary System

Minimally Invasive Therapy of the Liver and Biliary System

James G. McNulty

with contributions by:
Andrew S. B. Chua
Michael G. Courtney
Brian G. Gazzard
John Keating
P. W. N. Keeling
Brian E. Lane
D. Henry Osborne

328 illustrations

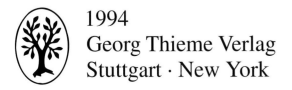
1994
Georg Thieme Verlag   Thieme Medical Publishers, Inc.
Stuttgart · New York   New York

Deutsche Bibliothek Cataloging-in-Publication Data

Minimally invasive therapy of the liver and biliary system /
James G. McNulty. With contributions by: Andrew S. B.
Chua ... – Stuttgart ; New York : Thieme ; New York :
Thieme Med. Publ., 1994
NE: McNulty, James

Cover drawing by Renate Stockinger

Important Note: Medicine is an ever-changing science un-
dergoing continual development. Research and clinical experience are continually expanding our knowledge, in particular our knowledge of proper treatment and drug therapy. In-
sofar as this book mentions any dosage or application, read-
ers may rest assured that the authors, editors and publishers
have made every effort to ensure that such references are in
accordance with the state of knowledge at the time of production of the book.

Nevertheless this does not involve, imply, or express any
guarantee or responsibility on the part of the publishers in
respect of any dosage instructions and forms of application
stated in the book. Every user is requested to examine carefully the manufacturers' leaflets accompanying each drug
and to check, if necessary in consultation with a physician or
specialist, whether the dosage schedules mentioned therein
or the contraindications stated by the manufacturers differ
from the statements made in the present book. Such examination is particularly important with drugs that are either rarely
used or have been newly released on the market. Every
dosage schedule or every form of application used is entirely
at the user's own risk and responsibility. The authors and
publishers request every user to report to the publishers any
discrepancies or inaccuracies noticed.

© 1994 Georg Thieme Verlag,
Rüdigerstraße 14, D-70469 Stuttgart, Germany
Thieme Medical Publishers, Inc., 381 Park Avenue South,
New York, N.Y. 10016

Typesetting by Druckhaus Götz GmbH,
D-71636 Ludwigsburg
(CCS-Textline [Linotronic 630])
Printed in Germany by K. Grammlich GmbH

ISBN 3-13-117901-5 (GTV, Stuttgart)
ISBN 0-86577-514-1 (TMP, New York)   1 2 3 4 5 6

To Linda, for all her help

Preface

> "A Man would do nothing if he waited until he could do it so well that no one could find fault with what he had done" –
> JOHN HENRY NEWMAN

The interventional physician requires the assistance, stimulation, and support of many colleagues and paramedical staff to successfully practice interventional or minimally invasive techniques. Competition and adversity stimulate the highest endeavor. Patient wellbeing and a successful outcome are the aims of minimally invasive therapy. These can only be achieved with practice, which leads to perfection. The continuing development and refinement of techniques improve the chance of success. Percutaneous procedures and endoscopic techniques have complications, and neither technique is supreme in the biliary tract. It is important to know when to refer patients to colleagues or to seek assistance when difficulties arise with the individual patient. We work closely with surgeons and endoscopists. This is essential for safe minimally invasive therapy. Diagnostic techniques in the liver and biliary tract should lead to interventional therapy immediately when abnormalities known to be treatable by these methods are discovered. Immediate therapy avoids known complications, such as sepsis, when biliary obstruction is demonstrated. The work of interventionalists over the past 10 years has shown that minimally invasive therapy, whether curative or palliative, has minimized patient discomfort, avoided unnecessary surgery, decreased morbidity, and reduced convalescent time. These are the aims of the procedures described in this text.

January 1994   James G. McNulty, Dublin

Acknowledgements

I wish to thank the contributors to this text for their support. I also thank my colleagues at the former Charitable Infirmary, Jervis Street, Dublin, Beaumont Hospital, Dublin and St. James's Hospital, Dublin, for referring patients for the procedures described in the various chapters. Without the expert assistance of the interventional nursing staff and the radiology technicians, the therapy described would not have been possible. The considerable help of Dr. Paul Brennan and Dr. Tony Farrell with editing and figure preparation is acknowledged. The expert assistance and help of Ms. Margaret Hadler, Ms. Betsy Solaro, and Mr. Helmut Schäfer of Thieme are gratefully acknowledged. Finally, I thank Ms. Clare E. McNulty for all her help in preparing the index.

Addresses

Andrew S. B. Chua, MD, MRCP
Department of Medicine & Gastroenterology
University of Dublin
Health Care Center
St. James's Hospital
Dublin 8, Ireland

Michael G. Courtney, MRCP,
Department of Medicine & Gastroenterology
Royal College of Surgeons in Ireland
Medical School
Beaumont Hospital
Dublin 9, Ireland

Brian G. Gazzard, MD, FRCP
Department of Gastroenterology
Chelsea & Westminister Hospital
London, SW10, U. K.

John Keating MD, MRCP
Department of Gastroenterology
Chelsea & Westminister Hospital
London, SW10, U. K.

P. W. N. Keeling, MD, FRCPI
Department of Medicine & Gastroenterology
University of Dublin
Health Care Center
St. James's Hospital
Dublin 8, Ireland

Brian E. Lane, FRCS, FRCS (Ed.), FRCSI
Department of Surgery
Royal College of Surgeons in Ireland
Medical School
Beaumont Hospital
Dublin 9, Ireland

James G. McNulty, MD, FRCR (Eng.)
Department of Radiology
University of Dublin
Health Care Center
St. James's Hospital
Dublin 8, Ireland

D. Henry Osborne, MD, FRCS
Department of Surgery
Royal College of Surgeons in Ireland
Medical School
Beaumont Hospital
Dublin 9, Ireland

Contents

Interventions for Benign Diseases of the Biliary Ducts 63

Introduction

Interventional radiology in the liver and biliary tract has much to offer the patient as an alternative to surgical treatment. It is now a well-established therapy for the hepatobiliary system. Generally radiologists are not primary-care physicians, and therefore patients are usually referred for interventional procedures by enlightened physicians and surgeons who consider such procedures more beneficial to certain patients than surgical therapy. Some interventions are curative, and some are palliative. Both types reduce morbidity and mortality, and success in one area leads to more referrals for similar procedures. Almost twenty years of interventional hepatobiliary procedures have shown that using care, acquired skills, high-quality imaging technology, modern needles, catheters and guide wires, and up-to-date endoscopic equipment, as well as having adequate nursing and technical personnel and working in a happy atmosphere, is best for successful results in individual patients and for the promotion of interventional radiology as a speciality within diagnostic radiology.

Within interventional radiology there is more than adequate material for development of the subspeciality of interventional hepatobiliary radiology. This group of interventional procedures is best promoted by good relations among physicians—surgeons, internists, and gastroenterologists. In hepatobiliary radiology the radiologist is supreme in imaging diagnosis and should be aware of all current advances in all modalities concerning the hepatobiliary system. If interventional radiologists wish respect for their speciality, they must have a good knowledge of the surgical and gastroenterologic literature of the hepatobiliary system and understand the pros and cons of both surgical and endoscopic procedures, which at times compete in providing alternative forms of minimally, invasive therapy, to avoid the confrontational battles for patients that have recently been reported in the international press:

Need a Costly Procedure? Don't Be Surprised if Your Doctors Fight to Perform it

By Eric Eckholm
New York Times Service

NEW YORK – The brain surgeons are jousting with the bone surgeons, the dermatologists are rubbing plastic surgeons the wrong way and the radiologists are fighting with nearly all their medical colleagues... – International Herald Tribune, Paris, July 8, 1991.

Radiologists doing interventional work should be concerned with preprocedure patient evaluation and postprocedure care in all forms of interventional radiology.

Proper evaluation of the patient before a procedure is as important as the successful carrying out of the procedure. Similarly, postprocedure care is as important, if not more important, to ensure a successful outcome for the patient. Follow-up of patients is of vital importance in order to continually improve methods of minimally invasive therapy. The referring clinician must never feel that the patient is being removed from his or her care but should be advised as to the possible immediate or delayed complications of procedures and how to best deal with them.

As mentioned elsewhere, external drainage catheters inserted in the interventional unit are not a high priority for nursing staff on a busy surgical ward. Therefore arrangements must be made for interventional staff to attend to such procedures as necessary in the wards or patient's room. A ward specially devoted to patient care in interventional radiology with a trained nursing staff who provides 24-hour cover is an ideal situation that exists in very few hospitals and clinics at present. An interventional ward close to the interventional suite would undoubtedly reduce morbidity, and complications could be dealt with before they become disasters for the patient. This ward would be used only while interventional work and immediate follow-up was being carried out and not for longer than 72 hours. The patient's physician would then continue to monitor progress. Consultations with gastroenterologists and surgeons could be held at the bedside with nurse and patient participation. Such consultations are more difficult in the surgical or internal medicine wards or units.

Short hospital stays are the ideal for patients, bed turnover times, increasing the number of patients treated, and cost saving, and are therefore to be desired as part of minimally invasive therapy. At all times, internal drainage is preferable for biliary interventions, and single-visit procedures are more welcome for the patient and his or her attending physician. It is also important to know when an interventional procedure is not indicated in a particular patient. Lack of awareness by physicians, surgeons, patients, and hospital administrators that an interventional service exists and that it has great importance in therapy of specific disorders hinders establishment of a sufficient workload to enable difficult procedures to be performed frequently enough that proficiency in a particular technique may be learned, improved, taught to radiologists in training, and maintained at a high level of success. Without sufficient referrals, proficiency in interventional techniques cannot occur, and if the success rate in any particular procedure is low, referrals even from pro-interventional clinicians soon cease. Radiologists who cannot practice self-referral have to align themselves with surgeons and internists and enlightened gastroenterologists if they wish to develop an efficient interventional service. Radiologists can benefit most from close interaction with these clinicians. A skilled and interested pathologist is a vital member of an interventional or minimally invasive therapy unit. The rivalries between gastroenterologists and interventional radiologists must be settled at a local level. This is best carried out by establishing protocols for specific interventions in a rational fashion with due regard to the respect one physician should show another in a different but competing speciality. Criticism of colleagues must be avoided. It must always be remembered that surgical colleagues should always be aware of the plans and consulted, if necessary, before major interventional procedures are performed.

The Anatomy of the Liver and Biliary System

1   The Anatomy of the Liver, Biliary Tract, and Pancreas

Gross Anatomy of the Liver

The liver, the largest glandular organ in the body, lies
in the right upper abdomen inferior to the diaphragm.
It occupies all of the right hypochondrium, most of the
epigastrium, and often extends into the left hypochondrium as far as the left mammary line. The liver
functions as an exocrine organ for bile secretion and
as a complex endocrine gland. It is brown-red and normally has a smooth surface due to the presence of a
thin connective covering (Glisson capsule). It has the
consistency of a soft solid (Goss 1971). The normal

adult liver weighs 1.2–1.6 kilograms. It is highly
vascular and easily lacerated. A knowledge of its surface anatomy is essential for all percutaneous diagnostic and interventional procedures involving the liver
and intrahepatic biliary ducts (Fig. 1.**1**).

The liver is shaped like an irregular hemisphere
with a relatively smooth convex diaphragmatic surface, which is protected laterally by the ribs, and a
more irregular concave visceral surface (Fig. 1.**2**).
The diaphragmatic area of the liver has four surfaces:
(1) anterior, (2) superior, (3) posterior, and (4) right.

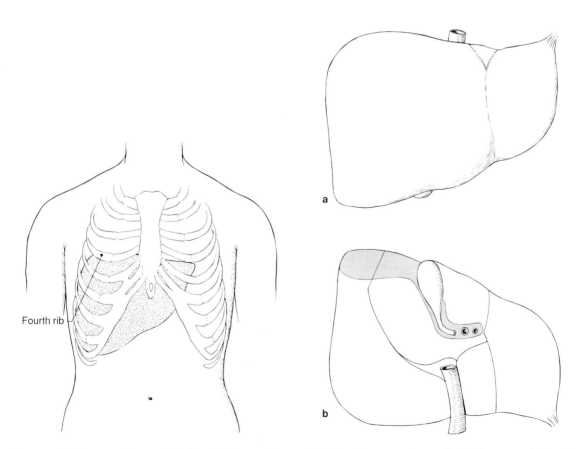

Fig. 1.**1**   **Surface markings of the liver** in the anterior–
posterior plane with the patient supine

Fig. 1.**2**   **Gross anatomy of the liver. a** anterior view.
b posterior view

1. The anterior surface is separated by the diaphragm from the sixth to tenth ribs and their costal cartilages on the right, and from the seventh and eighth costal cartilages on the left. In the median region it lies posterior to the xiphoid process of the sternum and the part of the muscular abdominal wall that is between the diverging costal margins. It is completely covered by peritoneum except along the line of attachment of the falciform ligament.

2. The superior surface is separated by the domes of the diaphragm from the pleura and lung on the right, and by the pericardium and heart on the left. The area near the heart is marked by a shallow concavity, the cardiac fossa. This surface is mostly covered by peritoneum, but along its dorsal part it is attached to the diaphragm by the superior reflection of the coronary ligament, which separates the part covered with peritoneum from the so-called bare area.

3. The posterior surface is broad and rounded on the right but narrow on the left. The central part presents a deep concavity that is molded to fit against the vertebral column and crura of the diaphragm. Close to the right of this concavity, the inferior vena cava lies almost buried in its fossa. Two or 3 centimeters to the left of the vena cava is the narrow fossa for the ductus venosus. The caudate lobe lies between these two fossae. To the right of the inferior vena cava, and partly on the visceral surface, is a small triangular depressed area, the suprarenal impression for the right suprarenal gland. To the left of the fossa for the ductus venosus is the esophageal groove for the cardiac antrum of the esophagus. A large area of the dorsal part of the diaphragmatic surface is not covered by the peritoneum. It is attached to the diaphragm by loose connective tissue. This uncovered area, frequently called the bare area, is bounded by the superior and inferior reflections of the coronary ligament.

4. The right diaphragmatic surface merges with the other three diaphragmatic surfaces and continues inferiorly to the right margin, which separates it from the visceral surface.

The visceral surface of the liver is concave and faces posteriorly, inferiorly, and to the left. It contains several fossae and impressions for neighboring viscera. A prominent marking of the left central part is the porta hepatis, a fissure for the passage of the blood vessels and main bile duct. The visceral surface is covered by peritoneum except where the gallbladder is attached to it and at the porta hepatis. The right lobe, which lies to the right of the gallbladder, has three impressions. On the right is the colic impression, a flattened or shallow area for the right colic flexure. More dorsally, a large and deeper hollow is the renal impression for the right kidney; and the duodenal impression is a narrow and poorly marked area lying along the neck of the gallbladder.

Between the gallbladder and the fossa for the umbilical vein is the quadrate lobe, which is in relation with the pyloric end of the stomach, the superior part of the duodenum, and the transverse colon. The left lobe, which lies to the left of the umbilical vein fossa, has two prominent markings. A large hollow extending out to the margin is the gastric impression for the ventral surface of the stomach. To the right it merges into a rounded eminence, the tuber omentale, which fits into the lesser curve of the stomach and lies over the ventral surface of the lesser omentum. Ventral to the inferior vena cava is a narrow strip of liver tissue, the caudate process, which connects the right inferior angle of the caudate lobe to the right lobe. Its peritoneal covering forms the ventral boundary of the epiploic foramen. The inferior border is thin and sharp and is marked opposite the attachment of the falciform ligament by a deep notch, the umbilical notch, and opposite the cartilage of the ninth rib by a second notch for the fundus of the gallbladder. In adult males this border generally corresponds with the lower margin of the thorax in the right mammary line, but in women and children it projects below the ribs. In the erect position it often extends below the interiliac line. The left border of the liver is thin and flat from above downward.

There are six gross anatomical configurations of the normal liver as studied by modern sectional imaging.

1. The entire liver lies to the right of the spine with its inferior margin lying in the eleventh intercostal space and its superior inferior axis at an angle of 45 degrees with the sagittal plane.
2. This is similar to (1), but an additional small area of liver is visible to the left of the spine.
3. The liver has the classic triangular shape with the lateral pole of the left lobe extending to the left as far as the midclavicular line.
4. This is similar to (3), but the medial segment of the left lobe is larger.
5. The right and left lobes are of equal size—horizontal liver.
6. The vertical liver is a variation of (1).

There is great variation in the distribution and relative sizes of the lobes and segments in the normal liver. These variations are readily demonstrated in all ultrasonic, radionuclide, computed tomographic, and magnetic resonance studies of the liver. These anatomical configurations are of obvious importance in all percutaneous interventional procedures in the liver and intrahepatic bile ducts. The normal position of the diaphragm, and hence the diaphragmatic pleura, in the right costophrenic angle is also of great importance if serious complications are to be avoided. On moderate inspiration in the supine position, the normal upper border of the liver lies at the level of the posterior third of the ninth right rib.

Segmental Anatomy of the Liver
(Table 1.**1**)
(Figs. 1.**3** and 1.**4**)

Anatomists recognize the right and left lobes of the liver separated by the falciform ligament and the caudate and quadrate lobes. For many years physiological liver lobes have been recognized. These are of great importance for modern liver surgery, and the segmental nature of the liver lobes and intrahepatic biliary ducts are important for all types of biliary drainage procedures. The physiological right and left lobes of the liver are separated by a line extending from the gallbladder fossa to the groove of the inferior vena cava superiorly. No surface markings indicate this physiological interlobar fissure. Vinyl acetate casts of the liver in which the hepatic veins are not injected demonstrate this main boundary fissure—the Cantlie line or "Hauptgrenzspalte" of Hjortsjo. The physiological divisions of the liver follow the anatomical distribution of the hepatic arteries, bile ducts, and portal veins. *The main interlobar fissure is occupied by the middle hepatic vein.* No significant branches of the bile ducts, hepatic arteries, or portal veins cross this interlobar fissure (Figure 1.**4**). The physiological right and left lobes are each subdivided into segments by a right and left segmental fissure.

1. The physiological right lobe is divided into two segments by an oblique right segmental fissure. It runs from a posterior inferior position inferiorly and anteriorly to the hilum.
2. The physiological left lobe is divided by the left segmental fissure into two segments. This fissure lies in the plane where the falciform ligament is attached to the parietal surface and is in line with the ligamentum venosum on the visceral surface.

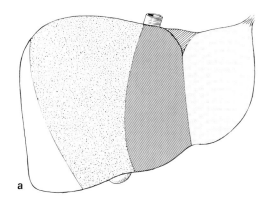

a

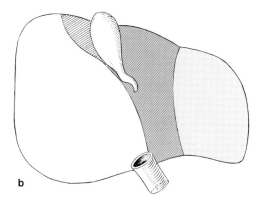

b

Fig. 1.**3** **Segmental anatomy of the liver**
a Anterior view showing the anterior and posterior segments of the right lobe, and the medial and lateral segments of the left lobe
b Posterior view showing the liver from below and behind the organ

Table 1.**1**   The segmental anatomy of the liver: a comparison of nomenclature

Couinaud	Reifferscheid	Healey and Schroy	Hjortsjo
Segment number			
I	Caudate lobe	Caudate lobe	Dorsal segment
II	Left lateralcranial	Lateralsuperior	Dorsolateral
III	Left lateralcaudal	Lateralinferior	Ventrolateral
IV	Left paramediocaudal (quadrate lobe)	Medialinferior	Dorsoventral
V	Right paramediocaudal	Anteriorinferior	Ventrocaudal
VI	Right lateralcaudal	Posteriorinferior	Dorsocaudal plus Intermediocaudal
VII	Right lateralcranial	Posteriorsuperior	Dorsocranial plus Intermediocranial
VIII	Right paramediocranial	Anteriorsuperior	Ventrocranial

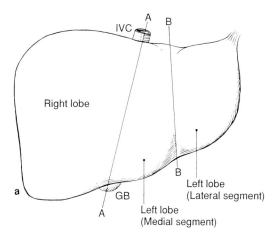

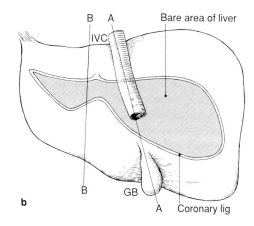

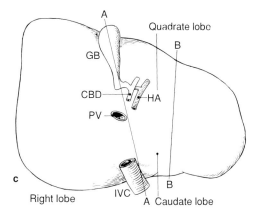

Fig. 1.**4 The physiological fissures and lobes of the liver**
a anterior view
b posterior view
c inferior view
A–A = the main interlobar fissure
B–B = the right segmental fissure
C–C = the left segmental fissure

PV   = portal vein
CBD = common bile duct
HA   = hepatic artery
IVC = inferior vena cava
GB   = gallbladder

Each segment is further divided into a superior and inferior area with one segemental bile duct and artery for that area except the medial segment of the left lobe, which has two bile ducts and two arteries for each area, and the caudate lobe, which has three bile ducts and two arteries—one bile duct for each part and one artery for the caudate process and the right half of the caudate lobe, and one artery for the left part of the caudate lobe.

The Intrahepatic Architecture (Fig. 1.5)

The human liver consists of columns of cells that radiate from a central vein and are interlaced in an orderly fashion by sinusoids. Each lobule has a portal tract at its periphery containing a biliary radicle, a hepatic artery, and a portal vein. Columns of cells extend between the systems of hepatic veins and portal triads. The two systems run in planes perpendicular to each other. The terminal portal radicle discharges blood into the sinusoids, and the direction of flow toward the central vein is determined by the higher pressure in the portal system. The sinusoid walls consist of endothelial cells, phagocytes of the reticuloendothelial system, and large granular lymphocytes (pit cells). The latter lie within the lumen but are attached to the sinusoidal wall. There is a potential space between the hepatocytes and the sinusoidal wall (the space of Disse), which contains tissue fluid that drains into lymphatic channels in the connective tissue of the peripheral areas. The hepatic arteries form a plexus around the bile ducts and supply the structures in the portal tracts. There are normally no direct arteriolar–portal vein anastomoses.

Bile secreted by hepatocytes passes through the network of bile canaliculi. It flows in the opposite direction to the plasma and enters small ductules or cholangioles. The junction between the hepatocyte and the adjoining bile ductule cell is called the canal of Hering. Cholangioles are less than 15 μm in diameter, are situated in the vascular area of an acinus at the periphery of a portal tract, and are not accompanied by vessels. They drain bile into interlobular bile ducts located in portal tracts. Interlobular ducts join to form septal ducts. Biliary columnar epithelium is lined by a basement membrane and surrounded by fibrous tissue containing many elastic fibers. All the bile ducts are supplied by a peribiliary vascular plexus that drains into the hepatic sinusoids. The biliary tract not only ex-

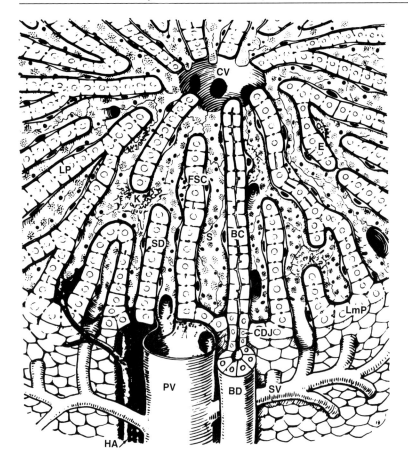

Fig. 1.**5   The intrahepatic architecture.** Three dimensional structure of the hepatic lobule (After Motta P, et al. The liver: an atlas of scanning electron microscopy. Tokyo: 1978 Igaku-Shoin.)

CV   = central vein
K   = Kupffer cell
FSC = fat storing cell
BC   = bile canaliculus
E   = endothelial cell
S   = sinusoid
SD   = space of Disse
HA   = hepatic artery branch
PV   = portal vein branch
CDJ = canal of Hering
BD   = interlobar bile duct
LmP = limiting plate
LP   = liver plate
SV   = septal branch of portal vein

cretes bile, but also is concerned with secretion and absorption. Bile leaves the liver in the extrahepatic biliary system. The bile ducts are lined by tall columnar epithelium and contain a subepithelial layer of connective tissue, elastic fibers, and some circular smooth muscle and mucous glands. The bile duct wall is 0.50 mm thick. In the gallbladder, bile is concentrated and stored. Concentration of bile is the result of complex processes that occur in the mucosa. The distal common bile duct has a thick wall and contains mucous glands within Beale saccules. Its lumen is narrow and villous, the muscular sphincter is formed by longitudinal and circular muscle fibers, and the duct is fixed to the duodenum by muscle fibers. The ampulla is lined with columnar epithelium arranged in long villous sheets and contains extensive smooth muscle fibers arranged in a circular fashion. The villous mucosa and the muscle fibers play antireflux roles.

The Intrahepatic Segmental Bile Ducts (Fig. 1. 6)

Recent studies have favored the terminology of Couinaud (1957) in describing segmental hepatic and bile duct anatomy.

The liver is divided into eight segments beginning with segment I—the caudate lobe, which lies posteriorly. Segment II is the superior lateral part of the left lobe. Segment III is the inferior lateral part of the left lobe. Segment IV is the quadrate lobe.

Segment V is the inferior part of the anterior segment of the right lobe. Segment VI is the superior part of the anterior segment of the right lobe. Segment VII is the superior part of the posterior segment of the right lobe, and segment VIII is the inferior part of the posterior segment of the right lobe. The bile ducts follow a lobar and segmental pattern, and anastomoses do not exist between the right and left lobe duct system except at the porta hepatis.

The segmental ducts in the anterior and posterior segments of the right lobe do not communicate within the liver.

seg
its
tra
live
to
joi
bile
late
the
ons
bla
var
bile
tion
pro
ves
duc
gall
peri
the
the
mai

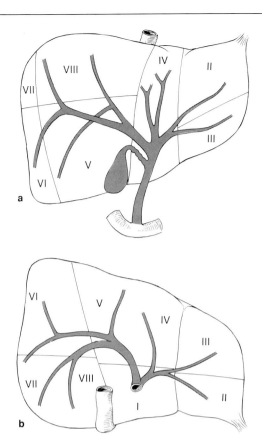

Fig. 1.**6**   **The segmental intrahepatic bile ducts**
a anterior view
b coronal view

a

b

c

d

Fig.
hepa

rately with the left hepatic duct to form the common hepatic duct, and in fact, that there are two right ducts, an anterior superior and a posterior inferior.

The Extrahepatic Bile Ducts
(Fig. 1.**7**)

Union of the right and left main ducts may occur within the liver or in the porta hepatis immediately after exit from the liver. The common hepatic duct descends in the free edge of the lesser omentum anterior to the foramen of Winslow.

The hepatic artery lies on the left, and the portal vein lies posteriorly. The common hepatic duct is 8 mm in diameter and varies in length from 1 cm to 5 cm depending on the position of the cystic duct junction. The common bile duct is formed by union of the cystic duct and the common hepatic duct. It descends in the hepaticoduodenal ligament, passes behind the first part of the duodenum, and lies in a groove in the head of the pancreas either wholly or partly covered by pancreatic tissue (Lytle 1959). The common bile duct varies from 15 mm to 90 mm in length depending on the site of cystic duct entry. The bile duct within the wall of the duodenum has a narrower lumen than the duct above the duodenum. The bile duct and pancreatic duct may join in the submucosa of the duodenum to form a common channel that opens into the papilla, or they may open separately into the duodenum. *The bile duct lies anterior or antero-lateral to the pancreatic duct.*

In 50%, the papilla of Vater is located in the middle of the descending duodenum on its posterior medial wall. In a few cases the papilla is located in the first

Variations in union of segmental ducts are common in both lobes of the liver. In 70% of cases the anterior and posterior segmental ducts of the right lobe unite to form the right hepatic duct at the porta hepatis. In 25% of cases the anterior or posterior segmental duct crosses the lobar fissure to join the left hepatic duct. The lateral segment of the left lobe is drained by two ducts, a superior and an inferior; the inferior duct is larger.

The medial segment drainage is more variable. In 60% of cases all four segmental ducts join to form a medial segmental duct, which is joined by the lateral segmental duct to form the left hepatic duct in the segmental fissure in 50% of cases, or to the right of the fissure in 45% of cases, or to the left of the fissure in 10% of cases. Caudate lobe bile ducts are difficult to demonstrate by direct cholangiography. The duct of the caudate process drains into the right hepatic duct. The duct of the left side of the caudate lobe drains into the left duct system.

The right hepatic duct is 9 mm long. The left hepatic duct is 17 mm long. Anatomical studies by Hjortsjo and Norman seem to indicate that the four segmental bile ducts from the right lobe join sepa-

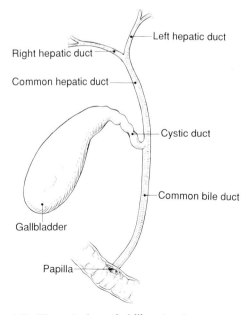

Fig. 1.**7**   **The extrahepatic biliary tract**

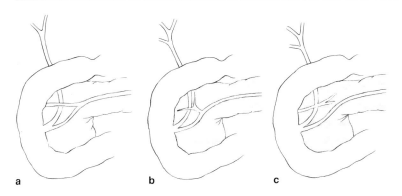

Fig. 1.12 Variations in pancreatic duct anatomy

a   b   c

ferior vena cava, the spine, the aorta, and the mesenteric artery and vein.

The tail extends to the splenorenal ligament. The organ averages 15.7 cm in length. Various shapes have been described. The organ may lie obliquely (50%), in an S shape (25%), or transverse (25%). Horseshoe and inverted V configurations have also been described. The annular pancreas encircles the descending duodenum.

Anteriorly, the pancreas is related to the lesser sac and posterior surface of the stomach. On the right is the duodenal loop and on the left the splenic hilum. Posterior to the head are the portal vein, the superior mesenteric vessels, and the common bile duct. The splenic artery and vein are behind the body. The inferior mesenteric vein, the inferior vena cava, and the aorta also lie posterior to the organ.

The Pancreatic Ductal System

There are two ductal systems for pancreatic drainage. The dorsal anlage is drained by the main duct. The ventral anlage is drained by the minor duct. The endocrine pancreatic tissue arises from the dorsal pancreas. In the head, the dorsal pancreas lies in front of the ventral anlage. The dorsal anlage forms the upper part of the head, the body, and tail. The ventral anlage forms the lower part of the head. The accessory duct may show many configurations. Figure 1.**11** shows the configuration in 50% of cases.

Other configurations are shown in Figure 1.**12**.

The main pancreatic duct runs from the tail through the body and head to the papilla. It lies near the posterior surface of the organ, and it is the only or most important duct in most cases.

The duct increases in width with age in the absence of disease. It measures 7.3 mm in diameter in the head, 5.7 mm in the body, and 2.5 mm in the tail.

The accessory duct may communicate with the main duct and with the duodenum via a minor papilla, or it may drain into the main duct or into the duodenum at the minor papilla without communicating with the main pancreatic duct (Fig. 1.**12c**).

References

1. Couinaud C. Le Foie, Masson, Paris, 1957.
2. Geber O. Surgical anatomy of the pancreas. In: Atlas of operative surgery: gallbladder, bile ducts, pancreas. Kremer K, Lierse W, Platzer W, et al., eds. Stuttgart: Thieme; 150–156, 1992.
3. Goss H. Gray's anatomy of the human body. 28th ed. Philadelphia: Lea and Febiger, 1971.
4. Healey JE, Schroy PC. Anatomy of the bile ducts within the human liver. Arch Surg 66 1953;599–616.
5. Hess W. Surgery of the biliary passages and pancreas. Princeton: D Van Nostrand, 1965.
6. Hjortsjo CH. The topography of the intrahepatic duct system. Acta Anat 1951;11:599–615.
7. Le Bail B, Balabaud C, Bioulac-Sage P. Anatomy and structure of the liver and biliary tree. In: Hepatobiliary Diseases. Prieto J, Rodes J, Shafritz DA, eds. Berlin: Springer, 1992:1–38.
8. Lytle WJ. The common bile duct groove in the pancreas. British J Surg 1959;47:209–212.
9. Mc Nulty JG. Radiology of the liver. Philadelphia: Saunders, 1977:1–26.
10. Norman O. Studies on the hepatic ducts on cholangiography. Acta Radiol (Suppl) 1951;84.
11. Reifferscheid M. Chirurgie der Leber. Stuttgart: Thieme, 1957.
12. Russell E, Yrizzary JM, Montalvo BM, et al. Left hepatic duct anatomy: Implications. Radiology 1990;174:353–356.

2 The Anatomy of the Arterial Supply to the Liver, Biliary Tract, and Pancreas

The arterial anatomy of the liver, pancreas, common bile duct, papilla of Vater, and head of pancreas is complex, variable, and important in the documentation of operability of neoplastic disease of these organs. Minimally invasive therapy involving endovascular procedures requires a detailed knowledge of the arterial supply of the liver, pancreas, bile ducts, and papilla. Anatomical variations often encountered during diagnostic studies involving ultrasound, computed tomography, or magnetic resonance imaging also require such knowledge.

The liver, biliary tract, and pancreas derive their entire arterial blood supply from the first and second branches of the abdominal aorta, the celiac artery and the superior mesenteric artery, and their branches.

The Celiac Artery

The classic celiac artery divides into the hepatic, splenic, and left gastric arteries. It arises from the front of the aorta at the level of the 12th thoracic first lumbar vertebrae, between the crura of the diaphragm a little below the aortic hiatus, and passes horizontally forward above the upper margin of the pancreas.

Anterior to the vessel is the lesser omentum, superior to it lies the left lobe of the liver and on either side lie the semilunar ganglia. The cardia of the stomach lies on the left and below are the upper borders of the pancreas and the splenic vein.

The Hepatic Artery (Fig. 2.1)

The common hepatic artery arises on the right side of the celiac artery and curves upward and to the right in the porta hepatis. Its terminal branches in the liver are a right, a left, and a middle hepatic artery. The latter supplies the quadrate lobe.

The common hepatic artery runs along the upper border of the head of the pancreas, forward and to the right behind the posterior layer of the peritoneum of the omental bursa. At the upper margin of the duodenum it courses anteriorly in the right hepatopancreatic fold. After passing through the two layers of the lesser omentum in the hepatoduodenal ligament, it ascends to the liver with the hepatic duct on its right and the portal vein posteriorly.

Most commonly, the hepatic artery arises from the celiac artery. However, in 18.5% of cases a partially or

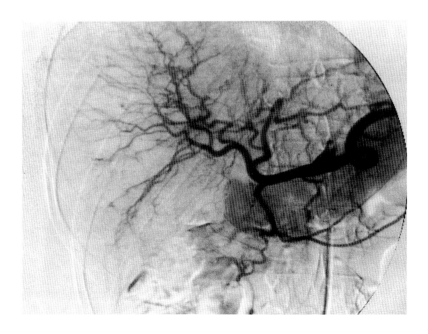

Fig. 2.**1** **Celiac axis arteriogram**

wholly replaced hepatic artery arises from the superior mesenteric artery (Fig. 2.**2**). Ten percent are replaced hepatic arteries; that is, there is no branch of the right hepatic artery arising from the celiac artery. Six percent are accessory right hepatic arteries; that is, they are present in addition to a corresponding right hepatic artery from the celiac artery. In 2.5% of cases, the common hepatic artery arises from the superior mesenteric artery.

Replaced or accessory hepatic arteries originating from the superior mesenteric artery behind the pancreas course upward to the right and behind or through the head of the pancreas before passing through the hepatopancreatic fold to the liver. Rarely, the left hepatic artery arises from the superior mesenteric artery.

The common hepatic artery ends with the origin of the gastroduodenal artery. The hepatic artery distal to the gastroduodenal artery is correctly termed the proper hepatic artery. This part of the artery ascends between the layers of the lesser omentum in the hepatoduodenal ligament. In most cases (85%) the right hepatic artery passes dorsal to the bile duct. Occasionally it is double; one artery crossing the duct anteriorly, the other posteriorly. A characteristic feature of the right hepatic artery is a caterpillar-like loop it often makes in the cystohepatic angle. The loop, in some instances, is sufficiently low to reach the cystic duct, where it may be injured easily during surgery.

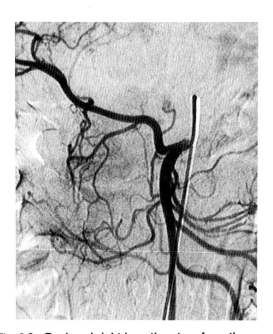

Fig. 2.**2** **Replaced right hepatic artery from the superior mesenteric artery.**

The Intrahepatic Segmental Arteries

The right hepatic artery divides into three to six branches. One branch supplies the caudate lobe; the other branches enter the liver superior to the point of entry of the portal vein.

The right hepatic artery supplies the physiological right lobe of the liver including the anterior and posterior segments and their superior and inferior divisions (segment V, VI, VII, and VIII). The anterior segmental artery lies close to the gallbladder fossa at its origin. It may be injured at cholecystectomy. The cystic artery may arise from the anterior segmental artery in some cases.

A branch of the right hepatic artery to the area above the caudate process of the caudate lobe may be mistaken at surgery for the cystic artery, especially when the right hepatic artery originates from the superior mesenteric artery and passes behind the bile duct. The left lobe of the liver has a more varied arterial supply. In 75% of cases the left hepatic artery is a single vessel arising from the proper hepatic artery. It enters the left lobe inferior to the left branch of the portal vein and then courses upward in the fissure for the ligamentum venosum, where it gives branches to both segments of the left lobe. In 25% of cases either the entire left hepatic artery or an accessory left hepatic artery originates from the left gastric artery. The left hepatic artery supplies the lateral segment of the left lobe (segments II and III) and most of the medial segment of the left lobe (segment IV) and part of the caudate lobe (segment I) in some cases. There is considerable variation in the segmental branching of the left hepatic artery.

The medial segmental branch of the left hepatic artery is termed the middle hepatic artery.

The middle hepatic artery supplies the medial segment of the left lobe (segment IV and part of segment I).

Hepatic artery branches in the liver are end arteries, and accessory hepatic arteries are vital to the area of liver tissue they supply. Corrosive cast studies of the hepatic arteries have failed to demonstrate direct arterial communications between lobes and segments within the liver, however, selective arteriography has demonstrated blood flow from the right or left hepatic artery by injecting one artery selectively. Cross flow from right to left or left to right is easily demonstrated when there are anomalous vessels, such as a replaced right hepatic artery.

Variations in the Origins of the Hepatic Arteries

Variations in the origins of the hepatic arteries are extremely frequent and include:

1. The textbook "normal." The right, middle, and left hepatic arteries originate from the common hepatic branch of the celiac artery.
2. A replaced right hepatic artery from the superior mesenteric artery and the left and middle hepatic arteries from the common hepatic branch of the celiac artery.
3. The right and middle hepatic artery arises from the celiac common hepatic, and the left hepatic from the left gastric artery (10%).
4. The right, middle, and left hepatic from the celiac common hepatic artery and a left hepatic accessory artery from the left gastric artery (8%).
5. The right, left, and middle hepatic arteries from the celiac common hepatic and an accessory right hepatic artery from the superior mesenteric artery (6%).
6. The right, middle, and left hepatic arteries from the celiac hepatic artery, an accessory right hepatic from the superior mesenteric artery, and an accessory left hepatic artery from the left gastric artery (1%).
7. The entire common hepatic artery replaced by the superior mesenteric artery (2.5%).
8. A replaced left hepatic artery from the superior mesenteric artery.

The Cystic Artery

The cystic artery arises from the right hepatic artery to the right of the hepatic duct in the triangle of Calot. In 20% of cases it arises from the common hepatic, left hepatic, middle hepatic, gastroduodenal, or retroduodenal artery crossing the hepatic duct in such cases. In 25% of cases it is double. These arteries may arise from the right hepatic, or, one branch from the right hepatic and one from the superior mesenteric artery (Figure 2.**2**). On reaching the gallbladder, it divides into a superficial and a deep branch. The former supplies the peritoneal surface of the gallbladder, the latter the nonperitoneal surface.

The cystic artery is important in endovascular interventional radiology since it must be identified prior to embolization in liver tumors or in hemobilia. Cystic artery occlusion leads to gallbladder necrosis. *Anomalous cystic arteries may be injured during laparoscopic cholecystectomy.*

The Gastroduodenal Artery

The gastroduodenal artery most commonly (75%) arises from the common hepatic artery but may arise from the right hepatic (7%), left hepatic (11%), or superior mesenteric artery via a replaced hepatic trunk (3.5%). It descends behind the first part of the duodenum, anterior to the pancreas, and divides into the right gastroepiploic and the anterior superior pancreaticoduodenal arteries.

In the majority of instances (90%) the gastroduodenal artery gives rise to the retroduodenal artery. This artery arises above or behind the duodenum and the head of the pancreas, where it gives rise to the blood supply of the common bile duct in the form of an epicholedochal plexus. It descends along the left side of the common bile duct, crosses its supraduodenal portion anteriorly (in some cases posteriorly), then runs along the right side of the common bile duct to the middle of the posterior surface of the head of the pancreas behind the intrapancreatic portion of the common bile duct and anastomoses with the posterior inferior pancreaticoduodenal artery to form the posterior pancreaticoduodenal arcade. Branches of this arcade supply the posterior surface of the duodenum, and to a lesser extent, the head of the pancreas (Figure 2.**3**).

The anterior superior pancreaticoduodenal artery arises from the gastroduodenal artery behind the first part of the duodenum, runs behind the peritoneum between the descending part of the duodenum and the pancreas into the head of the pancreas; on exiting from the head of pancreas posteriorly it anastomoses with the anterior inferior pancreaticoduodenal artery, which arises from the superior mesenteric artery to form the anterior pancreaticoduodenal arcade. The anterior and posterior arcades may vary from one to four in number. *The posterior arcades lie superior to the anterior arcades.* These arcade patterns are very complex, and one or both arcades may arise from, or terminate in a right hepatic artery arising from the superior mesenteric artery. The right gastroepiploic artery is the final termination of the gastroduodenal artery. It supplies the pylorus, passes along the greater curve of the stomach in the anterior layers of the great omentum, supplies the greater curve of the stomach, and anastomoses with branches of the right and left gastric arteries and the left gastroepiploic artery, a branch of the splenic artery. Anterior branches of the right and left gastroepiploic arteries descend between the two layers of the great omentum to its free edge and turn superiorly to become the posterior epiploic arteries, which join the large epiploic arcade in the posterior layers of the great omentum below the transverse colon. They may also anastomose with the descending posterior epiploic arteries derived from the transverse pancreatic artery.

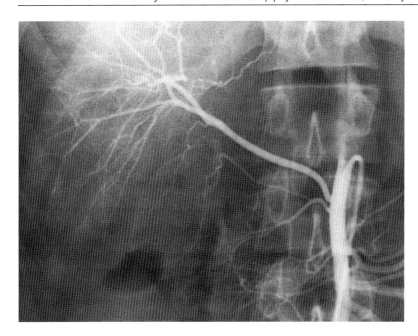

Fig. 2.**3** **Cystic arteries arising from the right hepatic and superior mesenteric arteries**

The posterior epiploic arcade is formed by the right and left epiploic arteries; the former from the right gastroepiploic branch of the gastroduodenal artery, the latter from the left gastroepiploic branch of the splenic artery. Branches from the omental arcades anastomose with branches from the middle colic artery, left colic artery, inferior pancreaticoduodenal artery, all branches of the superior mesenteric artery, and with the transverse pancreatic artery a secondary branch of the splenic artery. These omental arcades are important potential channels for collateral blood flow.

The Right Gastric Artery

The right gastric artery arises from the common hepatic or left hepatic in 80% of cases, or from the gastroduodenal artery (8%) or the middle or right hepatic artery (5%). It is small and often difficult to find on arteriography. It descends to the pylorus, turns to the left, and courses along the lesser curve of the stomach, where it has an inconstant anastomosis with the left gastric artery. The right gastric artery frequently gives rise to the supraduodenal artery, which supplies the first 3 centimeters of the duodenum and the transition zone between it and the pylorus of the stomach.

The Left Gastric Artery

The left gastric artery, after its origin from the celiac artery, courses upward and to the left toward the gastric cardia, where it turns sharply downward and passes along the lesser curve of the stomach to the pylorus to anastomose, in some cases, with the right gastric artery. It gives branches to the lower end of the esophagus, and in 3% of cases the left inferior phrenic artery arises from it. In 25% of cases the left gastric artery gives rise to an aberrant left hepatic artery. This is a replaced left hepatic artery in 12% of cases and an accessory left hepatic artery in 13% of cases.

The Splenic Artery

The splenic artery arises from the celiac artery, takes a short loop to the right, and then courses to the left in a tortuous manner along the upper border of the pancreas, above the splenic vein, and ultimately to supply the spleen. The artery is divided into four segments for descriptive purposes. The first segment lies above the pancreas and is 1–3 cm long. The second segment is usually also suprapancreatic. It is variable in length and very tortuous, especially in the aged. The third segment runs along the anterior surface of the pancreas. The fourth segment lies between the tail of the pancreas and the splenic hilum. It terminates in the spleen in several branches that are end arteries. In its course it carries the blood supply to the pancreas and stomach. The first important branch of the artery is the dorsal pancreatic artery, which arises from the first segment in 40% of cases. This artery arises from other sources in 60% of cases, such as the right hepatic (12%), superior mesenteric (14%), and celiac artery (22%). The dorsal pancreatic artery lies behind the junction of the superior mesenteric and splenic veins. It descends and supplies the posterior surface of the pancreas and gives off the transverse pancreatic artery, which courses to the left to supply the body and tail of the pancreas.

It gives off two branches to the right; one supplies the unicate process, the other anastomoses with the anterior superior pancreaticoduodenal artery, the gastroduodenal artery, or the right gastroepiploic artery. *A fourth important branch of the dorsal pancreatic artery descends in some cases below the border of the pancreas to anastomose with the superior mesenteric artery or to form the middle colic artery.*

The arteria pancreatica magna arises from the second segment of the splenic artery, descends behind the pancreatic duct, and joins the transverse pancreatic artery. The arteries to the tail of the pancreas are often multiple, arise from the third and fourth segments of the splenic artery and its terminal branches, enter the tail, and join branches of the arteria pancreatica magna and of the transverse pancreatic artery. The left gastroepiploic artery arises from the splenic artery near its termination and passes down and to the right along the greater curve of stomach. The superior and inferior terminal branches of the splenic artery supply the spleen. Superior and inferior splenic polar arteries arise from the splenic artery or the celiac artery (superior) giving two splenic arteries. The inferior polar artery commonly arises from the left gastroepiploic artery.

The Superior Mesenteric Artery

The superior mesenteric artery arises from the aorta below the celiac artery, usually at the level of the first vertebra posterior to the body of the pancreas and the splenic vein. It emerges from the lower border of the pancreas, passes forward to the upper border of the third part of the duodenum, and descends anteriorly over the uncinate process of the pancreas. Usually, the middle colic artery arises from it just before entering the mesentery. Within the mesentery the artery courses to the right lower quadrant of the abdomen, curving with a gentle convexity to the left. Reaching the cecum, it anastomoses with the ileocolic artery, thus forming the superior mesenteric loop. The superior mesenteric vein lies to the right of the artery in its course through the mesentery. An early right-sided branch of the superior mesenteric artery is the inferior pancreaticoduodenal artery. In 50% of cases this artery arises from or in common with the first jejunal artery from the left side of the superior mesenteric artery. Two inferior pancreaticoduodenal arteries occur in 60% of cases and a common inferior pancreaticoduodenal artery in 40% of cases. The inferior pancreaticoduodenal artery passes to the right behind the mesenteric vein to anastomose with the superior pancreaticoduodenal arteries dorsal to the head of the pancreas. The anterior inferior artery anastomoses with the anterior superior artery; the latter is a branch of the gastroduodenal artery.

The posterior inferior artery anastomoses with the posterior superior artery (retroduodenal artery), also a branch of the gastroduodenal artery. In 60% of cases a small artery joins the first jejunal artery to the inferior pancreaticoduodenal artery, thus providing an additional anastomosis if the superior mesenteric artery is occluded.

Collateral Arterial Pathways to the Liver

Mitchels (1955) described 26 collateral arterial pathways to the liver. By selective arteriography it is possible to demonstrate several of these arterial routes including:

1. By a replaced or accessory right hepatic artery from the superior mesenteric artery;
2. By a replaced or accessory left hepatic artery from the left gastric artery;
3. By the right and left gastroepiploic arteries, the gastroduodenal artery, and short gastric arteries;
4. By the right and left gastric arteries;
5. By the pancreatic arcade from the splenic to the gastroduodenal artery;
6. By the superior mesenteric artery via the pancreaticoduodenal arteries and the gastroduodenal artery to the hepatic branch of the celiac artery;
7. By the inferior phrenic arteries to peripheral branches of the intrahepatic arteries on the diaphragmatic surface of the liver;
8. By the ascending artery of the common bile duct from the gastroduodenal artery or retroduodenal artery;
9. By paraesophageal arteries, retroesophageal arteries and anastomoses in the porta hepatis.

References

1. Becker CD, Cooperberg PL. Sonography of the hepatic vascular system AJR 1988;999–1005.
2. Brash JC. Cunningham's Manual of Practical Anatomy. 11th ed. London: Oxford University Press, 1948:233–297. (Thorax and Abdomen; vol 2.).
3. Couinaud C. Le Foie. Paris: Masson, 1957.
4. Le Bail B, Balabaud C, Bioulac-Sage P. Anatomy and structure of the liver and biliary tree. In: Priesto J, Rodes J, Shafritz DA, eds. Hepatobiliary Diseases. Berlin: Springer, 1992:1–38.
5. Gans H. The anatomy of the intrahepatic structures and its repercussions on surgery. Amsterdam: Elsevier, 1955.
6. Lunderquist A. Arterial segmental supply of the liver. Acta Radiol 1967; (suppl. 272):14–80.
7. Michels NA. Blood supply of the upper abdominal organs. Philadelphia: Lippincott, 1955.
8. Nebesar RA, Kornblith PL, Pollard JJ. Celiac and superior mesenteric arteries. Boston: Little Brown and Company, 1969:9–34.
9. Liver, Biliary Tract, and Pancreas. In: Netter, FH. The Ciba Collection of Medical Illustrations. Ciba, New Jersey, 1964:14–19.

3 The Anatomy of the Portal Venous System of the Liver

The liver receives its blood supply from two sources, the portal vein and the hepatic artery. Normally the portal vein supplies 70–80% of the blood to the liver, and the hepatic artery supplies the remaining 20–30%. The hepatic artery is normally a high-pressure source of blood supply to the organ, and the portal vein is a low-pressure system. Occlusion of the hepatic artery increases portal vein flow, and occlusion of the portal vein markedly increases arterial flow to the organ. The portal system of veins includes all the veins that drain blood from the gastrointestinal tract and from the spleen, pancreas, and gallbladder. From these viscera, blood is conveyed to the liver by the portal vein. In the liver, the vein divides like an artery and ends in capillary-like vessels termed sinusoids. From the sinusoids, blood is conveyed to the inferior vena cava by the hepatic veins. In the adult, the portal vein and its tributaries are valveless (Fig. 3.1).

The Main Portal Vein

The portal vein is a short vein, about 8 cm long and 9–14 mm in diameter (3). It has a thick wall that contains more smooth muscle than a systemic vein of a corresponding caliber. The main portal vein is formed by union of the splenic and superior mesenteric veins behind the neck of the pancreas anterior to the inferior vena cava at the level of the second lumbar vertebra. It passes superiorly and to the right, at a 45 to 60 degree angle to the lumbar spine, behind the first part of the duodenum and ascends in the right border of the lesser (gastrohepatic) omentum to the right side of the porta hepatis, where it divides into a right and a left branch, which accompany the corresponding branches of the hepatic artery into the substance of the liver. In the lesser omentum it is placed posterior to and between the common bile duct and the hepatic artery, the former lying to the right of the latter. *The portal vein divides outside the parenchyma of the liver.* The right branch enters the right lobe after receiving the cystic vein. The left branch is longer and smaller in diameter and supplies branches to the caudate lobe and quadrate lobe before entering the left lobe of the liver. As it crosses the left sagittal fossa, it is joined anteriorly by a fibrous cord, the ligamentum teres (obliterated umbilical vein), and is united to the inferior vena cava by a second fibrous cord, the ligamentum venosum (obliterated ductus venosus).

The portal vein is surrounded by the hepatic plexus of nerves and is accompanied by numerous lymph vessels and some lymph nodes. There is some evidence for streaming of blood flow in the portal vein, with blood from the splenic vein passing preferentially to the left lobe, caudate lobe, and quadrate lobe and blood from the superior mesenteric vein going to the right lobe.

The Splenic Vein

The splenic vein commences by the union of many tributaries that carry blood from the spleen. These unite to form a single vessel that passes from left to right, making a groove on the superior and dorsal part of the pancreas inferior to the splenic artery, and ends

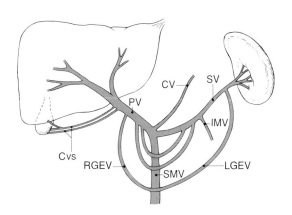

Fig. 3.**1** **The portal venous system**

SV   = splenic vein
PV   = portal vein
SMV = superior mesenteric vein
RGEV = right gastroepiploic vein
LGEV = left gastroepiploic vein
Cvs = cystic veins
IMV = inferior mesenteric vein

dorsal to the neck of the pancreas by uniting at a right angle with the superior mesenteric vein to form the main portal vein. The splenic vein is not tortuous like the artery. The tributaries of the splenic vein are:

1. *The short gastric veins.* These are four or five in number and drain the fundus and left part of the greater curve of the stomach. They pass between the two layers of the gastrolienal ligament to end in the splenic vein or one of its large tributaries.
2. *The left gastroepiploic vein* receives tributaries from both the anterior and posterior surfaces of the stomach, and from the greater curve of the stomach. It ends in the splenic vein.
3. *The pancreatic veins* consist of several small vessels that drain the body and tail of the pancreas and open into the trunk of the splenic vein.
4. *The inferior mesenteric vein* returns blood from the rectum, the sigmoid colon, and the descending colon. It begins in the rectum as the superior rectal vein, which has its origin in the rectal plexus. Through this plexus it communicates with the middle and inferior rectal veins. The superior rectal vein leaves the lesser pelvis, crosses the left common iliac vessels with the superior rectal artery and continues upward like the inferior mesenteric vein. This vein lies to the left of the artery and ascends under cover of the peritoneum and anterior to the left psoas major; it then passes dorsal to the body of the pancreas and enters the splenic vein, or in some cases, in the angle of union of the splenic and superior mesenteric veins, or drains into the superior mesenteric vein.
5. *The superior mesenteric vein.* The superior mesenteric vein carries blood from the small intestine, the cecum, the ascending colon, and the transverse colon. It begins in the right iliac fossa by union of the veins that drain the terminal ileum, cecum, and appendix and ascends between the two layers of the mesentery. In its course it passes anterior to the right ureter, the inferior vena cava, the inferior part of the duodenum, and the lower part of the head of the pancreas. Dorsal to the neck of the pancreas, it unites with the splenic vein to form the portal vein. The superior mesenteric vein receives blood from the jejunal veins, ileal veins, ileocolic, right colic, and middle colic veins, and from the right gastroepiploic vein and the pancreaticoduodenal venous arcade. The latter include the superior and inferior pancreaticoduodenal veins; the inferior group may join the right gastroepiploic vein, which receives blood from the greater omentum, from the anterior and posterior surfaces of the stomach, and anastomoses with the left gastroepiploic vein. It runs from left to right along the greater curve of the stomach between the layers of the greater omentum.
6. *The coronary (left gastric) vein.* The coronary vein receives veins from both surfaces of the stomach. It runs from right to left along the lesser curve of the stomach between the layers of the lesser omentum to the cardia, where it receives some esophageal veins. It then turns downward and passes from left to right dorsal to the peritoneum of the lesser sac and ends in the portal vein.
7. *The pyloric vein* is a small vein that drains the pyloric end of the lesser curve of the stomach. It runs from left to right in the lesser omentum and ends in the portal vein.
8. *The cystic veins* are several small vessels that drain blood from the gallbladder, accompany the cystic duct, and drain into the right branch of the portal vein.
9. *The paraumbilical veins* are several veins that establish an anastomosis between the veins of the anterior abdominal wall and the portal vein, and the internal and common iliac veins. The most important is a vein that commences at the umbilicus and runs posteriorly and superiorly in or on the surface of the ligamentum teres between the layers of the falciform ligament and terminates within the liver in the left branch of the portal vein. This vein is a frequent portal–systemic collateral route in portal hypertension (Juttner et al. 1982). Recent studies of the intrahepatic portal system of veins using Doppler ultrasound have documented important venous flow patterns within the intrahepatic veins and the development of new venous channels in the left lobe of the liver communicating with paraumbilical veins in severe portal hypertension with cirrhosis (13).

The Intrahepatic Distribution of the Portal Vein

The right branch of the portal vein is 2–3 cm in length. It passes laterally to the right, where it divides into anterior and posterior segmental veins. These subdivide further into superior and inferior subsegmental veins. The right anterior segmental vein may arise from the left branch of the portal vein. The left branch of the portal vein is longer and narrower than the right. Two parts of this branch have been described.

These are a transverse part, which lies in the liver hilum, and an umbilical part, which lies in the left segmental fissure. The transverse part is 2–4 cm long. The vein then bends anteriorly and laterally to form the umbilical segment, which immediately gives off to the superior part of the lateral segment of the left lobe. The distal end gives rise to the veins for the inferior part of both the medial and lateral segments.

The superior part of the medial segment receives a portal vein from the concavity of the umbilical segment.

The caudate lobe receives veins from the right portal vein close to the main division and veins from the

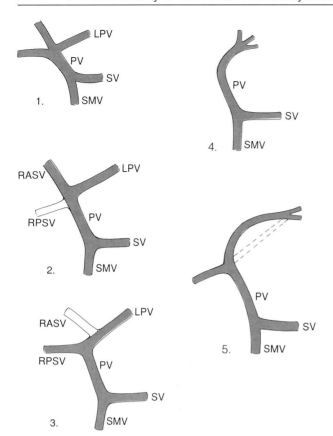

Fig. 3.**2** **The intrahepatic veins and their variations** (modified after 1)

PV   = main portal vein
SV   = splenic vein
RPSV = right posterior segmental branch
RASV = right anterior segmental branch

transverse part of the main branch of the left portal vein.

Atri et al. (1992) showed congenital anomalies of the intrahepatic portal veins in 20% of 507 patients examined using ultrasound (Fig. 3.**2**).

The main anomalies were: (1) Trifurcation of the main portal vein due to direct origin of the right anterior and posterior segmental veins from the portal vein (10.8%); (2) The right posterior segmental vein arose directly from the main portal vein before its bifurcation (4.7%); (3) The right anterior segmental vein arose from the left portal vein (4.3%); (4) Absent horizontal segment of the left portal vein (0.1%).

These authors noted that slight variations of the "normal" distribution are commonly seen. These include a short main right portal vein, a short horizontal segment of the left portal vein, segmental veins of varying disproportional size, and a segmental vein that often has the same size as the liver segment it supplies. Couinaud (1957) reported a 20% incidence of intrahepatic portal vein anomalies in anatomical studies. Such abnormalities may have significance for interventions within the liver that involve intrahepatic portal systemic stent shunts. Before stent insertions, careful ultrasonic studies of the portal system within the liver are necessary because of the high incidence of such anomalies.

Table 3.**1** Anomalies of the intrahepatic portal vein

1. Trifurcation	11.0%
2. RPSV from main vein	5.0%
3. RASV from the left portal branch	4.0%
4. Absent right branch portal vein	0.01%
5. Absent horizontal segment left portal branch	0.2%

RPSV right posterior segmental branch
RASV right anterior segmental branch
(Modified after 1)

Portal–Systemic Anastomoses
(Fig. 3.**3**)

Anastomoses normally exist between the portal and systemic systems of veins. Any of these anastomotic sites may play an important part in providing spontaneous portal decompression in the presence of por-

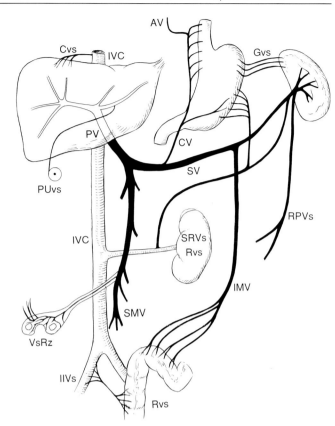

Fig. 3.**3**   **Portal systemic anastomoses**

Gvs = gastric veins
AV = azygos vein
IMV = inferior mesenteric vein
Rvs = rectal veins
IIVs = internal iliac veins
SRVs = suprarenal veins
RVs = renal veins
Vs Rz = veins of Retzius
IVC = inferior vena cava
SV = splenic vein
RPVs = retroperitoneal veins
PUvs = paraumbilical veins
Cvs = capsular veins

tal hypertension. The known anatomical communications are:

1. Anastomoses of the gastric veins and the esophageal veins that drain to the azygos system.
2. Anastomoses of the inferior mesenteric veins with the rectal veins and the internal iliac veins.
3. The veins of Retzius in the mesentery of the small intestine.
4. Anastomoses of the gastric veins with the left suprarenal and renal veins and the inferior vena cava.
5. Anastomoses of the splenic veins and the retroperitoneal veins.
6. Anastomoses of the left branch of the portal vein with the paraumbilical veins and the superficial epigastric veins and the iliac veins.
7. Anastomoses from the intrahepatic portal vein via capsular veins to the inferior vena cava especially via the bare area of the liver.

Portoportal Collaterals in Extrahepatic Portal Hypertension

The main portoportal collaterals are:

1. Splenic vein–short gastric veins–coronary vein–portal vein.
2. Splenic vein–left gastroepiploic–right gastroepiploic–portal vein.
3. Splenic veins–omental veins–superior mesenteric vein–portal vein.

4. Splenic vein–pancreaticoduodenal veins–cystic veins–portal vein.
5. Portal vein–pancreaticoduodenal veins–cystic veins–hilar portal veins.

The Anatomy of the Inferior Vena Cava and the Hepatic Veins

The Inferior Vena Cava (Fig. 3.**4**)

The common iliac veins are formed opposite the sacroiliac joints by the confluence of the external and internal iliac veins bilaterally. The inferior vena cava originates behind and to the right of the common iliac artery where the right and left iliac veins unite. The largest vein in the body drains all the blood from the lower limbs, pelvis, and abdomen into the right atrium. It runs superiorly and to the right from the fifth lumbar vertebra to the diaphragm, where it is separated from the aorta by the right, medial, and intermediate crura of the diaphragm and the caudate lobe of the liver. Posterior to the liver, it passes through the fossa venae cavae, pierces the diaphragm, and enters the right atrium. Anteriorly it is covered by peritoneum and crossed by the right spermatic artery, the transverse colon, the root of the mesentery, the duodenum, the head of the pancreas, the portal vein

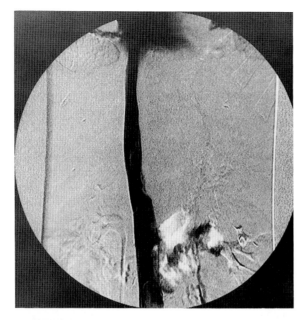

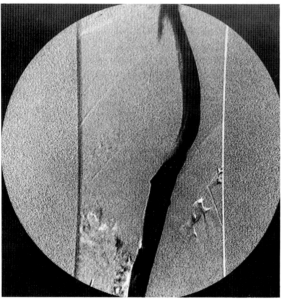

Fig. 3.**4**   **The inferior vena cava**
DSA study; **a** anterior **b** lateral view in hepatomegaly associated with hepatic vein thrombosis.

and the liver. Posteriorly it is related to the lumbar vertebrae, the psoas muscle, the right lumbar arteries, the right renal artery, and the right medial crus of the diaphragm.

On the left lies the aorta and on the right the peritoneum, ureter, right kidney, and liver.

The hepatic veins

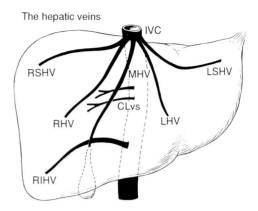

Fig. 3.**5**   **The hepatic veins**

RHV = right hepatic vein
LHV = left hepatic vein
MHV = middle hepatic vein
RSHV = right superior hepatic vein
RIHV = right inferior hepatic vein
LSHV = left superior hepatic vein
CLvs = caudate lobe veins

The Hepatic Veins (Figs. 3.**5** and 3.**6**)

The hepatic veins drain blood from the liver into the inferior vena cava within the posterior surface of the liver and are usually inserted into its anterior and lateral walls. Three main veins, the right, middle, and left, return most of the blood from the liver to the systemic circulation. In 50% the middle and left hepatic veins unite and enter the vena cava as a single channel. The caudate lobe has its own draining veins, which open directly into the vena cava anteriorly and to the left side. The right, middle, and left veins are valveless. They commence as filiform structures, draining the sinusoids, and intercommunicate at the segmental and subsegmental levels. They do not follow the segmental distribution of the intrahepatic arteries or biliary ducts. The hepatic veins lie in the major intersegmental fissures.

The right hepatic vein drains the posterior segment of the right lobe and most of the superior part of the anterior segment of the right lobe. It lies in the intersegmental plane and separates the anterior and posterior segments of the right lobe.

The middle hepatic vein lies mostly in the main fissure and separates the right and left lobes of the liver. It drains the inferior part of the anterior segment of the right lobe and the superior part of the medial segment of the left lobe.

The left hepatic vein drains the lateral segment of the left lobe and the superior part of the medial segment of the left lobe.

The right superior hepatic vein drains an area bound by the coronary ligament and usually joins the right hepatic vein, but may drain directly into the inferior vena cava.

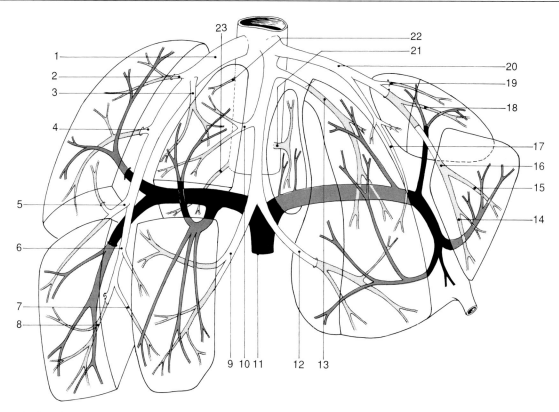

Fig. 3.**6** **Detailed anatomical study of the hepatic veins showing the left intermediate vein of Hess**
(Modified after 2)

1. Right hepatic vein
2. Right posterior vein
3. Posterior internal vein
4. Transversal vein
5. Right anterior transversal vein
6. Right anterior trunk
7. Right anterior internal vein
8. Right anterior external vein
9. Right anterior vein
10. Right posterior vein
11. Trunk of middle hepatic vein
12. Left anterior vein

13. Left posterior vein
14. Anterior branch
15. Transverse branch
16. Left saggital vein
17. Fissural vein
18. Left transverse vein
19. Posterior vein
20. Trunk of left hepatic vein
21. Left retrohepatic vein
22. Middle right retrohepatic vein
23. Inferior right retrohepatic vein

The left superior hepatic vein drains the area marked by the left triangular ligament and enters directly into the inferior vena cava. This vein may be injured during surgery at the esophageal hiatus.

Variations in liver shape affect the location of the hepatic veins. The right inferior hepatic vein drains the right inferior part of the posterior segment of the right lobe. This vein is important in the hemodynamics of the Budd–Chiari syndrome and in surgical resections of the right lobe of the liver.

The ultrasonic and angiographic anatomy of the inferior vena cava and the hepatic veins has assumed new importance with the stent shunt procedure for minimally invasive therapy of portal hypertension and in the assessment of liver tumor localization and operability.

The arrangement of right, middle, and left hepatic veins is present in 70% of cases. More than three main hepatic veins are present in 30% of patients. Twenty percent of cases have two left hepatic veins; three percent have two middle hepatic veins; and 8% have two right hepatic veins. Six percent have an accessory right hepatic vein draining directly into the inferior vena cava below the level of the normal hepatic veins. Hess (1965) described an additional vein that he termed an "intermediate vein" between the left and middle hepatic veins that drains an area of parenchyma about 4 cm wide in the area of the falciform ligament, and drains into the left hepatic vein or into the inferior vena cava directly. This vein was demonstrated by Masselot and Leborgne (1978) also and termed the small umbilical vein. This vein is single in 70% of cases and drains part of segment IV when the middle hepatic vein is ligated (Scheele 1989).

References

1. Atri M, Bret PM, Fraser-Hill MA. Intrahepatic portal venous variations prevalence with ultrasound. Radiology 1992; 184:157–158.
2. Baird RA, Britton RC. The surgical anatomy of the hepatic veins: variations and their implications for auxillary lobar transplantation. J Surg Res 1973;15:345–347.
3. Couinaud C. The hepatic pedicle. 1. The intrahepatic portal vein. In: Couinaud C, ed. The liver: anatomic and surgical studies. Paris: Masson, 1957:71–118.
4. Dawson P, Dunn G. Intraarterial digital subtraction venography (IA DSA) of abdominal vessels. Acta Radiol 1989;30:109–111.
5. Doehner G, Ruzicka F, Hoffman G, Rousselet L. The portal venous systems: its roentgen anatomy. Radiology 1951; 57:691–701.
6. Douglass BE, Baggenstoss AH, Hollinstead WH. The anatomy of the portal vein and its tributaries. Surg Gynecol Obstet 1950;91:562–576.
7. Elias H, Petty D. Gross anatomy of the blood vessels and ducts within the human liver. Am J Anat 1952;90:55–111.
8. Flament JB, Delattre JF, Palot JP, et al. Le foie, rappel anatomo-radiologique Ann Gastroenterol Hpatol 1985;21:3–11.
9. Franco D, Smadja C, Kahwaji F, et al. Segmentectomies in the management of liver tumours. Arch Surg 1988;123:519–522.
10. Hardy KJ. The hepatic veins. Aust NZ J Surgery 1972; 42:11–14.
11. Hess W. Surgery of the biliary passages and the pancreas. Princeton: Van Nostrand, 1965:31–32.
12. Hill MC, Dach JL, Shawker TH. Ultrasonography in portal hypertension. Clin in Gastroenterol 1985;14:83–104.
13. Juttner HU, Jenny JM, Ralls PW, et al. Ultrasound demonstration of portosystemic collaterals in cirrhosis and portal hypertension. Radiology 1982;142:459–463.
14. Lafortune M, Madore F, Patriquin H, Breton G. Segmental anatomy of the liver. Radiology 1991;181:443–448.
15. Makuuchi M, Hasegawa H, Yamazaki S, et al. The inferior right hepatic vein: ultrasound demonstration. Radiology 1983;148:213–217.
16. Marks CL. The portal venous system. Springfield: Thomas, 1973:1–39.
17. Masselot R, Leborgne J. Anatomical study of the hepatic veins. Anat Clin 1978;1:109–125.
18. McNulty JG. Normal anatomy. In: Radiology of the liver. Philadelphia: Saunders, 1977:19–22.
19. Morin C, Lafortune M, Pomier G, et al. Patent paraumbilical vein: Anatomic and hemodynamic variants and their clinical importance. Radiology 1992;185:253–256.
20. Mukai JK, Stack CM, Turner DA, et al. Imaging of surgically relevent hepatic vascular and segmental anatomy. Part 1, Normal anatomy. AJR 1987;149:287–292.
21. Nakamura S, Tsuzuki T. Surgical anatomy of the hepatic veins and the inferior vena cava. Surg Gynecol Obstet. 1981;152:43–50.
22. Norhagen A. Selective angiography of the hepatic veins. Acta Radiol 1963;(Suppl 221).
23. Scheele J. Segment orientated resection of the liver: rationale and technique. In: Lygidakis NJ, Tytgat GNJ, eds. Hepatobiliary and Pancreatic Malignancies. Stuttgart: Thieme, 1989:219–247.
24. Weinreb J, Kumari S, Phillips G, Pochaczevsky R. Portal vein measurements by real time sonography. AJR 1982;139:497–499.

4 Anatomy of the Duodenum and Duodenal Papilla

The duodenum is the shortest and widest part of the small intestine. It measures 25 cm to 30 cm in length and 3.5 cm to 5 cm in diameter. It forms a single curve in its course when the stomach is empty, and its termination in the jejunum is only a little to the left of its commencement. Distension of the stomach and movement of the pylorus to the right make the curve of the duodenum U shaped rather than circular. The loop of the duodenum does not all lie in one plane. The beginning of the duodenal bulb (first part) and the greater portions of the third and fourth parts occupy a coronal plane, while the termination of part one, the second part, and the beginning of the third part bend backward on the right of the inferior vena cava and occupy a sagittal plane. The duodenal loop surrounds the head of the pancreas. The duodenum has no mesentery and is only partly covered by peritoneum.

Anatomy textbooks describe four parts in the duodenum (Fig. 4.**1**).

1. The first part, or pars superior, is the most variable in length and direction. It extends from the mobile pylorus of the stomach to the region of the neck of the gallbladder. Posteriorly it is related to the head of the pancreas, the portal vein, the common bile duct, and the gastroduodenal artery. Anteriorly it is related to the liver and anterior abdominal wall.

2. The second part, or descending duodenum, commences below the neck of the gallbladder opposite the right side of the first lumbar vertebra and passes inferiorly to the level of the third or fourth lumbar vertebra, where it turns sharply inward to join the third part. Posteriorly it is related to the right kidney, the renal vessels, the right ureter, and the psoas muscle. Medially it is related to the head of the pancreas. The common bile duct descends behind the left border of this part of the duodenum, and the pancreatic duct accompanies it for a short distance.

3. The third, or horizontal part of the duodenum is 6–8 cm long. It begins on the right of the third or fourth lumbar vertebra, passes to the left and upward to the left side of the aorta and joins the ascending, or fourth part of the duodenum.
   Posteriorly it is related to the right psoas muscle, the inferior vena cava, the aorta and the left psoas muscle. Superiorly it is related to the head of the pancreas. The superior mesenteric artery and vein groove its anterior surface.

4. The fourth, or ascending part of the duodenum passes upward on the left side of the aorta to the level of the second lumbar vertebra, where it turns anteriorly to join the jejunum at the duodenojejunal flexure. It is related posteriorly to the left psoas muscle, the left renal vein and the medial side of the left kidney. Anteriorly it is related to the peritoneum and the stomach. The termination of the duodenum is suspended by the ligament of Treitz from the right crus of the diaphragm.

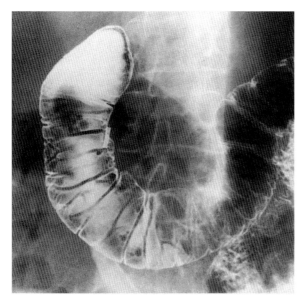

Fig. 4.**1 The anatomy of the duodenum.** The organ is distended and paralyzed with Buscopan (scopolamine)

The Duodenal Papilla and the Longitudinal Duodenal Fold

On the medial wall of the second part of the duodenum is a longitudinal fold of mucous membrane at the upper end of which is located the duodenal papilla (the major papilla with a central depression for the orifice of the bile and main pancreatic ducts). Inferiorly the longitudinal fold joins another landmark, the circular fold.

Proximal and anterior to the major papilla lies the minor papilla containing the orifice for the accessory duct of the pancreas (Fig. 4.2).

Periampullary Duodenal Diverticula

Duodenal diverticula are common in elderly patients. They are usually located in an arc extending from 9 o'clock to 3 o'clock on the face of the papilla, or the papilla may lie with a large diverticulum as visualized by endoscopy.

Endoscopic Anatomy of the Duodenal Papilla

A side-viewing endoscope is used to visualize the second part of the duodenum. After entering the duodenum, passing the superior duodenal angle, and viewing the mucosal folds of the descending duodenum, the papilla is visualized with the endoscope lens facing the medial wall of the descending duodenum. When the papilla is not visualized, the endoscope is usually too far into the duodenum, usually in the third part of the duodenum.

The endoscope is now straightened into the short scope position and the papilla is seen from below after withdrawing the endoscope slightly above the angle that separates the second and third parts of the duodenum where there is a bare shelf of mucosa without transverse folds. Above the shelf, a longitudinal fold or several oblique folds of different sizes lead directly to the papilla. The normal papilla varies in size, shape, and appearance from patient to patient.

Most often it is located in the second part of the duodenum. Rarely, the position of the common bile duct in the horizontal duodenum may be obvious, lying vertically a few centimeters above the papilla. The papilla may be surrounded superiorly by a horizontal cover that may hide the orifice. The orifice always lies at the apex of the papilla. It may be obscure and invisible or patulous with protruding mucosa. Most cases of failure to find the papilla with the endoscope in the duodenum by the short route occur because the instrument has been inserted too far into the duodenum (checked by fluoroscopy if necessary) and has not been withdrawn sufficiently to visualize the site of the papillary orifice.

The Duodenal Papilla after Partial Gastrectomy

While pyloroplasty and Billroth I gastrectomy do not alter the route to the duodenal papilla, gastroenterostomy (and pyloric stenosis) and Billroth II gastrectomy prevent access to the major duodenal papilla by the conventional route. In these circumstances the afferent loop must be found and the papilla catheterized from below after locating, first, the circular fold and then, the long vertical duodenal fold.

The Anatomy of Endoscopic Sphincterotomy
(Figs. 4.3)

Spincterotomy is performed with a standard side-viewing endoscope combined with an electrosurgical power source, which includes blend, coagulation, and

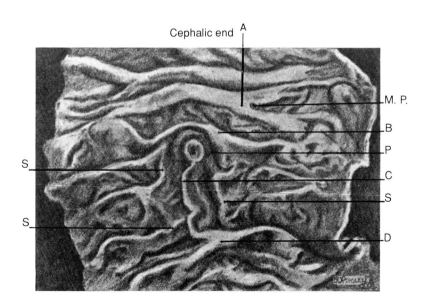

Fig. 4.2 **The second part of the duodenum opened.**
(Modified after 3)

MP = minor papilla
P = depression containing the major papilla at its center
C = longitudinal fold
D = horizontal shelf
B = horizontal hood
A = superior end
S,S,S = secondary folds

cutting modes. A short-nosed sphincterotome as developed by Demling and Classen (pull-type) is still most valuable. After catheterization of the common bile duct (not the pancreatic duct) confirmed by contrast medium injection and fluoroscopy, the sphincterotome is withdrawn slowly until the proximal end of the wire is visible outside the papilla and pointing between 11 o'clock and 1 o'clock. Using slight bowing and a short length of wire in contact with the mucosa (not more than 5–7 mm), a blend current setting of 2 or 3, and elevation of the sphincterotome to provide cutting pressure, the incision is performed slowly. A short length of cutting wire in contact with the mucosa concentrates the current and therefore the cutting density and effectiveness of the wire knife. The procedure is complete when the bile duct mucosa is visible. The incision length is determined by the previously documented duct diameter. Incision of the papilla in a dilated system is less risky than in an undilated bile duct. Usually, an incision is adequate when

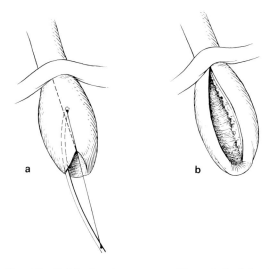

Fig. 4.**3** **Sphincterotomy a** position of "knife" at 11 o'clock. **b** completed procedure.
(After 2 with permission)

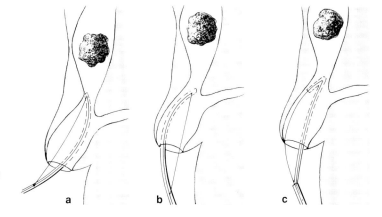

Fig. 4.**4** **a** Conventional knife position
b Incorrect position after Billroth II gastrectomy
c Correct position with special papillitome after Billroth II gastrectomy
(Modified after 2)

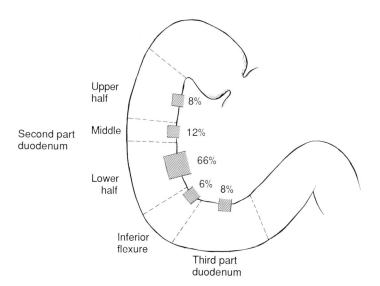

Fig. 4.**5** **Locations of the papilla in 2000 cases during cholangiography** by ERCP, FN, PTHC, and operative cholangiography

Second part duodenum

Upper half

Middle

Lower half

Inferior flexure

Third part duodenum

8%

12%

66%

6%   8%

the "knife" shoots into the bile duct as the upper sphincter is incised, and there is free flow of bile or the bowed "knife" passes easily in and out of the bile duct. Cutting down to the duodenal wall only is usually safe, but it may not reach the upper sphincter making cutting within the duct necessary to complete the sphincterotomy.

Precutting Sphincterotomy

Precutting means making an incision without having catheterized the bile duct. Cotton (1990) recommends two methods of doing this procedure and indicates that it should only be done by experienced endoscopists and should not be used for diagnostic access to the bile duct.

One method is to use a sphincterotome with the cutting wire extending to its tip. This is placed in the papillary orifice and, with upward pressure, a cutting current is applied; this carries the risk of pancreatitis from coagulation of the pancreatic duct.

A second method is to use a needle knife inserted into the papilla or into the wall of the dilated intramural bile duct to perform fistulotomy.

References

1. Cotton PB, Williams CB: Practical gastrointestinal endoscopy. Oxford: Blackwell Scientific, 1990:85–156.
2. Fruhmorgen P, ed. Diagnostische und therapeutische Endoskopie in der Gastroenterologie. Berlin: Springer, 1991:128–180.
3. Schapper EA, Symington J, Bryce TH. Quain's Elements of Anatomy, 11th ed. (Vol II. Part 11.) London: Longmans Green. 1914:97–113.
4. Siegel JH. Endoscopic retrograde cholangiopancreatography. New York: Raven Press, 1992:14–59.

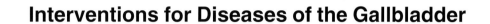

Interventions for Diseases of the Gallbladder

5 Laparoscopic Cholecystectomy

B. E. Lane

Cholecystectomy is the most common nonemergency abdominal operation carried out. In the United States of America approximately half a million cholecystectomies are carried out per year (11), and it is expected that this number will increase due to the aging population.

Open cholecystectomy was first carried out by Langenbuck in 1882. Since then, the results have improved making it an effective and extremely safe operation. Series have been reported with no mortality and minimal morbidity.

The first laparoscopy was performed by Kelling on a dog in 1902. Since then, the use of endoscopic methods has increased by gynecologic surgeons, orthopedic surgeons, and other specialists. In 1984 gynecologists performed over 300 000 laparoscopies in the United States (13). More recently, diagnostic laparoscopy has been used by general surgeons with a high diagnostic yield and a low morbidity and mortality (14).

Since 1987, when the first laparoscopic cholecystectomy was carried out by Mouret in Lyon, France (10), the demand for the operation by patients has increased at an unprecedented rate. Initially patient demand exceeded the ability of the manufacturers and suppliers to provide the equipment. The patient demand for laparoscopic cholecystectomy is driven by the absence of a large scar resulting in less postoperative pain and a good cosmetic result, a short hospital stay, and the ability to return to work relatively early. But any new surgical technique must be as safe as the operation it is replacing. Unfortunately laparoscopic cholecystectomy has a higher incidence of bile duct injuries then open cholecystectomy. Some authors suggest that this may be a manifestation of the "learning curve" with a new technique (16).

The results of financial analysis of laparoscopic cholecystectomy versus open cholecystectomy are not clear cut. The use of laser rather than electrocautery, of disposable trocar/cannula, disposable instruments, and routine operative cholangiography tend to increase hospital expenses. These expenses should be balanced against the financial implications of early return to work by the patients.

Indications and Contraindications for a Laparoscopic Cholecystectomy

The indications for laparoscopic cholecystectomy are the same as for traditional open cholecystectomy. Included are patients with symptomatic gallstones causing chronic calculous cholecystitis, biliary colic, acute cholecystitis of short duration, and gallstones pancreatitis.

Patients with suggested or known stones in the common bile duct are best deferred until they have had the stones extracted endoscopically, or a normal common bile duct has been demonstrated by ERCP. Common bile duct stones should be suspected if there is a history of recent jaundice, abnormal liver function tests, or a common bile duct greater than 7 mm in diameter on ultrasound.

Previous extensive abdominal operations are not an absolute contraindication to laparoscopic cholecystectomy. The presence of adhesions makes the procedure more difficult and increases the risk of injury to intraperitoneal organs when creating the pneumoperitoneum and when inserting the first trocar. If extensive troublesome adhesions are anticipated, the Hasson open laparoscopic technique is an alternative approach (6). Patients on anticoagulants and patients with coagulopathies should have their abnormal tests corrected before this procedure.

Obesity is also not a contraindication to laparoscopic cholecystectomy. The obese patient is at increased risk during open and laparoscopic cholecystectomy. These risks are less with the laparoscopic operation if the surgeon is aware of the difficulties. There may be difficulties in creating the pneumoperitoneum, inserting the trocars in the correct position, or the trocars and the operating instruments may be too short.

Patients who are unfit for general anesthesia are obviously unfit for a laparoscopic cholecystectomy. A patient with impaired respiratory function should have a lower postoperative morbidity with laparoscopic cholecystectomy than with open cholecystectomy.

Preoperative Preparation

Prior to laparoscopic cholecystectomy a complete history must be obtained and a full physical examination must be performed. The anesthetist must be aware of any cardiorespiratory problem. The operating surgeon must be aware of previous surgery and the presence of any intra-abdominal masses or organomegaly. The investigations normally performed before open cholecystectomy are carried out prior to laparoscopic cholecystectomy. Informed consent must be obtained. The patient must be aware of the complications and of the possibility of the need to convert to open cholecystectomy.

Laparoscopic cholecystectomy is performed under general anesthesia in an operating room with full monitoring facilities including pulse oximetry and end tidal–carbon dioxide monitoring. The patient is placed in the supine position and securely strapped to the operating table to allow table tilt. The stomach and bladder should be decompressed with a nasogastric tube and Foley catheter to lessen the risk of injury to these organs during the introduction of the Verres needle and trocars.

Position of Surgeon and Equipment

The surgeon, the assistant, and the instrument nurse must all have a clear view of the television monitor. The surgeon must also have a clear view of the carbon dioxide insufflator. He or she should be able to see and understand the significance of the different gauge readings, which include the volume of the gas in the tank, the insufflation pressure, the flow rate of the gas, and the volume of gas insufflated.

The surgeon stands on the patient's left with the television monitor opposite to him or her. On the stand under this monitor are the carbon dioxide insufflator, the light source, and the camera control unit. The assistant stands opposite the surgeon on the patient's right in full view of the second monitor, which is on the patient's left. Suction and electrocautery equipment are also positioned on the patient's left. The instrument nurse stands opposite the surgeon near the foot of the table (Fig. 5.1).

Insertion of Verres Needle and Trocars

A pneumoperitoneum is established by inserting a Verres needle into the peritoneal cavity. The patient is placed in a 10–20 degree Trendelenburg position. The patency of the Verres needle is checked. The Verres needle is held like a dart between the index finger and the thumb and inserted via a stab wound below the umbilicus while the abdominal wall is held up. The operator will notice a sudden "give" as the needle passes through the linea alba and peritoneum. A drop of saline placed on the hub of the Verres needle should disappear on lifting the abdominal wall, confirming that the tip of the needle is in the peritoneal cavity. The Verres needle should be aspirated to ensure the needle is not in a blood vessel. The Verres needle is connected to the electronic insufflator, which is preset to insufflate to an intra-abdominal pressure of 10–15 mmHg. The initial flow rate of carbon dioxide should not be greater than 1.5 L per minute. A higher flow rate may cause hypotension and bradycardia or both. Insufflation continues till 3–4 L have been infused.

The Verres needle is removed. The subumbilical stab wound is enlarged and a 10/11-mm trocar inserted. When inserting the trocar, the left hand grasps the shaft of the trocar to act as a brake to prevent sudden deep penetration and injury to intraperitoneal or retroperitoneal structures. The creation of a pneumoperitoneum and the insertion of the primary trocar/cannula are two of the most dangerous parts of this operation. A zero degree telescope attached to the

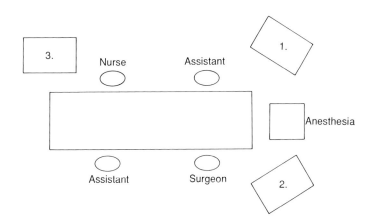

Fig. 5.**1 Operating theater positions**
1. Number 1. monitor, insufflator, light source, and camera control unit
2. Number 2. monitor, suction, and electro-cautery
3. Instruments

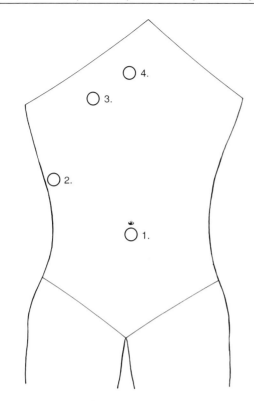

Fig. 5.2
1. Primary portal
2. Lateral portal
3. Midclavicular portal
4. Midline operating port

camera is inserted into the peritoneal cavity via the subumbilical port. The secondary ports are inserted under direct vision. A 10–11-mm operating port is inserted in the midline 4 cm below the xiphoid process entering the peritoneal cavity to the right of the falciform ligament. A 5-mm port is inserted on the midclavicular line just below the costal margin. The fourth port is inserted along the anterior axillary line midway between the anterior superior iliac spine and the costal margin (Fig. 5.2).

Dissection of Cystic Duct and Artery

The patient is now repositioned into the reverse Trendelenburg position with left-side-down lateral tilt. Through the anterior axillary port, a blunt grasping forceps is passed and applied to the fundus of the gallbladder. The fundus of the gallbladder is pushed above the liver and to the right. A second grasping forceps is inserted via the midclavicular port and applied to the neck or infundibulum of the gallbladder.

Downward traction on the neck of the gallbladder opens up Calot's triangle. With a dolphin-nose blunt dissector through the epigastric port, the peritoneum along the inferior and posterior aspect of the cystic duct is removed until the cystic duct is exposed and clean. This dissection starts at the neck of the gallbladder and is continued medially toward the common bile duct. The use of electrocautery and sharp dissection should be avoided until the cystic duct and cystic artery have been identified and divided.

When the cystic duct has been identified and a segment cleaned, three clips are applied to the cystic duct. The cystic duct is then divided. It is often easier to identify the cystic artery after division of the cystic duct. Care must be taken not to avulse the gallbladder from the cystic artery. The cystic artery is doubly clipped and divided. The gallbladder is now dissected off the liver from the neck to the fundus using diathermy scissors or a diathermy hook, first dividing the medial and lateral peritoneal reflexions of the gallbladder. During this dissection it may be necessary to reposition the grasping forceps to get maximum traction of the gallbladder away from the liver bed. Before the last attachment of the gallbladder to the liver is divided, the gallbladder bed is inspected for bleeding and bile leaks. It is difficult to inspect the liver bed after the gallbladder has been completely detached from the liver. The freed gallbladder, in one of the graspers, is placed between the liver and the diaphragm. The subhepatic space is irrigated with normal saline. This saline irrigation is best carried out with the patient repositioned in the Trendelenburg position and slight right side down lateral tilt. This allows the saline to collect between the diaphragm and the liver from where it is aspirated.

The final step is to remove the gallbladder through the abdominal wall. The gallbladder is firmly grasped by the neck and removed via the right iliac fossa port in preference to the subumbilical port as the shutter valve effect of the abdominal wall muscles in the right iliac fossa obviates the need to place a suture in the abdominal wall after the gallbladder has been removed. The telescope is removed. The abdomen is deflated of carbon dioxide and the ports removed. The skin incisions are closed with subcuticular suture and Steristrips.

Alternative Techniques

As with most open operations there are many ways of achieving the same result. A surgeon's choice of technique is often a personal choice or a result of his or her teachers' influence. In continental Europe, some surgeons position the patient in the lithotomy position. The assistant controlling the camera stands between the patient's legs. The positions of the ports may also be altered. A 5-mm trocar cannula may be inserted in the epigastric. Through this, rigid suction doubles as a liver retractor. A grasping forceps for the neck of the gallbladder is placed through the right iliac fossa 5-mm port while a 10-mm operating port is inserted to the left of the midline (5).

An additional port may be added at any time for liver retraction or for retraction of the colon and omentum. An additional 5-mm port can be inserted in the left midclavicular plane and may be necessary during laparoscopic cholecystectomy for acute cholecystitis.

Dissection Using Laser or Diathermy?

The explosive demand by the public for laparoscopic cholecystectomy is partially due to the concept that this operation is possible because of developments in laser technology. There have been few studies comparing the use of electrocautery versus laser in laparoscopic cholecystectomy. The main disadvantages of laser are the initial capital outlay and that the surgeon must learn how to use the equipment safely. Most surgeons are familiar with the use of electrocautery. This may be a disadvantage as the surgeon may inappropriately use diathermy while dissecting Calot's triangle, resulting in bile duct injury due to ischemia. Rossi et al. (12) found electrocautery was employed for dissection during laparoscopic cholecystectomy in nine of 11 patients who developed postoperative bile duct stricture.

Esther and Moossa (4) concluded that laser dissection was more dangerous than dissection with electrocautery. This conclusion was based on the finding that laser dissection had been used in five out of six patients with a postlaparoscopic cholecystectomy bile duct injury. The use of electrocautery dissection is associated with less blood loss, shorter operating time, and lower operating room charges (17).

Intraoperative Cholangiography

The routine use of operative cholangiography during open cholecystectomy has been controversial. Understandably, this controversy has continued with the introduction of laparoscopic cholecystectomy. The main benefits of operative cholangiography during open cholecystectomy were the detection of stones in the common bile duct and the lower incidence of bile duct injury in patients who had operative cholangiography (3). The detection of bile duct stones is less important during laparoscopic cholecystectomy because these patients are at low risk of having stones in the common bile duct due to preoperative evaluation of common bile duct status and preoperative clearance of ductal stones by ERCP and endoscopic sphincterotomy.

Operative cholangiography may help prevent bile duct injury and stricture (7). It may also help detect a bile duct injury at the time of the primary operation when the chances of a successful repair are higher than after delayed repair (9). It is our policy to routinely carry out intraoperative cholangiography during laparoscopic cholecystectomy.

The technique of intraoperative cholangiography during laparoscopic cholecystectomy is similar to that used at open cholecystectomy. Inserting the cannula into the cystic duct at laparoscopic cholecystectomy is more difficult than at open cholecystectomy. A success rate of 90% can be achieved (1).

The cystic duct is identified and cleared as described above. A hemoclip is applied to the cystic duct at its junction with the neck of the gallbladder. A microscissors is passed through the epigastric port and a small opening in the cystic duct is made. One of the many specifically designed laparoscopic cholangiography catheters or a ureteric catheter (4 Fr or 5 Fr with end hole) is introduced through the midclavicular port or percutaneously through a 14-gauge angiocath close to the midclavicular port. The cystic duct is cannulated and the catheter held in position by a clip or cholangiogram clamp. All radiopaque materials are removed where possible. The cholangiogram is performed in the standard fashion using a C arm with fluoroscopic freeze frame, digitized image and X-ray

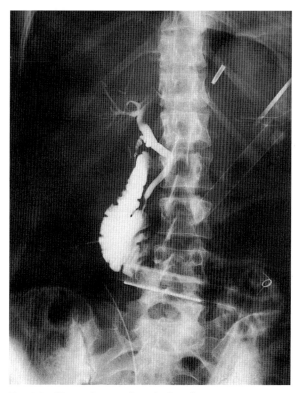

Fig. 5.**3** **Normal operative cholangiogram**

capabilities, or three static films. When good visualization of the ductal system has been obtained the catheter is removed. A double clip is applied to the cystic duct and the gallbladder removed as described above (Fig. 5.**3**).

Complications of Laparoscopic Cholecystectomy

Laparoscopic cholecystectomy is a safe and effective technique for the management of gallbladder disease in the vast majority of patients. Laparoscopic cholecystectomy is a new technique, and it can be expected that the increased complication rate will decrease with improved techniques, improved instruments, better recognition of high-risk patients, and acceptance by the public and by surgeons that the conversion to open cholecystectomy is in the interest of safe surgery. Surgeons have felt pressured to fulfil the patient's expectations of a pain-free operation and minimal scars, even in the presence of unsafe anatomy.

A low incidence of a wide range of complications have been reported in the literature. Complications can occur during the initial laparoscopy. Perforation of an intra-abdominal viscus or a major rectroperitoneal vessel can occur during the insertion of the Verres needle. These injuries are more likely to occur if the patient has had previous abdominal surgery resulting in adhesions.

During insufflation of the pneumoperitoneum, hypotension and/or bradycardia can occur. These are more likely to occur if the rate of insufflation is greater than 1.5 L per minute. Misplacement of the Verres needle results in surgical emphysema. Pneumothorax has also occurred.

The major operative complications include injury to the bile duct, hemorrhage, and viscus perforation by laser or electrocautery. Hemorrhage should be recognized during the surgery and, if serious, can be controlled by open operation if necessary. Bile duct injury during laparoscopic cholecystectomy is more frequent than during open cholecystectomy. The incidence of bile duct injury during open cholecystectomy is about 0.2%, and during laparoscopic cholecystectomy it is between 0.5% and 2% (2). The presence of obesity with excess fat in the porta hepatis, fibrosis of Calot's triangle, acute cholecystitis, and bleeding during surgery are factors that increase the risk of bile duct injury (3). A bile duct injury results in a lifelong risk of recurrent biliary problems. The use of routine intraoperative cholangiography, lateral traction rather than cephalic traction on the gallbladder neck, a 30-degree forward oblique telescope, and a low threshold for conversion to open cholecystectomy may help to reduce the high rate of bile duct injury during laparoscopic cholecystectomy (7).

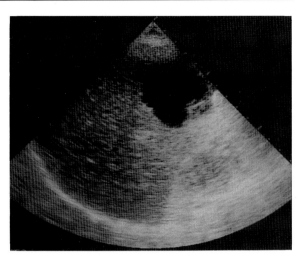

Fig. 5.**4 Biloma in the gallbladder bed after laparoscopic cholecystectomy.** This was aspirated with a fine needle and did not recur

A postoperative laparoscopic cholecystectomy bile leak is another complication. A bile leak may be due to dislodgement of the clip from the cystic duct. It may also be from a bile duct injury or directly from an accessory duct in the gallbladder bed on the liver. If a patient's serum bilirubin is elevated in the postoperative period, an ERCP and ultrasound scan of the upper abdomen should be performed. The ERCP demonstrates the bile duct and possibly the site of the leak. The ultrasound scan shows the presence of the leak and the size of the collection. If the ductal system appears to be intact on the ERCP, this bile collection can be aspirated under ultrasound control. A large bile leak may require a laparotomy.

Wound infections at the site of the trocar and cannula are a minor problem. Hernias at the port site are also infrequent. To lessen the risk of hernia at the trocar and cannula site, the abdomen should be deflated via the epigastric port with the tip of the cannula between the liver and diaphragm. The other cannulas should be removed with the valve in the open position. It is also advisable to repair the midline fascia after the cannulas are removed.

Laparoscopic Management of Common Bile Duct Stones

Endoscopic Transcystic Bile Duct Exploration

During open cholecystectomy, common bile duct stones are removed by choledochotomy. At the end of the exploration, a T tube is inserted into the common bile duct, and the common bile duct is closed with sutures on either side of the T tube. The difficulties with inserting the T tube and laparoscopic suture closure of the common bile duct have led to laparoscopic transcystic bile duct exploration. For this technique to be successful, the cystic duct should ideally be wide and should enter the right lateral side of the common duct.

Intraoperative cholangiography is carried out by inserting the cholangiogram catheter percutaneously in the standard fashion through a point on the abdominal wall close to the midclavicular port. If stones are seen in the common bile duct, a guide wire is passed through the cholangiogram catheter into the common bile duct until the tip of the guide wire is in the duodenum. A 8-Fr to 12-Fr sheath with a pneumostatic valve and a dilating introducer are inserted over the guide wire into the abdomen. The dilating introducer is removed from the sheath. With the guide wire safely in the duodenum, the cystic duct is dilated to a size large enough to allow extraction of the stone from the common bile duct through the cystic duct. This dilation is carried out using a balloon catheter. The balloon catheter is introduced over the guide wire. The balloon, 2–4 cm long, is positioned so that its distal end is just in the common bile duct.

The balloon is inflated to the recommended pressure for 5 minutes. When the cystic duct has been dilated to the desired size (4–8 mm), the deflated balloon catheter is removed, leaving the guide wire in situ. (Dilation with a 4-mm balloon would allow the cystic duct to take a 10-Fr sheath and a 9-Fr choledochoscope). The sheath and introducer are passed into the cystic duct. The introducer is removed, and the sheath acts as a conduit for a flexible 7-Fr to 11-Fr choledochoscope. Choledochoscopy and stone extraction are similar to open common bile duct exploration. Stones can be extracted using a stone removal basket.

Contact lithotripsy with electrohydraulic and pulsed dye laser equipment has also been used to fragment large stones.

If the cystic duct has been dilated, it is advisable to put a ligature rather than a clip on the cystic duct following transcystic endoscopic exploration of the common bile duct.

Fluoroscopic Transcystic Bile Duct Exploration

Fluoroscopic transcystic bile duct exploration and stone extraction similar to the Burhenne technique for removal of retained common bile duct stones has also been used at the time of laparoscopic cholecystectomy without cystic duct dilation (8).

A major disadvantage of endoscopic transcystic bile duct exploration and fluoroscopic transcystic bile duct exploration is that these techniques are usually only suitable for stones in the lower common bile duct.

The results of transcystic bile duct exploration show that a success rate as high as 93% can be achieved (15). The numbers in most published series are still small. Failures are due to unfavorable anatomy, impacted stones, or stones in the intrahepatic ducts.

Laparoscopic exploration of the common bile duct is possible, but few surgeons have the technical skills necessary. The main difficulty is suturing the common bile duct closed around the T tube.

References

1. Berci G, Sackier JM, Paz-Partlow M. Routine or selected intraoperative cholangiography during laparoscopic cholecystectomy? Am J Surg 1991;161:355–360.
2. Braasch JW. Laparoscopic cholecystectomy and other procedures. Arch Surg 1992;127:887.
3. Collins PG, Gorey T. Iatrogenic biliary stricture: presentation and management. Br J Surg 1984;71:980–1.
4. Easter DW, Moossa AR. Laser and laparoscopic cholecystectomy: a hazardous union. Arch surg 1991;126:423.
5. Grace AP, Quereshi A, Coleman J, et al. Reduced postoperative hospitalization after laparoscopic cholecystectomy. Br J Surg 1991;78:160 –162.
6. Hasson MH. Open laparoscopy vs closed laparoscopy. A comparison of complication rates. Adv Planned Parenthood 1978;13:41–43.
7. Hunter JG. Avoidance of bile duct injury during laparoscopic cholecystectomy. Am J Surg 1991;162:71–76.
8. Hunter JG. Laparoscopic transcystic common bile duct exploration. Am J Surg 1992;163:53–58.
9. Moosa AR, Mayer AD, Stabile B. Iatrogenic injury to the bile duct. Arch Surg 1990;125:1028–30.
10. Nathanson LK, Shimi S, Cuscheiri A. Laparoscopic cholecystectomy: the Dundee technique. Br J Surg 1991;78:155–159.
11. Olsen DO. Laparoscopic Cholecystectomy. Am J Surg 1991;161:339 –344.
12. Rossi RL, Schirmer WJ, Braasch JW, Sanders LB, Munson JL. Laparoscopic bile duct injuries. Risk factors, recognition and repair. Arch surg 1992;127:596–602.
13. Rutkow M. Surgical operations in the United States: 1979 –1984. Surgery 1987;101:192–200.
14. Sackier JM, Berci G, Paz-Parthlow M. Elective diagnostic laparoscopy. Am J Surg 1991;161:326–331.
15. Swanstorm L, Sangster W. Laparoscopic choledochoscopy [abstract]. Surg Endosc 1992;6:92.
16. The Southern Surgeons Club. A prospective analysis of 1518 laparoscopic cholecystectomies. N Engl J Med 1991; 324:1073–1078.
17. Voyles CR, Petro AB, Meena AL, Haick AJ, Koury MA. A practical approach to laparoscopic cholecystectomy. Am J Surg 1991;161:365–370.

6 Oral Dissolution of Gallstones and Extracorporeal Shock Wave Lithotripsy

Laparoscopic cholecystectomy is now the gold standard for the treatment of *all types of symptomatic gallbladder stones*. Reports from clinical studies and postmortem examinations show that gallstones are more common in Western Europe, the United States, and South American countries than in Africa and the East. Prevalence varies from 10% in the United States to 25% in Europe and 45% in females in Chile and rises to 70% in native American people over 50 years of age (2, 4, 6, 12). Ultrasound surveys in Italy showed that 9% to 11% of the population had asymptomatic gallstones (32, 33). In Western Europe and in North and South American countries cholesterol stones predominate, and gallstone incidence increases with age. Women have a higher incidence up to age 65 than men when the male : female incidence ratio is equal. Multiparity, obesity, and hypertriglyceridemia are associated with a higher incidence of gallstones (12, 34). Solitary large stones, multiple small stones, and floating gallstones more often cause symptoms and complications (15, 18, 34). Cholesterol stones contain bile acids, bile pigments, phospholipids, fatty acids, proteins, calcium salts, and 70% cholesterol and account for 80% of all gallbladder stones in Western countries. Pigment stones contain calcium bilirubinate.

The causes and the natural history of gallstones are poorly understood. A patient with silent gallstones who develops symptoms over 10 to 20 years cannot be identified so that preventive therapy cannot be undertaken (13). Gallstone treatment clinics should involve imaging and clinical evaluation prior to therapy. Ideally, surgeons, gastroenterologists, and radiologists should work as a team to provide optimal imaging of the gallbladder and biliary tract, improve patient care, and promote clinical research. Nonsurgical therapy should only be undertaken in a setting in which there is close cooperation between an informed, competent biliary surgeon, an interventional endoscopist, and a competent interventional radiologist interested in the biliary tract and its diseases.

Oral Dissolution of Gallstones

Cholesterol gallstones are present in 80% of patients with gallbladder stones; these stones may be treated by nonsurgical techniques including oral dissolution, contact dissolution, combined therapy with oral and contact dissolution, or combined oral therapy with extracorporeal shock wave lithotripsy (ESWL). Oral dissolution therapy reduces cholesterol saturation of the bile and causes gradual dissolution of cholesterol gallstones. Two bile acids have been used to dissolve cholesterol stones. Chenodeoxycholic acid and ursodeoxycholic acid (URSO) are both efficacious in dissolving cholesterol stones and, given together at a reduced dose, may be more effective than ursodeoxycholic acid alone. Chenodeoxycholic acid has side effects that now preclude its use as a single drug for stone dissolution including dose-related diarrhea, raised aminotransferases, and moderate elevation of cholesterol. Ursodeoxycholic acid 10 mg/kg/day or combined therapy with the two acids at a reduced dose each of 5 mg/kg/day slowly dissolves cholesterol gallstones in selected patients.

Selection of Patients
(Table 6.1)

Proper selection of patients determines the success of therapy. Patients with normal functioning gallbladders containing small (less than 5 mm diameter) floating gallstones show a 90% success rate of complete stone dissolution within 1 year. If this treatment is limited to small floating stones, only 10% of patients with gallstones are eligible for this form of therapy (29).

The drug should not be used for patients with recurrent biliary colic since such patients would not be able to endure the course of therapy. Patients who decline surgery and have suitable gallstones that are considered responsible for their symptoms are potential candidates for this form of therapy. Calcification in the wall of the calculi as demonstrated by plain film or CT of the gallbladder *before any contrast medium is*

Table 6.1 Oral Dissolution of gallstones. Favorable factors for dissolution

Normally functioning gallbladder
Small gallstones (less than 5 mm diameter)
Floating gallstones
Absence of calcification
Excellent patient compliance

administered is a contraindication to therapy. The cystic duct must be patent as shown by a normal functioning gallbladder on oral cholecystography. The latter is also the best method of determining the diameter of the gallstones visualized. The stones should be less than 20 mm in diameter, preferably less than 15 mm, and optimally less than 5 mm. Stone diameter is critical for success; stone numbers are less important. Stones more than 20 mm in diameter are a contraindication to therapy.

Patient compliance is also very important for success.

Mechanism of Stone Dissolution

Bile salts dissolve gallstones by removing the cholesterol on the stone surface. Bile supersaturated with cholesterol is desaturated increasing the carrying capacity of bile for cholesterol. The latter is removed from the stones by micelles and evacuated via the cystic duct. Liquid crystals of cholesterol plus bile salt are less dense than bile and are excreted from the gallbladder as it contracts and empties. Ursodeoxycholic acid is thought to decrease cholesterol absorption from the intestine, decrease hepatic synthesis, and decrease cholesterol transport across the bile canalicular membrane. It does not prevent hepatic synthesis of bile salts from cholesterol. Ursodeoxycholic acid increases from 2% to over 50–60% concentration in the bile during therapy and does not attain a higher concentration with larger doses. This drug concentration is reached within 2 weeks of beginning therapy. The optimal dose of URSO is 10 mg/kg/day. The following drugs should not be used during URSO therapy since they bind bile salts and prevent URSO absorption from the intestine: antacids (particularly aluminum-containing drugs), cholestyramine, colestipol, sucralfate, and charcoal.

URSO therapy does not prevent hepatic production of bile salts, and cholesterol continues to be converted into bile salts during therapy. Therapy with URSO is a prolonged form of treatment because, with good compliance, stone diameters decrease 0.7–1 mm per month. A combination of URSO and a new class of lipid-lowering agents that inhibit the enzyme 3-hydroxymethyl-glutaryl coenzyme A reductase may produce faster dissolution of cholesterol stones or fragments of stones. These agents lower the cholesterol saturation index in bile and lower serum lipoprotein cholesterol (5, 20).

Stone composition is the most important factor in dissolution with URSO. Pigment stones do not dissolve, and 10% of these are radiolucent but do not float on oral cholecystography. Cholesterol stones shown to be calcium free on CT dissolve best on URSO therapy. If this form of therapy is used, calcium must be excluded by pretreatment CT scanning of the gallbladder, ideally after ultrasound has been used to diagnose gallstones and before oral cholecystography or any other contrast study of the gallbladder.

Monitoring Oral Dissolution Therapy

Serum transaminase levels are checked before therapy is commenced and after 1–2 months. If the initial results are normal, six monthly checks are adequate for the duration of the therapy.

Monitoring of stone dissolution is performed initially by cholecystography. Stones of 5 mm diameter are checked at 6 months; smaller stones or fragments are checked at 3 to 4 months. Failure of stone size reduction at 6 months indicates failed therapy while a decrease in stone size is a favorable sign.

At 6 months, therapy is either continued or abandoned.

If stones are decreasing in size, ultrasound is performed at 6 monthly intervals until dissolution is complete. URSO therapy is continued for 3 months after the gallbladder is stone free as indicated by ultrasound in an attempt to dissolve microstones or crystals, which could form the nidus for reformation of stones.

Recurrence of stones occurs in 60% of patients after 10 years reduced to 30% recurrence by giving low-dose URSO therapy (300 mg/day for prevention of stone recurrence. Elderly and other high-risk patients should be treated with prevention therapy.

Contraindications to Oral Dissolution Therapy

Contraindications include acute cholecystitis and recurrent acute biliary colic. Because of the lack of information, the drug should not be used during pregnancy or in women who may become pregnant. Intrahepatic or extrahepatic cholestasis, hepatitis, and cirrhosis are contraindications (14, 15, 18).

Complications of Oral Dissolution Therapy

URSO therapy has few side effects. Diarrhea is rare, transient, and resolves on continued therapy. Rarely, there is mild elevation of serum transaminase. Serum cholesterol levels are unaffected. Twenty percent of patients develop biliary pain, cystic duct obstruction, acute cholecystitis, or acute pancreatitis during URSO therapy. These may represent at least in part the natural history of symptomatic gallstones rather than direct complications of therapy.

Extracorporeal Shock Wave Lithotripsy

Extracorporeal shock wave lithotripsy (ESWL) may be used to disintegrate gallbladder stones. Lithotripsy may be based on electrohydraulic, piezoceramic, or electromagnetic principles. Lithotripsy of gallstones was originally introduced with two objectives: first, to facilitate stone dissolution particularly of large gallstones and second, to allow passage of gallstone fragments into the intestine (26, 27, 29). Results of gallstone therapy with this form of treatment depend on the type of lithotripsy used, stone size, number of stone present, presence or absence of calcification, energy level of shock waves used, number of shock waves generated, number of treatment visits, and addition of adjuvant therapy. Only 10–15% of patients with symptomatic gallstones are ideal patients for this form of gallstone therapy if the treatment is restricted to patients with single solitary gallstones (29).

Indications for Lithotripsy of Gallstones
(Table 6.2)

Gallbladder stone lithotripsy is an *elective procedure* performed most often in combination with oral dissolution drugs in the presence of normal extrahepatic bile ducts. Stone size may be less critical than formerly considered, when a stone diameter of 30 mm or two–three stones up to 15 mm in diameter or four stones 10–12 mm in diameter were considered to be maximum sizes.

Specific indications for this therapy are still poorly defined. In general, they are similar to the indications for URSO therapy. Unsuitability for general anesthesia in a patient with radiolucent gallstones in a *normally functioning and contracting gallbladder* is a recognized indication. Refusal of surgery by the patient with symptomatic gallstones is a current main indication.

Table 6.**2** Indications for lithotripsy of gallbladder stones

A single gallstone or stones up to 30 mm diameter
Absence of acute symptoms
Normally functioning gallbladder
General anesthesia contraindicated
Refusal of surgery
Radiolucent stone(s)

Contraindications to Lithotripsy of Gallstones

Contraindications to this form of symptomatic gallstone therapy include the presence of associated choledocholithiasis, the presence of anticoagulant therapy or significant uncorrected coagulopathy, aneurysm of the upper abdominal aorta or its branches, intrahepatic or extrahepatic cholestasis, acute gallbladder diseases, acute cholangitis, chronic cholecystitis, acute pancreatitis, pregnancy, presence of a pacemaker, history of significant arrhythmia, gallbladder wall calcification, gallstones with a nonfunctioning gallbladder, or failure of the gallbladder to respond to a fatty meal.

Techniques of Gallstone Lithotripsy

The technique of ESWL comprises stone imaging by ultrasound or contrast and X-rays, fragmentation by physical methods, clearance of fragments from the gallbladder by gallbladder evacuation with or without dissolution by oral bile salts or intracholecystic methyl tert butyl ether. Stone size is determined by oral cholecystography. The latter may be as good as or better than ultrasound for counting gallstones or gallstone fragments. The gallstone matrix is softer than that of most renal stones and, because of this, a gallstone absorbs shock wave energy and requires a larger amount of shock wave energy for stone fragmentation. The cystic duct and common bile duct passage of stone fragments presents a more difficult problem than the "stone street" after ESWL of a kidney stone. After ESWL the often large gallstone fragment volume also has to pass through narrow biliary passages to reach the duodenum.

With one exception, the gallstone is localized by ultrasound for targeting. Fluoroscopic targeting is necessary for ductal stone lithotripsy. Lithotripsy systems use either electrohydraulic (spark gap), electromagnetic, or piezoelectric mechanisms of shock wave generation. Current lithotriptors require only patient sedation and analgesia and neither submersion in a water bath nor admission to hospital. Spark gap technology has the highest fragmentation rate. Retreatment rates are greater with the piezoelectric system than with the electromagnetic system. Regardless of the source of shock waves generated, they pass practically unimpeded through the soft tissues of the body, which have an acoustic impedance similar to that of water. On striking a gallstone in the gallbladder, there is a change in acoustic impedance, and part of the shock wave is reflected creating a compressive force on the surface of the stone. The rest of the pulse travels through the stone to its posterior surface where it is reflected; it then travels back through the stone as a tensile pulse. These stress fields combined with cavitation on the stone surface, and perhaps within cracks in the stone, cause stone destruction (21, 22, 26, 27).

Lithotripsy Procedure

This involves:

1. *Positioning the patient*

Treatment may be performed in the supine or prone position. Good gallbladder visualization is essential for stone targeting and fragmentation. Bowel gas, fecal masses, and obesity may hinder gallbladder stone visualization. Most patients are positioned prone according to clinical reports. In the supine position the gallbladder is easier to visualize with ultrasound, stones may fragment more easily, and it is more comfortable for the patient.

2. *Targeting the gallbladder stone(s)*

Some current lithotriptors have two types of transducers, in-line and out-of-line transducers, to aid in gallbladder and stone localization for targeting and monitoring of fragmentation. The "in-line" transducer is best for stone targeting and fragmentation. Targeting must be precise for successful fragmentation and in order to avoid the lung, liver, and pancreas. Targeting of stone fragments or a small stone is much more difficult than targeting an individual large gallstone. Changes in targeting delay stone fragmentation. Only medical personnel competent in the use of ultrasound should use lithotripsy for gallstone therapy.

3. *The gallstone fragmentation process*

Two processes are involved in stone fragmentation: first, the stone breaks at microfissures on the surface opposite the shock wave; second, cavitation occurs in which microbubbles produced by the shock waves produce pitting of the stone surface, and a cloud of dust appears on the ultrasound image that obscures targeting of individual stones and fragments. The cavitation effect occurs when a shock wave strikes gallbladder bile and causes a collection of microbubbles to form, which mimics gallstone fragments in motion. Cavitation phenomenon occurring remote from the site of gallstones may be confused with fragmentation of stones. Gallstone "dust" particles may obscure large stone fragments, or they may mimic a stone. The latter may be excluded by rotating the patient through 360 degrees (the rollover maneuver). An "out-of-line" ultrasound probe is also valuable for assessing stone fragmentation. Stone lamination, especially with pigment or cholesterol, more than 1 mm thick influences the mechanism of fragmentation by delaying pulverization, especially fine pulverization. The number, size, composition, and volume of stones influence fragmentation by lithotripsy. Patients with large single gallstones or multiple large stones require more than one session for fragmentation. Stone fragmentation is also negatively influenced by the size of the gallbladder at initial targeting. A single stone is also more easily fragmented than multiple stones of the same volume (7, 8, 10, 11, 22, 24, 25).

Efficacy of ESWL of Gallstones
(Fig. 6.**1**)

The aim of lithotripsy is to produce small, 3–5-mm fragments of gallstones that will clear the gallbladder via the cystic duct and common bile duct. Adjuvant therapy is usually needed to achieve this stone-free state in the gallbladder, however the use of high-energy shock waves and multiple treatment visits may produce gallbladder clearance of fragments without other therapy. More sessions of therapy are required using piezoelectric lithotripsy than electrohydraulic therapy for stone fragmentation. More analgesia or intravenous sedation and analgesia are necessary with high-energy electrohydraulic or electromagnetic therapy. The global results of lithotripsy of gallbladder stones are difficult to compare because of differences of technique with different therapy units and the use of adjuvant therapy. Solitary, noncalcified gallstones 2 cm in diameter respond best to ESWL (1, 3, 7, 11, 26, 27). Gallbladder clearance is most successful when gallstone sand particles are 2 mm in diameter or less. This is achieved by an increased number of shock waves and higher energy shock waves. Results for calcified stones are mostly poor unless high energies or multiple treatments are used (8, 25).

Stone Recurrence after ESWL

Early recurrence is reported by Shackmann et al. in 9% of cases after 1 year. Recurrences are less after single stone therapy and after a stone-free period of 9 months after therapy of a single gallstone. Therapy with oral dissolution drugs does not prevent stone recurrence. Stone recurrence is higher in the first year after stopping bile acid therapy (11%) than in subsequent years.

Complications of ESWL

Severe side effects occur in 3–5% of cases. These required sphincterotomy or gallbladder removal in 5% of cases.

Paumgartner (1989) reported that 33% of patients developed one or more episodes of biliary colic caused by passage of stone fragments. One percent of patients developed mild pancreatitis, and 0.5% developed cholestasis. If stone clearance from the gallbladder is incomplete after ESWL, biliary colic occurs in 30% to 70% of cases for 2–3 months after therapy. Studies of gallbladder motility failed to demonstrate any short- or long-term effects of gallbladder lithotripsy (31), but in 33% of cases prolonged gallbladder luminal narrowing was detected, and these patients eventually required cholecystectomy (37).

Skin petechiae at the site of shock wave entry occurs in some patients. Hematuria and hemobilia have been reported (22, 25).

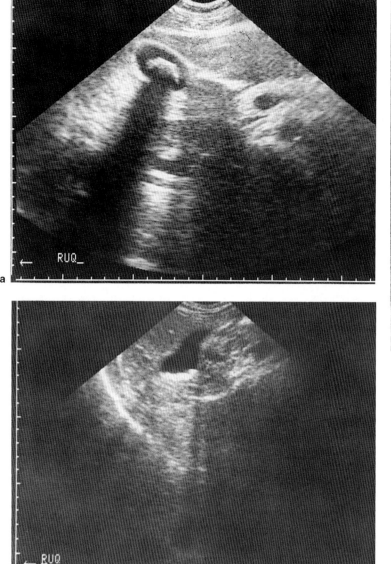

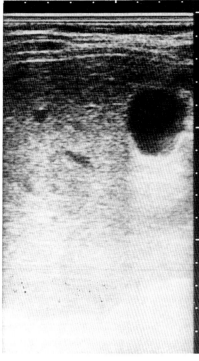

Fig. 6.**1 ESWL of gallstones**
a before and **b** after therapy
c at 3 months

Gallbladder stone lithotripsy is without doubt a valuable addition to nonoperative therapy of gallstones especially as adjuvant therapy to oral dissolution with bile acids combined with HMGCoA reductase inhibitors or monoterpenes, or combined with contact dissolution of gallbladder stones with MTBE (20).

References

1. Albert MB, Fromm H, Borstelmann R, et al. Successful out patient treatment of gallstones with piezoelectric lithotripsy. Ann Intern Med 1990;113:164–166.
2. Barbara L, Sama C, Morselli Labate AM, et al. A population study on the prevalence of gallstone diseases. The Sirmione study. Hepatology 1987;126:914–917.
3. Barkun AN, Valette PJ, Montet JC, et al. Physicochemical determinants of in vitro shock wave biliary lithotripsy. Gastroenterology 1991;100:222–227.
4. Bateson MC, Bouchier IAD. Prevalence of gallstones in Dundee. A necropsy study. BMJ 1975;4:427,429.
5. Bateson MC. Simvastatin and ursodeoxycholic acid for rapid gallstone dissolution. Lancet 1990;336:1196.
6. Brett M, Barker DJP. The world distribution of gallstones. Int J Epidemiol 1976;5:335–341.

7. Burnett D, Ertan A, Jones R, et al. Use of external shock wave lithotripsy and adjuvant ursodiol for treatment of radiolucent gallstones. A national multicenter study. Dig Dis Sci 1989;34:1011–1015.

8. Darzi A, Monson JRT, O'Morain C, et al. Extension of selection criteria for extracorporeal shock wave lithotripsy for gallstones BMJ 1989;299:302–303.

9. Diehl AK, Rosenthal M, Hazuda HP, et al. Socioeconomic status and the prevalence of clinical gallbladder disease. J Chronic Dis 1985;38:1019–1026.

10. Ell CH, Kerzel W, Heyder N, et al. Piezoelectric lithotripsy of gallstones. Lancet 1987;2:1149–1150.

11. Ferrucci JT. Biliary lithotripsy AJR 1989;153:15–22.

12. Freiherr G. Gallstones: Statistical considerations. In: Ferrucci JT, Delius M, Burhenne HJ. Biliary lithotripsy. Chicago: Year Book Medical 1989.

13. Friedman GD, Kannel WB, Dawber TR. The epidemiology of gallbladder disease. Observations in the Framingham study. J Chronic Dis 1966;19:273–292.

14. Fromm H. Gallstone dissolution therapy: current studies and future prospects. Gastroenterology 1986;91:1560–1567.

15. Gleeson D, Ruppin DC, Saunders A, et al. Final outcome of ursodeoxycholic acid treatment in 126 patients with radiolucent gallstones. Q J Med 1990;279:711–729.

16. Gracie WA, Ransohoff DF. The natural history of silent gallstones. N Eng J Med 1982;307:798–800.

17. Hood KA, Keighley A, Dowling HR, et al. Piezoelectric lithotripsy of gallstones. Experience in 38 patients. Lancet 1988;2:1322–1324.

18. Howard PJ, Gleeson D, Murphy GM, et al. Ursocholic acid: Bile acid and bile lipid dose response and clinical studies in patients with gallstones. Gut 1989;30:97–103.

19. Lanzini A, Jazrawi RP, Kupfer RM, et al. Gallstone recurrence after medical dissolution: An overestimated threat? J Hepatol 1986;3:241–246.

20. Logan GM, Duane WC. Lovastatin added to ursodeoxycholic acid further reduces biliary cholesterol saturation. Gastroenterology 1990;98:1572–1576.

21. Lubock P. The physics and mechanics of lithotripters. Dig Dis Sci 1989;34:999–1005.

22. Mosnier H, Guivarch M, Voinchet B, et al. Extracorporeal shock wave lithotripsy of gallstones: Tolerence, complications and preliminary results. Gastroenterol Clin Biol 1989;13:482–488.

23. O'Donnell LDJ, Heaton KW. Recurrence and re-recurrence of gallstones after medical dissolution: A long-term follow up. Gut 1988;29:241–246.

24. Paumgartner G. Shock wave lithotripsy of gallstones. AJR 1989;153:235–242.

25. Ponchon T, Barkun AN, Pujol B, et al. Gallstone disappearance after extracorporeal shock wave lithotripsy and oral bile acid dissolution. Gastroenterology 1989;97:457–463.

26. Rawat B, Burhenne JH. Extracorporeal shock wave lithotripsy of calcified gallbladder stones. Radiology 1990;175:667–670.

27. Sackmann M, Delius M, Sauerbruch T, et al. Shock wave lithotripsy of gallbladder stones: The first 175 patients. N Eng J Med 1988;318:393–397.

28. Sackmann M, Ippisch E, Sauerbruch T, et al. Early gallstone recurrence after successful shock wave therapy. Gastroenterology 1990;98:392–396.

29. Sackman M, Pauletzki J, Sauerbruch T, et al. The Munich gallbladder lithotripsy study: results of the first five years with 711 patients. Ann Int Med 1991;114:290–296.

30. Sauerbruch T, Paumgartner G. Gallstones: management. Lancet 1991;338:1121–1124.

31. Schoenfield LJ, Berci G, Carnoval RL, et al. The effect of ursodiol on the efficacy and safety of extracorporeal shock wave lithotripsy of gallstones. The Dornier National Biliary Lithotripsy Study. N Eng J Med 1987;323:1239–1245.

32. Sprengler U, Shackmann M, Sauerbruch T, et al. Gallbladder motility before and after extracorporeal shock wave lithotripsy. Gastroenterology 1989;96:860–863.

33. The Rome Group for the epidemiology and prevention of cholelithiasis (GREPCO) Prevalence of gallstone disease in an adult female population. Am J Epidemiol 1984;119:796–805.

34. The Rome Group for the epidemiology and prevention of Cholelithiasis (GREPCO). The epidemiology of gallstone disease in Rome, Italy Part 1. Prevalence data in man. Hepatology 1988;8:907–913.

35. Thistle JL, Cleary PA, Lachin JM, et al. The natural history of cholelithiasis. The National Cooperative gallstone study. Ann Int Med 1984;101:171–175.

36. Torres WE, Steinberg HV, Davis RC, et al. Extracorporeal lithotripsy of gallstones: Results and 6-month follow up in 141 patients. Radiology 1991;178:509–512.

37. Torres WE, Baumgartner BR, Casarella WJ. Abnormalities of the gallbladder after extracorporeal shock wave lithotripsy: imaging findings. AJR 1992;159:325–327.

38. Villanova N, Bazzoli F, Taroni F, et al. Gallstone recurrence after successful oral bile acid treatment. Gastroenterology 1989;97:726–731.

39. Zeman RK, Davros WJ, Goldberg JA, et al. Cavitation effects during lithotripsy. Part II. Clinical observations. Radiology 1990;177:163–166.

7 Percutaneous Cholecystostomy

Transhepatic Cholecystostomy for Gallbladder Stone Dissolution with Methyl Tert Butyl Ether (MTBE)

Indications

The advent of laparoscopic cholecystectomy has reduced, but has not eliminated the need for nonsurgical treatment of gallbladder stone disease, whether by stone dissolution (cholesterol stones) or stone removal (all stone types). This technique is indicated for patients with symptomatic gallstones who are unfit for surgery and patients who refuse surgery. We have used the technique in morbid obesity, when abdominal girth precluded laparoscopic cholecystectomy.

MTBE lysis of stone debris after ESWL is also a valid indication for gallbladder catheterization (44).

Technique of Transhepatic Catheterization of the Gallbladder

Percutaneous catheterization of the gallbladder is easier when a transhepatic route from the right axilla is used.

Usually only a short segment of the inferior part of the right lobe of the liver is traversed (Fig. 7.1). If the right lobe is slender inferiorly, the area of liver traversed is minimal. The presence of the liver track prevents bending of the catheter or guide wire during the catheter's introduction over a guide wire into the gallbladder lumen. Traversing the liver also helps to maintain the catheter in its original position within the gallbladder during dissolution therapy. An axillary approach to the gallbladder is easier than an anterior one and involves less radiation to the radiologists hands, which are not working directly within the radiation beam when a conventional undercouch fluoroscopy unit is used. Puncture of the colon is also avoided. The aim is to puncture the body of the gallbladder in its middle third where it is attached to the undersurface of the liver and hence, to avoid the peritoneal cavity. The track of the catheter should be parallel to the fluoroscopic tabletop.

A gallbladder on a mesentery is more difficult to puncture, and it shifts medially to lie anterior to or just to the right of the lumbar spine when attempts are made to puncture it. This type of gallbladder puncture is more painful presumably because of traction on its mesentery.

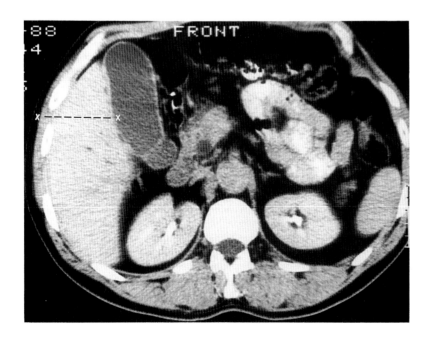

Fig. 7.**1** **CT scan of the gallbladder showing the transhepatic route to the gallbladder** (– – – –)

Preparation of the Patient

Dissolution of gallstones by MTBE is *a planned procedure*. The patient is admitted to the hospital on the evening before treatment. A routine hematological examination including coagulation screening and liver function tests is performed. Details of the technique are explained to the patient and written consent is obtained.

Technique of Gallbladder Catheterization

The technique is performed in the radiology department. Single plane fluoroscopy is adequate for the gallbladder in most patients. Digital imaging during the procedure produces poorer images than conventional units but it has the advantage of screening in multiple planes if necessary.

The fasting gallbladder has a large surface area in comparison with an intrahepatic bile duct at FN PTHC, and there is seldom difficulty in puncturing the organ. For catheterization, the gallbladder is opacified by oral cholecystography. Biloptin or Telepaque is given in standard dosage on the evening prior to the procedure.

The patient fasts overnight and has nothing to eat or drink until the procedure is completed. An intravenous line for hydration of the patient is set up on the morning of the procedure.

Pethidine and midazolam are given i. v. with the patient positioned supine on the radiographic table. All clothing is removed from the upper abdomen. The lead apron protection is removed from the right side of the radiographic table. The puncture site is chosen in the right axilla using metal forceps, and the opacified gallbladder and posterior–anterior fluoroscopy. The site of skin puncture chosen is that which is closest to the correct site on the lateral wall of the gallbladder (Fig. 7.**2a**).

The AP depth is judged by consulting the CT scan of the gallbladder. The site is marked on the skin of the axilla. The site of skin puncture is usually a little anterior to the midaxillary line. Next, the skin of the upper abdomen, right axilla, and chest is cleaned with antiseptic solution and the puncture area surrounded by sterile towels. Using an aseptic technique, the skin puncture site is infiltrated with local anesthetic, and the intercostal muscles and tissues are infiltrated down to the liver capsule. A small incision is then made in the skin at the puncture site, and a track is made with mosquito forceps down to the liver capsule.

The gallbladder is easiest to puncture with a fine needle (for cholecystocholangiography), but we have found that it is also easiest to lose this needle (during catheterization) because it is necessary to change guide wires before successful eventual catheterization with a 5-Fr Thistle catheter (Fig. 7.**3**).

Some authors enhance gallbladder opacification using contrast medium injected via a fine needle and change later to a larger needle/catheter system that accepts an .038 guide wire (5). The purpose of this is to retain gallbladder opafication, and, in the event of loss of the gallbladder or perforation of the gallbladder during insertion of a guide wire or catheter, to enable further attempts at needling the opacified organ. Although we prefer to use a catheter needle (needle 19 gauge × 190 mm; catheter 4.8 Fr × 170 mm Surgimed, Denmark) to puncture the gallbladder, there are several alternative needle catheters available that allow change from a fine needle and guide wire to a standard guide wire and a 5-Fr catheter for eventual catheterization (Hawkins Introducer Set, Cook, Denmark; Accustick, Medi-tech, USA; Desilet–Hoffman introducer, Cook).

Pain during gallbladder needling with the 19-gauge catheter needle is similar to the pain caused by the 5-Fr dilator used to introduce the 5-Fr catheter using fine needle introducer systems. We insert the catheter/needle through the skin incision parallel to the tabletop, through the liver under fluoroscopic control, toward the site of puncture in the lateral wall of the gallbladder. Penetration of the gallbladder wall is easier when a site is chosen close to the neck of the organ in the upper third of the body, where there is more fixation of the gallbladder to the undersurface of the liver. When the catheter needle tip reaches the wall of the opacified gallbladder, it indents the wall on pressure if it is correctly positioned. Next, a stab is made with the catheter needle into the lumen of the gallbladder. The movement is similar to that used for puncturing the femoral artery at angiography. Simply pushing the catheter needle into the wall does not result in penetration into the lumen.

The stylet of the catheter needle is now removed, and black bile drips slowly from the catheter (Fig. 7.**2b**). Next, a semistiff guide wire is passed through the catheter into the lumen of the gallbladder, and the wire is coiled two or three times within the gallbladder (Fig. 7.**2c**).

This is the critical point; correct looping of the wire within the gallbladder lumen is essential for successful catheterization. It increases the stability of the transhepatic wire, and adequate looping of the wire aids looping of the drainage catheter.

Next, the catheter introducer is removed over the wire and a 5-Fr pigtail catheter (Thistle, Cook, Denmark or Hellstern, Angiomed, Germany) with 32 side holes in the loop is inserted over the wire. (Fig. 7.**2d**).

It is passed rapidly through the liver into the gallbladder and coiled over the wire until three or four loops of catheter lie within the gallbladder lumen. Chilling the catheter increases its rigidity and assists its passage through the liver and through the gallbladder wall. Sometimes, looping of the catheter over the coiled wire in the gallbladder is more difficult than de-

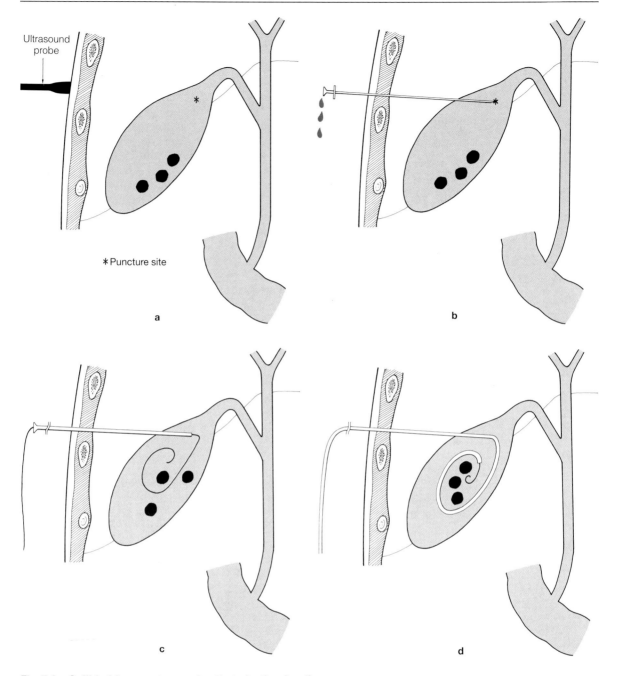

Ultrasound probe

*

* Puncture site

a

b

c

d

Fig. 7.**2**   **Gallbladder puncture and catheterization (a–d)**

scribed above. In this case it may help to slowly with-draw the wire one loop while advancing the catheter into the gallbladder and to repeat this maneuver until three or four catheter loops lie within the gallbladder lumen.

Occasionally, the semistiff guide wire is not rigid enough to enable passage of the pigtail catheter over it without bending the catheter and the wire between the skin surface and the gallbladder wall. This may be due

to a hard liver, or because the original track to the gall-bladder did not traverse the liver owing to the configu-ration of the right lobe, or because the gallbladder, al-though apparently in contact with the right lobe, is in fact lying free and has its own mesentery. When the semistiff wire fails as an introducer, a rigid Lunder-quist wire is used. The pigtail catheter is withdrawn, and an attempt is made to pass the catheter introducer back into the gallbladder lumen, and the semistiff

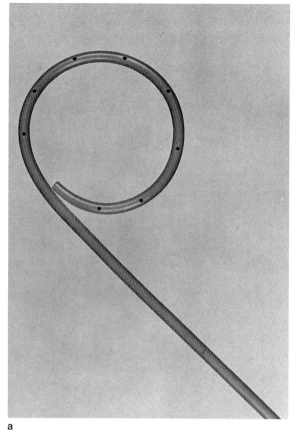 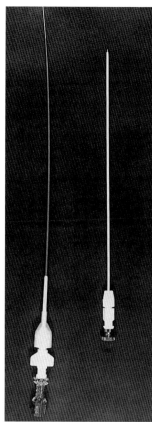

Fig. 7.**3** **a** Thistle catheter (5 Fr, Cook, Denmark) **b** Puncture catheter needles (Angiomed, Germany; Cook, Denmark)

a   b

wire is removed and replaced by the Lunderquist wire. Only the soft length of this wire is coiled in the gallbladder, and the pigtail is inserted over it into the lumen of the gallbladder using external fixation of the wire to prevent it from perforating the organ. When one loop of the pigtail is introduced into the gallbladder, the Lunderquist wire is replaced by the semistiff guide wire that is coiled in the gallbladder. The pigtail catheter is now advanced over the looped guide wire as before.

When the gallbladder is not in contact with the liver, puncture is more difficult. The catheter needle is inserted to indent the lateral gallbladder wall and to displace it to the left until it no longer moves on pressure. At this stage, it is punctured successfully by a stabbing motion of the catheter needle.

When this attachment anomaly of the gallbladder is recognized, additional analgesia is given i. v. to alleviate the pain caused by the gallbladder mesentery that is attached to the liver. After correctly positioning the pigtail catheter in the gallbladder, all bile is aspirated from the organ, and a water-soluble contrast medium is injected in order to determine the gallbladder capacity, demonstrate the number of gallstones present, outline the bile ducts down to the duodenum, and demonstrate any bile duct stones.

The pigtail catheter is now securely fixed to the skin of the axilla and connected to a closed drainage system.

The patient is now transferred to a special treatment room fitted with a ventilation system and an extractor outlet close to the patient's bed, the lower end of which is elevated 20 degrees. Treatment is commenced immediately if catheterization is uneventful. When the gallbladder wall is normal, leakage of contrast medium or bile does not occur around the catheter insertion. When a single large gallstone is present, it is essential to move the stone into the fundus of the gallbladder and position the pigtail loop around the stone before commencing dissolution. It is always best to locate the pigtail in the fundus of the gallbladder to prevent spill of MTBE during dissolution into the cystic duct and duodenum. Stones should always be dissolved, if possible, while the pigtail loop lies in the fundus. As dissolution proceeds, the gallbladder capacity diminishes, probably due to an irritant effect of the MTBE. This may cause escape of MTBE into the bile duct and duodenum unless extreme care is taken with MTBE injections. If multiple small stones are present, the pigtail catheter distributes the MTBE through its multiple side holes and perfuses around the calculi with rapid stone dissolution.

Catheter manipulations and stone displacements within the gallbladder are carried out using a straight or angled-tip glide wire (Terumo, Japan). It is often necessary to uncoil the catheter loops to achieve fundal stone placement or to move the pigtail catheter around within the gallbladder. To position the catheter around a stone, the guide wire is first positioned around the stone, and the catheter is coiled over the wire around the stone.

Complications

Serious complications are rare when a careful technique is used. *Perforation of the gallbladder* with the guide wire may occur during attempts at coiling the guide wire. It is of no significance when it is recognized, and the gallbladder wall is normal as the puncture hole closes off almost immediately. It is usually necessary to withdraw the guide wire completely and begin again with a fresh puncture of the gallbladder. Loss of gallbladder opacification may occur, or the opacification may be too faint for fluoroscopic gallbladder puncture. This is avoided by fine needle cholecystography before catheterization. Alternatively, ultrasound may be used to visualize puncture of the organ and catheterization continued as above. A single perforation of the wall is not an indication for termination of the procedure. Following successful catheterization of the gallbladder, a percutaneous cholecystogram is performed after a delay of 24 hours; it is very rare to still find leakage from the perforation site at this time, provided the wall of the organ is normal. Stone dissolution is commenced if there is no leakage of contrast medium.

Cholesterol Gallstone Dissolution with MTBE

Properties of the Solvent MTBE

Cholesterol stones are known to dissolve rapidly in diethyl ether. The ether vaporizes at 34.5 degrees C. MTBE has physical properties almost identical to those of diethyl ether but its boiling point is higher (55.2 degrees C). It thus remains a liquid at body temperatures. The physical properties of MTBE are:

Formula	$C_5 H_{12} O$
Mol. wt.	88.14
Specific gravity	0.741
Boiling point	55.2. degrees C
Ignition temperature	224 degrees C
Viscosity	0.27
Oral toxicity	4000 mg/kg (mouse)

MTBE dissolves gallstones rapidly in vitro. Our in vivo studies in dogs in whom human cholesterol gallstones were implanted surgically showed rapid dissolution of the stones by MTBE instilled into the gallbladder via a surgically implanted catheter. Histology of the gallbladder later showed no evidence of gallbladder wall injury from the MTBE.

MTBE is a flammable solvent with explosive properties. It requires careful storage in a flameproof cabinet. It is kept in glass containers, which are tightly capped, or in metal cans. It is a strong solvent that affects many plastics such as those used in disposable syringes and specimen containers. Plastic syringes or bottles cannot be used to house this solvent. It must be injected using glass syringes that do not have rubber stoppers as rubber is also dissolved by the MTBE. The catheter used for stone dissolution is manufactured from low-density polyethylene, which resists dissolution by MTBE. MTBE is used as an octane enhancer in petrol. It is 97% pure. Distillation and microfiltration are used to sterilize the solvent prior to instillation into the gallbladder.

MTBE floats on bile while most cholesterol stones sink. Adequate contact of the solvent with the stone requires continuous mixing by injection and withdrawal through the pigtail catheter. Stone solvent contact is a critical factor in determining the rate of gallstone dissolution. Ideally an infusion pump that allows rapid injection of MTBE followed by slow aspiration would shorten dissolution time. When used clinically, great care is necessary to prevent accidents with this potentially explosive solvent. After gallstone dissolution the ether/bile/cholesterol mixture should be disposed of as a toxic waste product.

Technique of Gallstone Dissolution

This is carried out in a special treatment room, which, at all times, has good ventilation including an extractor for removal of ether vapor. The extractor is located close to the patient's abdomen.

A number of all glass syringes containing increasing volumes of MTBE are prepared and stored (capped) in a rack in the treatment room. Infusion and aspiration of solvent is commenced with 2 mL for 30 minutes increasing to 10 mL volumes over 2–3 hours with frequent syringe changes as the MTBE becomes saturated with cholesterol. Treatment sessions last 3 hours followed by an interval of 3–4 hours and a second 3-hour treatment session.

Twice-daily treatment sessions are continued until cholesterol is absent from the aspirate. Most gallstones are dissolved within 6–9 hours of MTBE infusion (Fig. 7.**4**). At the first 2-mL injection of MTBE, right upper quadrant pain may be felt by the patient. If this happens, non-narcotic analgesics are given. Continuous light sedation is maintained throughout the stone dissolution periods. When the stone(s) are clinically dissolved the patient is returned to the radiology department, and percutaneous cholecystography is performed with dilute contrast medium to confirm total stone dissolution. If the pigtail catheter is in situ

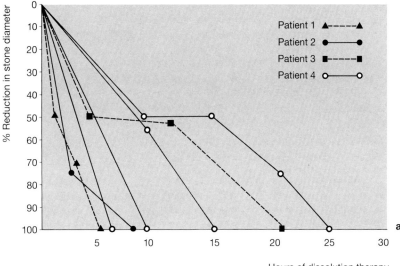

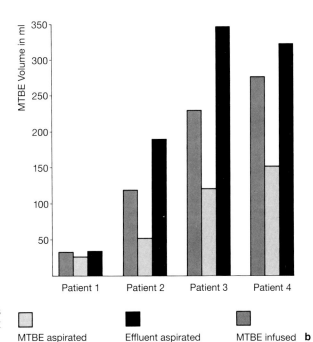

Fig. 7.**4** **a** Times of gallstone dissolution in four patients **b** Volumes of MTBE infused, aspirated, and effluent aspirated

☐ MTBE aspirated   ■ Effluent aspirated   ▨ MTBE infused **b**

overnight, percutaneous cholecystography is used to check catheter position in the gallbladder before dissolution is again commenced. A stone-free gallbladder at percutaneous cholecystography is an indication for continued therapy for a further 3 hours to dissolve any debris not detected by contrast study of the gallbladder. During MTBE infusions the therapy room is frequently visited by a staff member to test by sniffing if the patient is expelling MTBE from the lungs. Between treatment sessions the pigtail catheter is connected to a closed drainage system. Nausea during dissolution sessions is treated symptomatically. As treat-

ment progresses, the gallbladder capacity decreases, and it is essential not to overinject the gallbladder capacity with MTBE, reducing MTBE volumes if necessary. It is best if the patient does not eat during the period of stone dissolution. Hydration is maintained by i. v. fluids. Multiple small stones dissolve rapidly in 3 or 4 hours with MTBE therapy while a large solitary stone may take 6 hours or more to fissure or break into fragments; after this, dissolution is rapid. Other multiple large stones may dissolve rapidly.

Repositioning the Pigtail Catheter during Stone Dissolution
(Fig. 7.**5**)

It may be necessary to reposition the catheter when:

1. *Multiple stones are present in a septate gallbladder*
This occurs if the gallbladder contains a septum with stones in both compartments. When stones are dissolved in one compartment, the catheter loop must be placed in the second compartment to complete stone dissolution. To achieve this the guide wire is inserted into the coiled catheter until its lies free in the lumen. The catheter loops are uncoiled over the wire without removing the catheter totally from the lumen. The guide wire is now positioned in the required area where the remaining stones lie, and the catheter is advanced over it into the required position, and the wire is removed.

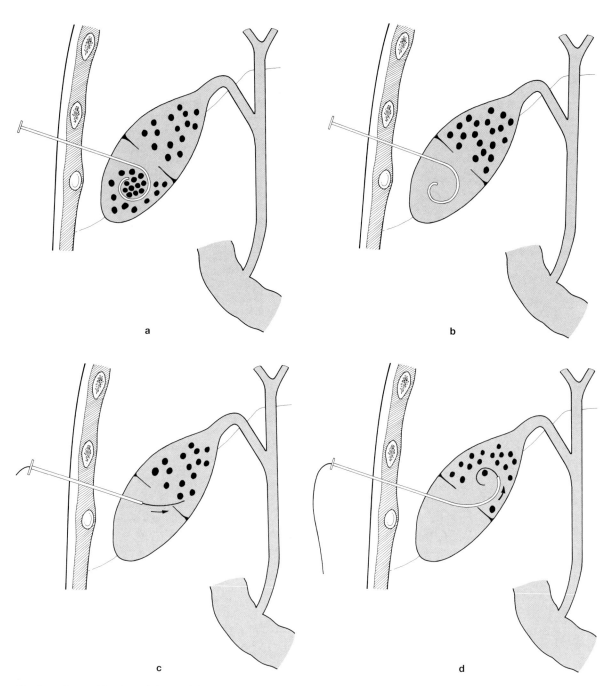

Fig. 7.**5**   **Repositioning of the gallbladder catheter for stone dissolution**

2. The catheter is partly dislodged

This occurs occasionally during an overnight interval between dissolution sessions. This may occur if an insufficient length of catheter has been inserted into the lumen of the organ at the original catheterization in the presence of a long narrow gallbladder or large hypotonic gallbladder, in the presence of morbid obesity, if the catheter has not been inserted transhepatically when a narrow thin right lobe of liver is present, or if it is pulled out by the elderly patient during sleep; therefore, fixation to the abdominal wall must be secure. A gallbladder on a mesentery should have a sufficient length of catheter within the organ to allow for excess mobility on patient movement to the left during sleep. Partial dislodgement of the catheter is discovered during a morning check of catheter position before continuing dissolution. Contrast medium is noted to leak from a side hole in the loop of the pigtail as well as opacify the gallbladder. If this happens, the guide wire is carefully inserted into the catheter until its tip reaches the lumen of the gallbladder. While the catheter is fixed on the skin by an assistant to prevent it being dislodged further by the guide wire, the wire is carefully inserted into the gallbladder lumen and coiled within it. The catheter is now pushed over the wire and looped within the lumen. The wire is removed, and after 2–3 hours and predissolution cholecystography shows absence of leakage, treatment is continued. Often it is easier, if the catheter is partly dislodged and it is possible to insert a guide wire into the gallbladder through it, to replace the catheter with a new catheter.

3. An undissolved stone is present in the neck of the gallbladder

(Fig. 7.**6**)

A guide wire is inserted through the lysis catheter into the gallbladder lumen. A loop of catheter or catheter wire is pushed into the neck of the gallbladder to surround the stone, and withdrawal of the loop pulls the stone into the body or fundus of the gallbladder.

Removal of the Transhepatic Catheter from the Gallbladder

The catheter is always removed in the radiology department over a guide wire using fluoroscopy under sterile conditions with analgesia. The catheter is freed at the skin and slowly withdrawn over the guide wire leaving the wire tip within the lumen. The guide wire is used to uncoil the catheter loops, which prevents these sticking together. The final cholangiogram should demonstrate the bile ducts, cystic duct, and gallbladder, and should show that no stone fragments have passed into the cystic duct or common bile duct during dissolution. Dilute contrast is used to study the gallbladder lumen.

Contrast medium is aspirated from the gallbladder completely, if possible, before catheter removal. The track in the liver is plugged with Gelfoam (5) by inserting a small dilator of 4–5 Fr over the wire 4–5 cm from the skin. The wire is removed, and compressed Gelfoam strips are inserted down the dilator as it is removed from the liver. The patient is kept in the hospital overnight while vital signs are monitored. The next morning, ultrasound of the gallbladder is performed (Fig. 7.**7**). This may show nonshadowing debris if all stones are dissolved. Most patients are symptom free at this stage; some experience mild upper abdominal pain for 24 hours. Only patients who are symptom free are permitted to leave the hospital. None of our patients have required readmission for any reason related to MTBE therapy. Ultrasound is repeated at 3 and 6 months to look for stone recurrence.

Stone Recurrence after MTBE Dissolution

When gallstones occur again in the gallbladder after oral dissolution, ESWL, or contact dissolution with MTBE they may originate as new stones or from residual debris left in the gallbladder at treatment termination. Resolution of fluoroscopic direct contrast injection cholecystography and even high-quality radiography with dilute contrast medium is poor for small stone-fragment detection. The contrast study may be normal, while ultrasound reveals residual debris often without acoustic shadowing. Repeat ultrasound examinations in the short term (1–6 weeks) fail to show clearance of this debris perhaps because the gallbladder is unable to expel the fragments because of an abnormality of motility. There is a good case for direct removal of any debris remaining in the gallbladder immediately after dissolution therapy is completed. We believe from the study of removed pigtail catheters after dissolution therapy with MTBE that flushing with saline may expel cholesterol fragments back into the gallbladder since these fragments accumulate around the 32 side holes in the pigtail in every patient in whom MTBE therapy is used (Fig. 7.**4**). Detection of residual debris by ultrasound is impossible while the catheter remains in the gallbladder, so preventive lavage should be undertaken using a new catheter inserted through the gallbladder fundus that allows direct access to the cystic duct also for thermal occlusion.

The Becker catheter (Cook, Denmark) is ideal for this purpose and for ablation of the gallbladder mucosa.

Cystic duct occlusion is essential prior to gallbladder ablation since the gallbladder mucosa regenerates from the cystic duct if it is not occluded by endoluminal coagulation by a bipolar 7-Fr catheter (Becker 1989). Before gallbladder ablation, catheter cholecystography is performed to confirm permanent cystic duct occlusion 2 weeks after thermal cystic duct occlusion. Conventional occlusive agents used in vascular system interventions do not produce permanent occlu-

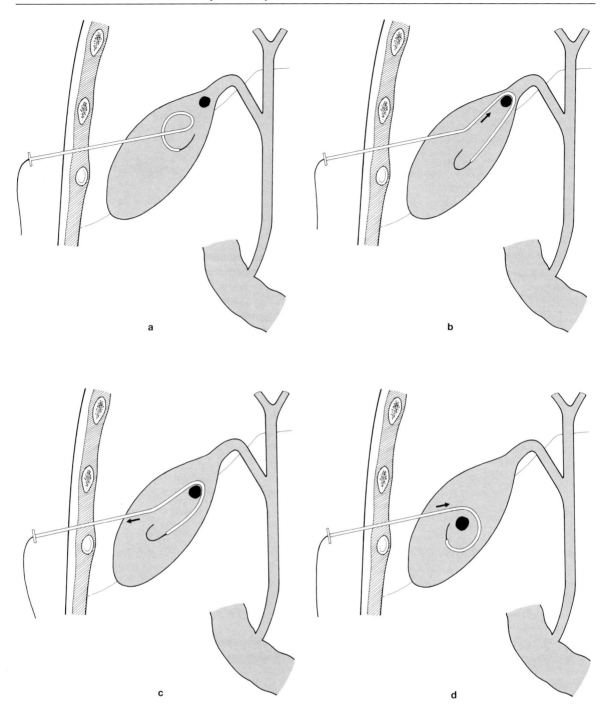

Fig. 7.**6**   **Retrieving a stone from the neck of the gallbladder**

sion in the cystic duct. Gallbladder mucosal ablation is achieved by injecting the equivalent of the gallbladder volume of absolute alcohol into the gallbladder and leaving it in situ for one hour (3, 4). Cystic duct occlusion without gallbladder mucosal destruction leads to formation of a gallbladder mucocele or a mucous

Fig. 7.**7   Gallstone dissolution with MTBE a** before ▶ and **b** after dissolution solitary stone **c** before and **d** after dissolution of multiple gallstones **e** gallbladder ultrasound post–stone dissolution of multiple stones. The gallbladder is stone and echo free at 24 hours post dissolution

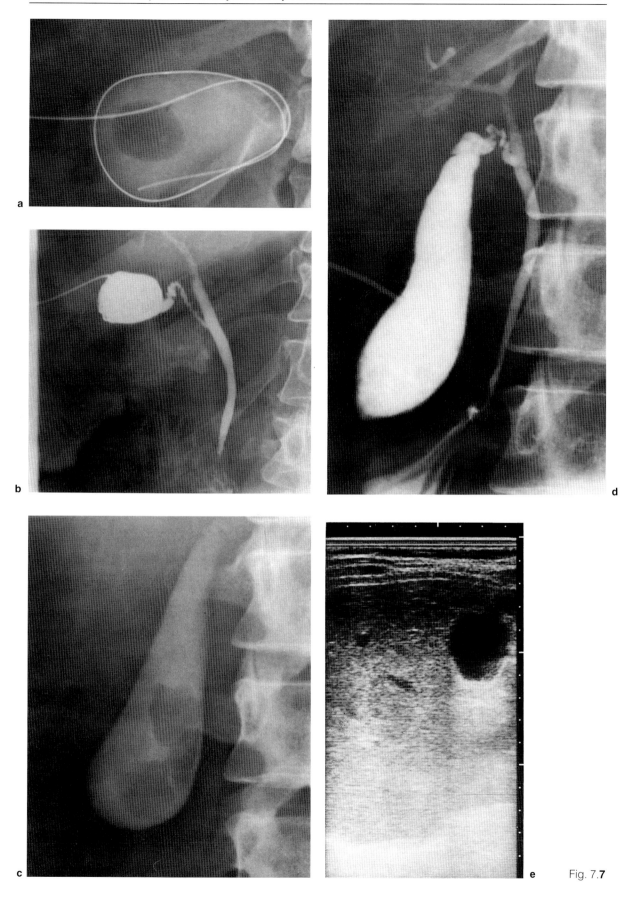

Fig. 7.**7**

fistula from the percutaneous cholecystostomy track. Exclusion of the gallbladder by these techniques prevents gallstone recurrence in the gallbladder.

Percutaneous Cholecystostomy for Gallbladder Stone Removal (Percutaneous Cholecystolithotomy)
(Fig. 7.**8**)

Indications

The indications for percutaneous cholecystolithotomy include patients who refuse surgery or are unfit for surgery because of cardiac or pulmonary disease, the very old patient with gallstones, severe obesity, religion (13), previous complicated abdominal surgery, failed fragmentation of gallstones at ESWL, acute gallbladder disease (mucocele or empyema with gallstones, but not in florid acute cholecystitis; drainage in acute cholecystitis is approached by the transhepatic route as an emergency procedure) or calcified gallstones unsuitable for ESWL, oral, or contact dissolution. The advantage of this technique is that all the gallstones are removed immediately regardless of composition size or the number of calculi present. It may also be used to remove stone fragments after ESWL and hence, to avoid complications of stone fragments passing into the cystic duct and common bile duct. The route is also valuable for gaining access to the common bile duct for stone removal (31) or stent insertion in selected cases of malignant biliary obstruction (30).

Contraindications

Contraindications to percutaneous cholecystolithotomy include very large gallstones, calcified gallbladder, gangrene or perforation of the gallbladder, chronic cholecystitis with contracted gallbladder, pregnancy, ascites, and bleeding disorders.

Preparation of the Patient

Percutaneous cholecystolithotomy is a *planned procedure*. We prefer that the patient for percutaneous cholecystolithotomy have a normally functioning gallbladder with a normal wall thickness as determined by CT and ultrasound. Normal function is not necessary for successful stone removal, but a diseased gallbladder wall is more likely to leak bile if the gallbladder is lost during track preparation or after catheter removal, and thickening of the wall by fibrosis may make puncture more difficult and dilatation of a track to the lumen less easy.

Ultrasound and CT are used to study the relationship of the gallbladder to the liver and colon, to

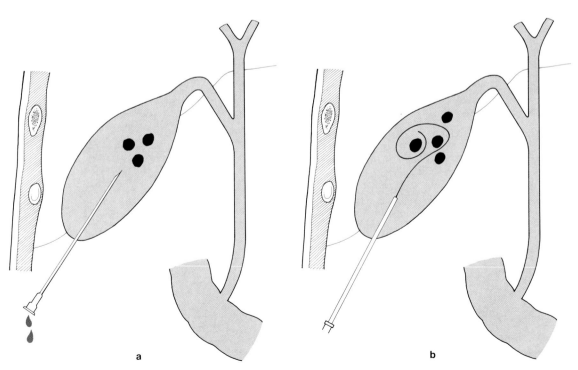

a   b

Fig. 7.**8**   **Subcostal cholecystostomy for gallstone removal. a** to **e** percutaneous procedure

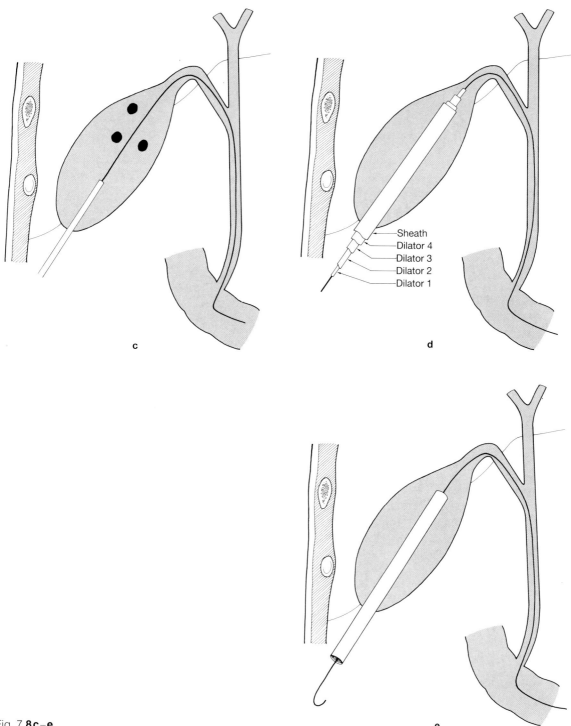

c

d

Sheath
Dilator 4
Dilator 3
Dilator 2
Dilator 1

e

Fig. 7.**8c**–**e**

choose a safe puncture site, and to choose the direction of angulation of the needle to puncture the gallbladder fundus. Coagulation and bleeding indices should be normal.

Technique

The examination is carried out in the radiology department under sterile conditions with local anesthesia, i. v. sedation, and analgesia. Preprocedure i. v. antibiotics are given. The examination is performed in the fasting patient with i. v. fluids for hydration. The right subcostal route is chosen for stone removal. A transhepatic route is used for external drainage or stent insertion into the bile duct. The patient is positioned supine on the fluoroscopy table. Adequate covering of the patient is necessary to maintain body heat if lithotripsy is being considered. The abdomen is cleaned with antiseptic and covered with waterproof surgical sheets, which protect the radiographic table from endoscopic irrigation fluid if lithotripsy is employed. Fluid is drained into a suitable container to prevent electrical hazards. The skin and abdominal wall over the gallbladder fundus are infiltrated down to the peritoneum with local anesthetic using sterile procedures. A 15-mm incision is made in the skin over the gallbladder fundus and a track extended down to the peritoneum with mosquito forceps. A 19-SWG catheter needle (Medi-tech, USA) is inserted into the fundus of the gallbladder with a stabbing motion, and the needle is withdrawn. Puncture of the wall may be observed by placing an ultrasound probe in the right lower subcostal or intercostal area. If the catheter lies in the gallbladder lumen, bile drips from its external tip. Next, a guide wire is inserted through the catheter and coiled in the lumen of the gallbladder. We next insert a 5-Fr pigtail catheter over the wire into the gallbladder and pass several loops into the lumen. The wire is now removed. The gallbladder is emptied of bile, and contrast medium is inserted to outline the gallbladder, cystic duct, and common bile duct to the duodenum. The gallbladder is irrigated with saline until the return is clear of bile. A small amount of contrast medium is now introduced into the gallbladder. The gallbladder volume is kept as small as possible by aspiration after the organ is irrigated. We now replace the pigtail catheter over a guide wire by a 5-Fr dilator. This dilator is now used to attempt to insert a guide wire (Amplatz Torque Teflon coated) into the cystic duct, common bile duct, and duodenum. If this is achieved, it greatly increases the stability of the guide wire during subsequent dilator insertion. When the guide wire cannot be inserted with the 5-Fr dilator, the smallest steerable catheter is used to direct the guide wire into the cystic duct and common bile duct. We now insert biliary dilators or a balloon dilator to 18 Fr, and a Teflon sheath is inserted into the gallbladder lumen. Coaxial dilators or coaxial metal dilators are best for track dilatation with less risk of losing the track than individual dilator replacements over the wire.

During dilator insertion the dilators should always be pointed toward the patient's head and held in place manually close to the skin at an acute angle with the skin of the abdominal wall.

If catheterization is easy and a wire is present in the bile duct, we proceed with stone removal following dilatation of the track to 25 Fr. A 25-Fr working sheath is now inserted into the gallbladder. Stone removal is carried out through this sheath. This may be performed by basket, forceps, suction, or irrigation if stones are small. Larger stones require fragmentation. This may be performed by (1) electrohydraulic lithotripsy using a 3-Fr electrode and direct vision with a flexible choledochoscope. Great care should be taken to avoid contact with the wall of the gallbladder. The gallbladder is irrigated with N/6 saline during lithotripsy. (2) A Kensey–Nash lithotrite (Baxter, Irvine, USA) may be introduced into the gallbladder via a 12-Fr sheath to pulverize stones rapidly to particles of less than 1 mm in size within 20–30 minutes or less depending on stone size. We use a transhepatic route to the gallbladder with this instrument. When the gallbladder is free of stone debris, a 12-Fr or 14-Fr Foley catheter is inserted down the sheath and inflated *before the sheath is removed.* The Foley catheter is connected to a closed biliary drainage bag. At 24 hours a contrast study is made of the gallbladder. If the gallbladder, cystic duct, and bile ducts are stone free, the catheter is removed after emptying the gallbladder completely. The patient is discharged at 24 hours if vital signs are normal.

Complications

Loss of the gallbladder is the major complication during this procedure. It is prevented by passing a guide wire via the cystic duct into the duodenum and using coaxial dilators or an angioplasty balloon catheter to dilate the track rather than replacement dilators. The guide wire in the cystic duct may prevent *escape of a stone fragment into the bile duct* during the procedure. If this happens, stone removal by endoscopic sphincterotomy is necessary.

Perforation of the gallbladder during stone fragmentation may occur. Immediate catheter drainage of the gallbladder is necessary if this occurs. Drainage may prevent the need for cholecystectomy.

Cholecystostomy by Minilaparotomy

This is a planned procedure for the removal of gallstones in the elderly (16). Under local anesthesia the fundus of the gallbladder is exposed by minilaparotomy. An incision is made in the wall of the fundus, and a large Foley catheter is inserted and inflated within the lumen. The gallbladder fundus is fixed to the abdominal wall by suturing so there is no danger of loss of the gallbladder with this technique. The gallstones are removed from the gallbladder subsequently. It is best if the catheter is inserted via the fundus rather than through its anterior wall since the latter makes it difficult to perform further manipulation within the organ or the bile duct.

Stone removal from the gallbladder is best performed with a Nitinol basket (Fig. 7.**9**).

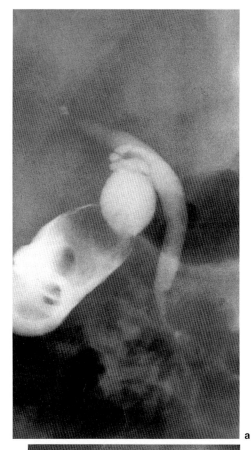

Fig. 7.**9 Percutaneous catheter cholecystography
after minilaparotomy**
a Showing gallstones and common bile duct stones
b Nitinol basket open
c Nitinol basket partly closed
d Cholangiogram via the gallbladder after gallbladder
and duct stone clearance

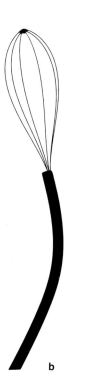

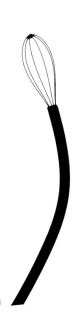

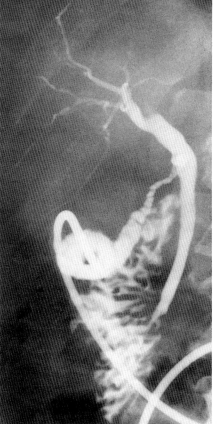

We have used this technique in patients, remote from the minilaparotomy period, for successful removal of gallstones, but we prefer to use a percutaneous catheterization technique for stone removal or gallbladder drainage.

References

1. Akiyama H, Ozazaki T, Takashima I, et al. Percutaneous treatments for biliary diseases. Radiology 1990;176:25–30.
2. Allen MJ, Borody TJ, Bugliosi TF, et al. Rapid dissolution of gallstones with methyl tert butyl ether. N Engl J Med 1985;312:217–220.
3. Asfar S, Al-Refai FI, Al-Mokhtar NY, Baraka A. Percutaneous sclerosis of the gallbladder. Lancet 1989;2:387.
4. Becker CD, Burhenne HJ. Percutaneous ablation of the cystic duct and gallbladder: Experimental and early clinical results. Semin Roentgenol 1991;26:259–266.
5. Bender CE, Williams HJ. Technical aspects of percutaneous gallstone dissolution. Semin Intervent Radiol 1988;5:186–194.
6. Bogan ML, Hawes RH, Kopecky KK, et al. Percutaneous cholecystolithotomy with endoscopic lithotripsy by using a pulsed dye laser: Preliminary experience AJR 1990; 155:781–784.
7. Conaway CC, Schroeder RE, Snyder NK. Tetatology evaluation of methyl tert butyl ether in rats and mice. J Toxicol Environmental health 1985;16:797–809.
8. Carrick J, Doust B, Coleman M, et al. Methyl tert butyl ether cholelitholysis of calculi in the gallbladder and bile ducts. Aust NZ J Med 1987;17:435–440.
9. Cope C. Percutaneous subhepatic cholecystostomy with removable anchor AJR 1988;151:1129–1132.
10. Cope C, Burke DR, Meranze SG. Percutaneous extraction of gallstones in 20 patients. Radiology 1990;176:19–24.
11. Cope C. Percutaneous cholecystolithotomy. Semin Roentgenol 1991;26:245–250.
12. Cope C. Novel ninitol basket instrument for percutaneous cholecystolithotomy. AJR 1990;155:515–516.
13. D'Agostino HB, van Sonnenberg E, Hofmann AF, et al. Contact dissolution for gallstones. Lippincott's Reviews: Radiology 1992;1:73–84.
14. Foerster EC, Matek W, Domschke W. Endoscopic retrograde cannulation of the gallbladder: direct dissolution of gallstones. Gastrointest Endosc 1990;36:444–450.
15. Gillams A, Curtis SC, Donald J, et al. Technical considerations in 113 percutaneous cholecystolithotomies. Radiology 1992; 183:163–166.
16. Hamilton S, Leahy AL, Darzi A, Keane FBV. Biliary intervention via minicholecystostomy Clin Radiol 1990;42:418–422.
17. Hellstern A, Leuschner U, Fisher H, et al. Percutane transhepatische Lyse von Gallenblasensteinen mit Methyltertbutyläther. Dtsch Med Wochenschr 1988;113:506–510.
18. Hoffman AF, Schteingart CD, vanSonnenberg E, et al. Contact dissolution of cholesterol gallstones with organic solvents. Gastroenterol Clin N Amer 1991;20:183–199.
19. Kellet MJ, Russell RCG, Wickham JEA. Percutaneous cholecystolithotomy. Endoscopy 1989;21:365–366.
20. Kellet MJ, Wickham JEA, Russell RCG. Percutaneous cholecystolithotomy Br Med J 1988;296:453–455.
21. Kerlan RK, LaBerge JM, Ring EL. Percutaneous cholecystolithotomy. Preliminary experience. Radiology 1985; 157:653–565.
22. Hellstern A, Leuschner M, Frank H, et al. Gallstone dissolution with methyl tert butyl ether: how to avoid complications. Gut 1990;31:922–923.
23. Hwang MH, Mo LR, Chan LR, et al. Percutaneous transhepatic cholecystic ultrasonic lithotripsy. Gastrointest Endosc 1987; 33:301–302.
24. Hruby W, Stackl W, Urgan M, et al. Percutaneous endoscopic cholecystolithotripsy. Work in progress. Radiology 1989; 173:477–479.
25. Larssen TB, Gothlin JH, Jensen D, et al. Ultrasonic and fluoroscopic therapeutic percutaneous catheter drainage of the gallbladder. Gastrointest Radiol 1988;13:37–41.
26. Lee LL, Mc Gahan JP. Dissolution of cholesterol gallstones: Comparison of solvents. Gastrointest Radiol 1986;11:169–171.
27. Leuschner U, Hellstern A. Perkutan-transhepatische Litholyse (PTL) mit Methyltertbutyläther. Aktueller Stand und Zukunftsperspektiven. Internist 1989;29:788–791.
28. Leuschner M, Hellstern A, Schmidt K, et al. Gallstone dissolution with methyl tert butyl ether in 120 patients: efficacy and safety Dig Dis Sci 1991;36:193–199.
29. Lindeman SR, Tung G, Silverman SG, Mueller PR. Percutaneous cholecystostomy. Semin Intervent Radiol 1988; 5:179–185.
30. Mc Nulty JG. Interventional radiology of the gallbladder. Berlin: Springer, 1990:21–65.
31. Mc Nulty J, Chua A, Ah-Kion S, Weir DG, Keeling PWN. Dissolution of cholesterol gallstones using methyl tert butyl ether: a safe effective treatment. Gut 1991;32:1550–1553.
32. May GR. Solvent dissolution of gallstones. Radiology 1988; 186:331–332.
33. Miller FJ, Rose SC. Intervention for gallbladder disease. Cardiovasc Intervent Radiol 1990;13:264–271.
34. Miller FJ, Rose SC, Buchi KN, et al. Percutaneous rotational contact biliary lithotripsy: initial clinical results with the Kensey–Nash lithotrite. Radiology 1991;178:781–785.
35. Peine CJ, Peterson BT, Williams HJ, et al. Extracorporeal shock wave lithotripsy and methyl tert butyl ether for partially calcified gallstones. Gastroenterol 1989;97:1229–1235.
36. Picus D, Marx MV, Hicks ME, et al. Percutaneous cholecystolithotomy: Preliminary experience and technical considerations. Radiology 1989;173:487–491.
37. Picus D. Percutaneous gallbladder intervention. Radiology 1990;176:5–6.
38. Ponchon T, Baroud J, Pujot B, et al. Renal failure during dissolution of gallstones by methyl tert butyl ether. Lancet 1988;2: 276–277.
39. Ponchon T, Baroud J, Mestas JL, Chayvialle JA. Gallstone lithotripsy: retrograde dissolution of fragments. Gastrointest Endosc 1988;34:468–469.
40. Schumacker KA, Swobodnik W, Janowitz P, et al. Radiographic aspects in transcatheter dissolution of calcified gallbladder concretions. Eur J Radiol 1990;10:28–34.
41. Simeone JF, Mueller PR, Ferrucci JT Jr. Nonsurgical therapy of gallstones: Implications for imaging. AJR 1989;153:11–17.
42. van Sonnenberg E, Hofmann AF, Neoptolemos J, et al. Gallstone dissolution with methyl tert butyl ether via percutaneous cholecystostomy: Success and caveats AJR 1986;146:865–867.
43. vanSonnenberg E, Hofmann AH. Horizons in gallstone therapy. AJR 1988;150:43–46.
44. vanSonnenberg E, D'Agostino HB, Casola G, et al. Interventional radiology in the gallbladder: Diagnosis drainage, dissolution, and management of gallstones. Radiology 1990;174:1–6.
45. vanSonnenberg E, Zakko S, Hofmann AF, et al. Human gallbladder morphology after gallstone dissolution with MTBE. Gastroenterol 1991;100:1718–1723.
46. vanSonnenberg E, D'Agostino HB, Goodacre BW, et al. Percutaneous gallbladder puncture and cholecystostomy: Results, complications and caveats for safety. Radiology 1992; 83:167–170.
47. Vogelzang RL, Nemcek AA. Towards painless percutaneous biliary procedures: new strategies and alternatives. J Intervent Radiol 1988;3:131–134.
48. Vogelzang RL, Nemcek AA. Percutaneous cholecystostomy: diagnostic and therapeutic efficacy. Radiology 1988;168:29–34.
49. Teplick SK. Diagnostic and therapeutic interventional gallbladder procedures. AJR 1992;152:913–916.
50. Thistle JL, May GR, Bender CE, et al. Dissolution of cholesterolgallstones by methyl tert butyl ether administered by percutaneous transhepatic catheter. N Engl J Med 1989;320:633–639.
51. Wenk H, Thomas ST, Schmeller N, et al. Percutaneous transhepatic cholecystic ultrasonic lithotripsy. Endoscopy 1989;21:221–222.
52. Wolpers C. Gallenblasensteine Ihre Morphogenese und Auswahl zur litholyse. Basel: Karger, 1987:202.
53. Zakko SF, Hofmann AF. Microprocessor-assisted solvent transfer system for effective contact dissolution of gallbladder stones. IEEE Trans Biomed Eng 1990;37:410–416.

8 Percutaneous Cholecystostomy for Gallbladder Drainage, Endoscopy of the Gallbladder, and Percutaneous Endoluminal Gallbladder Biopsy

Percutaneous Cholecystostomy for Gallbladder Drainage

Percutaneous gallbladder drainage is used in the treatment of acute cholecystitis, in drainage of a mucocele or empyema of the gallbladder, and in drainage of the extrahepatic biliary tract obstruction when the obstruction lies below the insertion of the cystic duct and ERCP drainage is unsuccessful, drainage after FN PTHC fails and the anatomy of the cystic duct insertion is unsuitable for stent insertion via the gallbladder. Emergency cholecystostomy may be used in addition to endoscopic biliary drainage in infective cholangitis when infection of the gallbladder is also suggested.

Preparation of the Patient

Preparation of the often very ill patient for emergency percutaneous cholecystostomy should include hydration of the patient with intravenous fluids, correction of coagulation defects, reversal of anticoagulant therapy if necessary, and treatment of cardiac failure since rapid respiration by the patient is a contraindication as there is a danger of causing a tear in the gallbladder wall during catheterization.

Preprocedure antibiotics are necessary in patients who are at risk because of heart valve replacements or other cardiac defects that may lead to bacterial endocarditis. *All patients with a history of heart disease are given 0.5 mg of atropine intramuscularly* before percutaneous gallbladder puncture. The diagnosis of acute cholecystitis is made from clinical and laboratory findings, ultrasound of a gallbladder and HIDA scanning. Ultrasound and HIDA scanning may have a low diagnostic accuracy in the fasting hospitalized patient or the patient receiving parenteral nutrition. In these patients fine needle percutaneous transhepatic gallbladder puncture may be used for diagnosis before drainage. The diagnosis of mucocele or empyema of the gallbladder is made by clinical examination and ultrasound. Percutaneous cholecystostomy in acute cholecystitis or mucocele is performed under ultrasonic control. We prefer to do the procedure in the radiology interventional unit, but it has been performed at the bedside (4, 8, 9, 10, 12). Percutaneous cholecystostomy for external biliary drainage of the bile ducts is used only when endoscopic and percutaneous transhepatic biliary drainage fail. The biliary tract in such cases is usually already opacified by previous direct cholangiography, which also establishes the diagnosis of lower common bile duct obstruction. It is of no value to drain the gallbladder when the obstruction lies above the common bile duct. These patients are often very ill with cholangitis or liver failure secondary to biliary obstruction, and percutaneous gallbladder drainage causes immediate relief of biliary obstruction.

Technique of Percutaneous Cholecystostomy

1. *Mucocele or empyema of the gallbladder* (Fig. 8.**1**) The gallbladder is almost always palpable in the presence of mucocele or empyema of the organ, and it may be visible on inspection of the abdomen during respiration. An anterior direct puncture of the gallbladder in the right upper abdomen may be performed, but we prefer transhepatic gallbladder puncture. Under local anesthesia, sedation, and analgesia, and using a sterile technique, a 19-guage catheter needle is inserted transhepatically into the upper third of the body of the gallbladder. The needle is removed and replaced by semistiff guide wire, which is looped in the gallbladder for stability of the wire during catheter insertion. Dilators, 5 Fr and 7 Fr, are now inserted over the wire. Next, a 9-Fr pigtail catheter is inserted and coiled over the guide wire within the gallbladder. A sufficient length of catheter is inserted into the gallbladder so that when the obstruction is removed and the organ returns to normal size, the catheter and its side holes are within the lumen. The wire is removed, and the catheter is fixed securely to the skin and attached to a closed drainage system.

The causal lesion in mucocele or empyema of the gallbladder is often a calculus. This may fall back into the organ when the gallbladder is drained. Following 24–48 hours drainage, the gallbladder is markedly reduced in size, and transcatheter cholecystocholangiography may be performed to assess the cause of the mucocele, the patency of the cystic duct, and the extrahepatic bile ducts. Manipulation within the gallbladder should not be performed for at least 1 week following drainage. At this time a stone in the neck of the gallbladder may be retrieved into the gallbladder lumen using a loop of guide wire. A stone in the cystic duct

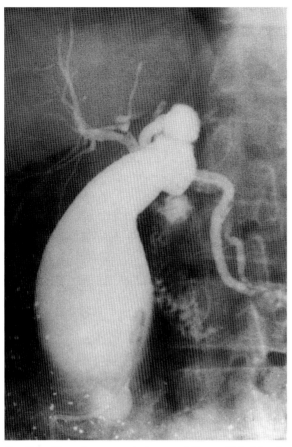

Fig. 8.**1**   **Percutaneous drainage of the gallbladder in mucocele**

may be removed using a Dormia basket introduced via the drainage catheter.

The percutaneous track may also be used to insert instruments to remove ductal stones as described in Chapter 10.

2. *Acute cholecystitis* (Fig. 8.**2**)

The gallbladder is a fragile organ in the presence of established acute cholecystitis. A small contracted gall-

---

Fig. 8.**2   Percutaneous gallbladder drainage in acute** ▶ **cholangitis with cholecystitis in an 87-year-old woman.** ERCP failed because of periampullary diverticula obscuring the papilla
a FN PTHC revealed stones in the bile ducts. The intrahepatic ducts are not dilated and transhepatic duct catheterization was not attempted
b The gallbladder was punctured and catheterized
c A 5-Fr pigtail catheter is coiled in the gallbladder for external drainage
d At 24 hours the fundus of the gallbladder was punctured and a guide wire inserted via the cystic duct into the duodenum
e A 10-Fr double pigtail teflon stent was inserted over the guide wire into the duodenum for internal drainage. The patient was too ill to attempt stone removal from the bile duct. Both cholangitis and cholecystitis resolved. She remained well for 3 months after the procedure
f The gallbladder catheter was removed. Multiple gallstones are present in the gallbladder. There was no leak of bile from the catheter
▼

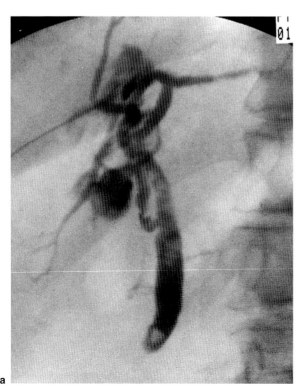

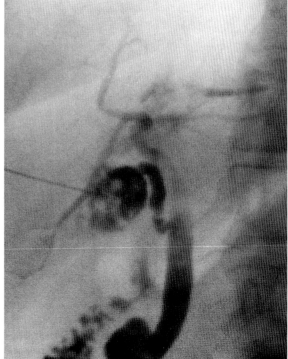

a   b

Fig. 8.**2a** u. **b**

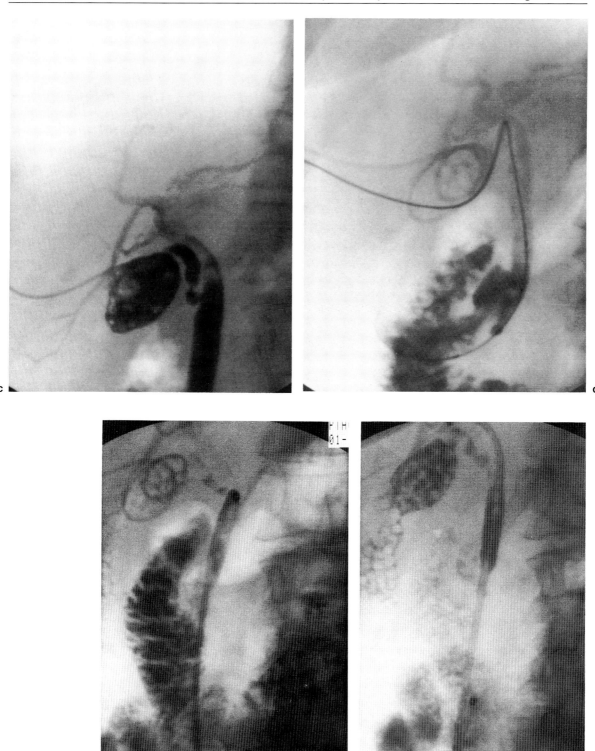

Fig. 8.**2c–f**

bladder is not suitable for this procedure. A gallbladder packed full of gallstones is difficult to catheterize, and the technique is likely to prove unsuccessful. Gentle percutaneous cholecystostomy with minimal intraluminal manipulations may be used to drain the inflamed gallbladder in acute cholecystitis with or without gallstones. The patient who is unfit for surgery because of advanced age, cardiac failure, liver failure, sepsis, renal failure, or immunosuppression benefits most from percutaneous gallbladder drainage. Our experience is that the patient who is fit for surgery should have surgical cholecystectomy as soon as the diagnosis of acute cholecystitis is established.

Sectional imaging is valuable for successful emergency gallbladder drainage. Ultrasound is essential for gallbladder localization in the emergency situation, and CT scanning is valuable in selecting the best site for percutaneous gallbladder puncture in order to avoid intervening intestine. A transhepatic route to the gallbladder is safest.

The gallbladder is punctured transhepatically via the axilla using a Chiba needle. When gallstones are present, the organ should be punctured if possible on the cystic duct side of the stones (i.e., above the stones). A guide wire is inserted through the needle and coiled within the gallbladder lumen. An Accustick catheter is inserted over the guidewire. The wire is removed with the inner catheter from the Accustick sets and a semistiff guide wire is now introduced in the gallbladder lumen.

A 5-Fr pigtail catheter is now inserted over the guide wire into the gallbladder lumen and coiled within the gallbladder. A small amount of dilute contrast medium is injected to conform catheter position only. The catheter is fixed to the skin and attached to a closed drainage system. Bile is sent for culture. At 48 hours, cholecystocholangiography is performed to study the cystic duct and bile ducts. Catheter drainage is continued until cholecystitis resolves. A decision as to the form of treatment of any gallstones present is then made. Cholesterol stones may be dissolved with MTBE, calcified stones may be fragmented by ESWL and removed or dissolved, or the gallbladder and its contents may be removed by surgery immediately or within 3 months after infection has resolved. When symptoms resolve and the patient requests nonsurgical therapy of the gallstones, this should be delayed for 3 months.

3. *Extrahepatic biliary obstruction*
Percutaneous cholecystostomy in extrahepatic biliary obstruction is a palliative procedure in the very ill patient. We have also used the technique in gross biliary sepsis with suppurative cholangitis when choledocholithiasis was present with gallbladder stones and ERCP and percutaneous biliary drainage had failed. We have also used the procedure in the therapy of acute biliary and pancreatic duct obstruction in acute pancreatitis after endoscopic sphincterotomy and stone removal and as a short term form of drainage in jaundice secondary to pancreatic head carcinoma (Fig. 8.**3**). The technique is of no value when the obstruction lies above the junction of the cystic and common bile duct. The technique of gallbladder drainage is similar to that described for mucocele of the gallbladder with anterior puncture of the dilated gallbladder under clinical or ultrasound control followed by catheterization of the lumen with a pigtail catheter that is fixed firmly by sutures to the skin of the anterior abdominal wall and connected to a closed drainage system (Fig. 8.**4**).

Endoscopy of the Gallbladder

Endoscopy of the gallbladder is a valuable procedure for inspection of the gallbladder lumen after all methods of stone removal. The technique, if performed routinely after stone dissolution or removal of gallbladder stones, could help establish whether recurrence of gallbladder stones is due to stone fragments being left behind after treatment or to the formation of new gallstones.

The technique has also been used for direct removal of gallstones and endoluminal tumor biopsy under direct vision. Biopsy is performed after inspection of the lumen is complete because bleeding after biopsy may make clear endoscopic inspection impossible. Complications are mostly related to track formation. These include loss of the gallbladder during initial catheterization and track dilatation. This does not occur if a guide wire is inserted through the cystic duct into the common bile duct as an initial procedure using a steerable catheter and Terumo glide wire. Tracks mature more quickly through the liver than following subcostal catheterization. Infection is minimized by continuing antibiotic therapy as long as external drainage is present.

Percutaneous Transhepatic Endoluminal Gallbladder Biopsy

Indications

The main indication for this procedure is the demonstration of a fixed filling defect in the gallbladder by imaging with ultrasound, oral cholecystography or CT scanning, or the presence of undiagnosed localized thickening of the wall of the gallbladder on ultrasound or CT scanning.

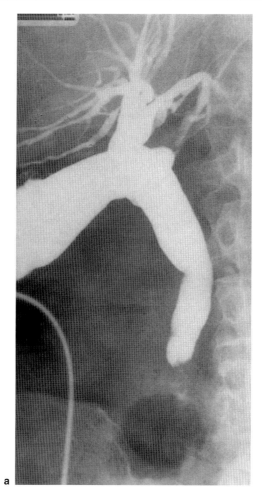
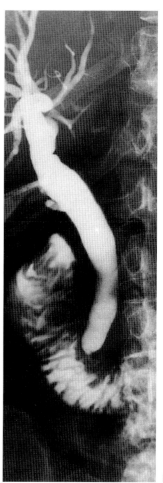

Fig. 8.**3 a External
drainage via the gallbladder
after perforation of the
lower CBD at endoscopic
sphincterotomy and stone
removal.** No contrast medium entered the duodenum.
The patient was very ill with
jaundice pyrexia and a palpable gallbladder
b Cholangiogram at 5 days
showing a stone-free duct
and free drainage to the
duodenum. The patient, a
75-year-old woman, had
deep jaundice, which re-
solved completely   a

b

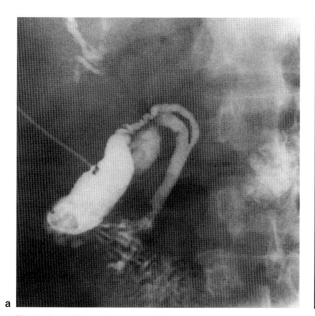
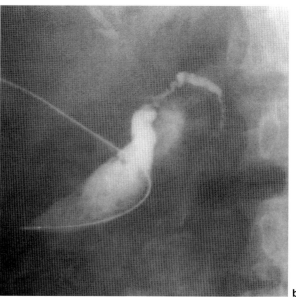

a

b

Fig. 8.**4 a Percutaneous cholecystostomy for stone
dissolution** revealed gallstones, a normal extrahepatic
biliary tract, and a fixed filling defect attached to the gallbladder wall.

b A 3-Fr biopsy forceps was inserted via the 5-Fr catheter,
and the endoluminal mass was biopsied and shown to be
due to cholesterol deposits

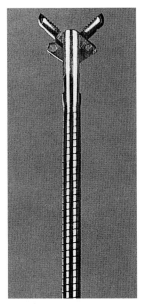

Fig. 8.**5** **3-Fr biopsy forceps (Cook, Denmark) for use with a 5-Fr catheter**

Contraindications

Contraindications include bleeding or coagulation disorders, hemobilia, and acute gallbladder disease.

Technique

Using an aseptic technique in the fasting patient and under i. v. sedation with analgesia and local anesthesia, a 5-Fr pigtail catheter is inserted transhepatically into the lumen of the gallbladder from the right axilla under ultrasound control (or fluoroscopy if there is a functioning gallbladder at oral cholecystography) using the technique described in Chapter 6. Only one loop of catheter is inserted into the gallbladder, and the catheter tip is positioned adjacent to the intraluminal mass using a guide wire to change catheter position if necessary. All gallbladder bile is removed from the organ, and the lumen is opacified with dilute contrast medium to visualize the intraluminal mass. A forceps biopsy needle is now inserted through the 5-Fr catheter until the lumen lies at the catheter tip (Fig. 8.**5**). While the biopsy forceps is being inserted, the catheter is fixed in position at the skin by an assistant to prevent it becoming dislodged or changing position within the gallbladder. After bite biopsy the biopsy forceps are withdrawn through the catheter and one loop of catheter coiled within the gallbladder lumen. The procedure is repeated until three fragments of the intraluminal lesion are obtained for histology.

Successful biopsy is evident during fluoroscopy as its pulls on the wall of the gallbladder during grasping of the lesion.

Complications of Percutaneous Endoluminal Biopsy

Following successful biopsy there is usually some venous bleeding from the catheter that ceases following irrigation with saline.

We have not encountered any incidences of perforation of the wall during the procedure. Following biopsy a cholecystocholangiogram is performed to exclude biliary obstruction, and the gallbladder is emptied of contrast medium and withdrawn over a guide wire.

References

1. Eggermont AM, Lameiras JS, Jeekil J. Ultrasound guided percutaneous transhepatic colecystostomy for acute acalculous cholecystitis. Arch Surg 1985;120: 1354–1358.
2. Hawkins JF. Percutaneous cholecystostomy. Semin Intervent Radiol 1985; 2:97–103.
3. Klimberg S, Hawkins IF, Vogel SB. Percutaneous cholecystostomy for acute cholecystitis in high risk patients. Amer J. Surg 1987; 53:125–128.
4. Lindemann SR, Tung G, Silverman SG, Mueller PR. Percutaneous cholecystostomy. Sem Intervent Radiol 1988; 5:179–185.
5. Lohela P, Soiva M, Suramo I, et al. Ultrasonic guidance for percutaneous puncture and drainage in acute cholecystitis. Acta Radiol 1986; 27:543–546.
6. Longmaid HE, Bassett JG, Gottlieb H. Management of gallbladder perforation by percutaneous cholecystostomy. Crit Care Med 1985; 13:686–687.
7. Mc Gahan JP, Lindfors KK. Acute cholecystitis: diagnostic accuracy of percutaneous aspiration of the gallbladder. Radiology 1988; 167:669–671.
8. Mc Gahan JP, Lindfors KK. Percutaneous cholecystostomy: an alternative to surgery for acute cholecystitis. Radiology 1989; 173:481–484.
9. Pearse DM, Hawkins IF, Shaver R, Vogel S. Percutaneous cholecystostomy in acute cholecystitis and common duct obstruction. Radiology 1984; 152:365–367.
10. Taylor S, Rawlinson J, Malone DE. Technical Report: Percutaneous cholecystostomy in acute acalculous cholecystitis. Clin Radiol 1992; 45:273 –275.
11. Teplick SK, Harsfield DL, Brandon JC. Percutaneous cholecystostomy in the critically ill patient. Gastrointest Radiol 1990; 16:154–158.
12. Vogelzang RL, Nemecek AA Jr. Percutaneous cholecystostomy: diagnostic and therapeutic efficacy. Radiology 1988; 168:29–34.
13. van Sonnenberg E, D'Agnostino HB, Casola G, et al. The benefits of percutaneous cholecystostomy for decompression of selected cases of obstructive jaundice. Radiology 1990; 176:15–18.
14. Werbel GB, Nahrwold DL, Joehl RJ. Percutaneous cholecystostomy in the diagnosis and treatment of acute cholecystitis in the high risk patient. Arch Surg 1989; 124:782–786.

Interventions for Benign Diseases of the Biliary Ducts

9 Endoscopic Sphincterotomy in the Treatment of Common Bile Duct Stones

D. H. Osborne and M. G. Courtney

The major application of therapeutic endoscopic retrograde cholangiopancreatography (ERCP) is endoscopic sphincterotomy (ES), and though this procedure has gained wide and increasing acceptance, it is associated with several potentially fatal complications. To minimize procedure-related risk to the patient, it is essential that the operator is thoroughly competent in the performance of ES. To this end, there can be no substitute for "hands-on" experience in the technique. ES can only be safely mastered by a prolonged and interactive apprenticeship with a practitioner already accomplished in the procedure. In the subsequent discussion, a high degree of familiarity with the subject is assumed. As with any invasive and/or potentially hazardous procedure, the reasons for performing the investigation and the possible risks involved should be fully explained to the patient, who must freely give informed written consent. Remember, zeal is no substitute for skill.

ES has been a major advance in the treatment of common bile duct stones (3). Although 80–90% of common duct stones can be successfully cleared after routine ES, the procedure carries significant morbidity (5–10%) and a small mortality (0.5–1.0%), even when performed by experienced operators (1). ES remains the method of choice for removing common duct stones in the majority of patients, but identification of those who are suitable is crucial. Controversy exists as to the use of this technique in young, fit patients with known cholecystitis/cholelithiasis and choledocholithiasis who may be treated alternatively by a surgical approach.

Endoscopic Sphincterotomy: Suitable Patients

Patients in whom ES is clearly indicated include:

1. The elderly or infirm with significant medical disease who present with obstructive jaundice secondary to gallstones (Fig. 9.1). ES is particularly useful in avoiding the appreciable operative morbidity and mortality in this group of patients.

2. ES is widely used prior to or following laparoscopic cholecystectomy in patients presenting with common bile duct stones (Fig. 9.2). Clearance of the common duct allows the laparoscopic pro-

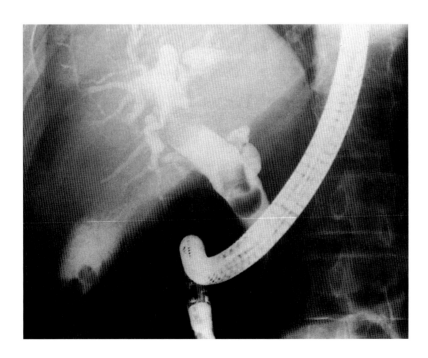

Fig. 9.**1** **Multiple common bile duct stones**

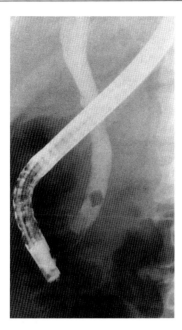

a

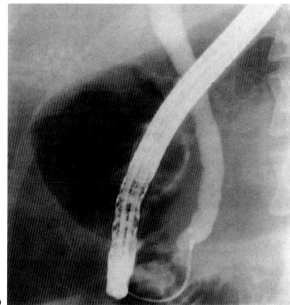

b

Fig. 9.**2 a ERCP before laparoscopic cholecystectomy** showing one stone in the bile duct and gallbladder stones.
b The duct is clear after ES and stone removal

3. Recurrent common bile duct stones following a previous cholecystectomy, whether performed recently or years previously, is an ideal indication for ES. In view of the previous cholecystectomy, there are usually few recurrent problems following ES and duct clearance.

4. ES has been advocated for patients with gallstone-associated acute pancreatitis (9). Those patients who fail to settle within 72 hours of the onset of stone-associated pancreatitis appear to benefit following removal of common bile duct stones in terms of improved survival and reduced hospital stay. Depending on the clinical indications, the gallbladder can subsequently be electively removed using a laparoscopic approach.

Technique of Endoscopic Sphincterotomy

An ample supply of well-maintained and reliable equipment is an essential prerequisite to a safe ES. Worn or malfunctioning equipment must be discarded and replaced without delay. A smoothly functioning team operating to clearly defined and practiced protocols is the hallmark of a "good" ERCP unit and ensures a high probability of successful intervention.

Following endoscopy with a side-viewing duodenoscope, cholangiography is obtained to confirm the presence of ductal stones. The caliber and configuration of the lower common bile duct is also noted. The cannula is removed and a sphincterotome is then inserted into the common bile duct. The position of the sphincterotome should always be confirmed on screening as it is possible to cannulate the pancreatic duct inadvertently. The wire of the bowed sphincterotome should be partially withdrawn so that only 50% remains inside the ampulla, lying approximately in the 12-o'clock position. This orientation ensures that a safe cut may be extended through the portion of the common bile duct that is traversing the duodenal wall. The safe extent of the incision superiorly is frequently delineated by the superior duodenal fold. However, there is an enormously varied morphology to the greater ampulla, and not infrequently, the superior fold is absent, in which case experience alone guides the extent of the cut. The incision should be fashioned by using the wire cautery in a "sawing" technique applied by alternatively withdrawing the sphincterotome a few millimeters and elevating the "bridge" of the duodenoscope. All the fibers of the sphincter should be divided when performing an adequate ES, and the sudden appearance of a "gush" of bile usually indicates the division of the internal sphincter. Experts differ in recommendations regarding the diathermy source, power setting, and whether blended or cutting current should be used. However, unhurried,

cedure to be performed without the need to perform the difficult technique of laparoscopic common bile duct exploration. When ERCP is performed prior to laparoscopic cholecystectomy, an additional benefit accrues: the precise anatomy of the common bile duct, cystic duct, and gallbladder can be ascertained, which may offer the surgeon greater latitude in the subsequent laparoscopic procedure.

methodical cutting for short periods is advisable to ensure optimal coagulation and to avoid a rapidly extended ("zipper") cut, which is associated with a greater incidence of bleeding and perforation. A sound understanding of the principles of tissue electrocautery is essential to perform ES safely.

The operator must be thoroughly familiar with the wide range of sphincterotomes available. Although it is acceptable to be more comfortable with a preferred range of equipment, it is advisable to extend one's experience to a wide range of "knives." The secret of success lies frequently in the correct choice of the most appropriate "knife" for a particular situation.

Endoscopic Sphincterotomy: Technical Modifications

Other technical refinements have been developed to overcome difficulties in cannulation of the common bile duct with a conventional sphincterotome (Fig. 9.**3a**). A long leading portion of cannula distal to the cutting wire on the sphincterotome (Fig. 9.**3b**) is a simple modification that reliably maintains insertion during ES. The "nose" anchors the knife in the lower common bile duct and facilitates repeated reinsertion of the wire portion to maintain correct orientation and to extend the cut in stages. A wire (previously inserted through a catheter into the common bile duct) can guide a suitably modified sphincterotome into the duct allowing subsequent ES. Alternatively a "precut" sphincterotome with no leading "nose" (Fig.

9.**3c**) can be employed to enlarge the ampullary orifice to a sufficient degree to allow conventional ES. A "needle-knife" sphincterotome (Fig. 9.**3d**) may be employed to carefully cut through the ampulla into the common bile duct, an event marked by a spurt of bile. Once a small opening has been fashioned, a conventional sphincterotome may be inserted easily via the choledochoduodenal fistula and the fistulotomy extended.

A Bilroth II (Polya) gastrectomy makes ERCP/ES technically very difficult, and a special push-type sphincterotome (Fig. 9.**3e**) has proved useful in performing ES in such circumstances.

When routine insertion of the sphincterotome into the ampulla is not possible for whatever reason, ES can be achieved after the percutaneous placement of a wire through the ampulla into the duodenum. The endoscopist can pick up the end of the wire with a forceps or snare and withdraw it through the endoscope. The insulated, low friction wire of 4 m then runs from the radiologist through the skin, liver, bile ducts, ampulla, and endoscope to the endoscopist. A specially adapted sphincterotome can then be advanced over the wire, through the endoscope, and positioned across the ampulla. It is advisable to remove even insulated guide wires prior to ES to obviate any risk of electrocution. ES can then be performed safely. It is also possible to use the "rendezvous" technique to place a stent across the ampulla, which aids the subsequent insertion of a conventional sphincterotome for ES. Alternatively, a "needle-knife" can be employed to cut down onto the stent. Fistulotomy-over-

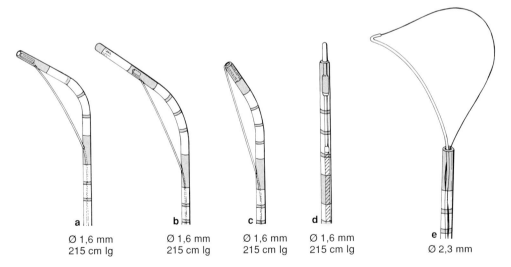

a   Ø 1,6 mm   215 cm lg

b   Ø 1,6 mm   215 cm lg

c   Ø 1,6 mm   215 cm lg

d   Ø 1,6 mm   215 cm lg

e   Ø 2,3 mm

Fig. 9.**3**
a Conventional sphincterotome
b "Long nose" sphincterotome
c Precut sphincterotome
d Needle-knife sphincterotome
e Push-type sphincterotome

the-stent is safer than conventional fistulotomy especially where the anatomy is unclear (e.g., unapparent intramural segment or ampulla buried inside a diverticulum).

ES can also be employed for other useful interventions, such as incision of a choledochocele or ampullary tumor, to establish biliary drainage per se and to facilitate the insertion of a stent, or both.

The foregoing techniques demand additional skills and are associated with a prolonged procedure time and greater risks of perforation, pancreatitis, and bleeding than with conventional ES.

Endoscopic Sphincterotomy: Problems

In the past, stones greater than 2 cm in diameter posed a particular challenge for endoscopists in view of the difficulty of extracting such large stones through the sphincterotomy. Conventional baskets are too small or too weak for large stones and, moreover, may impact in the sphincterotomized ampulla. Rarely, this may necessitate cutting through the basket handle to remove the scope before requesting surgery, though it is usually possible to use the "needle-knife" endoscopically to cut down on and retrieve the basket and stone. However, new mechanical lithotripsy baskets (Fig. 9.**4a**) are larger, stronger, and open more effectively. These are used for stones of 2 cm or more in diameter and increase duct clearance rates to 93%. Such baskets are able to crush the stones within the duct (Fig. 9.**4b**), and subsequently, small portions of stones can be removed using balloon retrieval (Fig. 9.**4.c**) or standard wire basket (Fig. 9.**4d**) retrieval. Owing to the size of these mechanical lithotripters, a large channel duodenoscope (4.2-mm diameter) is required.

Electrohydraulic, ultrasonic (6), and laser (2) lithotripsy via endoscopically or choledochoendoscopically deployed catheters and ESWL have also been used to disrupt large stones (10). Common bile duct stones may also be dissolved using chemical agents introduced into the biliary tree via a nasobiliary drain (8). These techniques are available only in specialized centers.

It is our usual practice to attempt to remove all stones following a sphincterotomy unless they are very small, as these pass spontaneously. Stones greater than 1 cm in diameter should be removed if at all possible because they may impact after the ERCP and cause deepening jaundice, cholangitis, or both.

Duodenal diverticula have a strong association with biliary calculi, and since they are present in up to 20% of patients, they present a challenge to endoscopic cannulation of the common bile duct. The major ampulla may be located deep inside the diverticulum, or more commonly situated at the edge of the diverticulum. This poses increased hazards during ES as the anatomy of the lower common bile duct and duodenal wall is altered.

Complications of Endoscopic Sphincterotomy and Stone Extraction

When performed by experienced personnel, ES has a 30-day mortality rate of approximately 1% and a morbidity rate of 10%. The complication rate decreases with greater operator experience and increases with patient age. Other factors relating to increased risk include the extension of a preexisting sphincterotomy, coagulopathy, high serum bilirubin, and low serum albumin levels.

Hemorrhage

There is a continuum of bleeding that may occur with ES. A sudden "red out" followed by the steady and continuing aspiration of a large volume of bright red blood indicates that the gastroduodenal artery or a branch of this vessel has been severed, usually by extending the ES beyond the horizontal duodenal fold. Immediate institution of appropriate resuscitative measures and early surgical intervention by laparotomy to control the bleeding is indicated. Fortunately, such catastrophic hemorrhage following ES is rare, and it is more usual for bleeding, if it occurs, to ooze from the sphincterotomy site with or without a pulsatile quality. This kind of bleeding may be controlled by local injection of several milliliters of 1:10 000 adrenaline via a variceal sclerotherapy needle. This may be combined with endoscopic balloon tamponade of the lower common bile duct immediately adjacent to the bleeding area. The site can be observed to ensure that the bleeding has ceased for several minutes before the endoscope is removed, and, if in doubt, the area can be washed by saline injected via a cannula. Hemorrhage occurs in 3–5% of patients (7), but minor degrees of bleeding, which do not require intervention, may occur in up to 20%.

All patients who have undergone ES irrespective of any degree of bleeding should be admitted overnight and carefully monitored for symptoms and signs of hemorrhage since bleeding may be delayed for several hours or even days due to late sloughing of the primary clot.

Pancreatitis

Endoscopic sphincterotomy for gallstone-associated acute pancreatitis in high-risk patients who are likely to have considerable problems following open surgery is now a well–recognized technique.

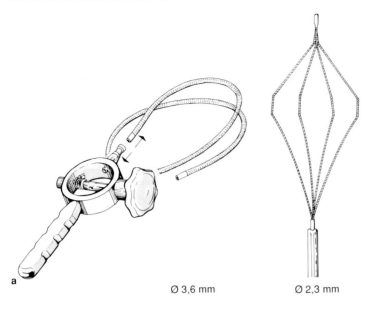

Ø 3,6 mm   Ø 2,3 mm

Fig. 9.**4 a Mechanical lithotriptor**
b Lithotriptor engaging stone
c After stone crushing
d Endoscopic baskets for stone removal

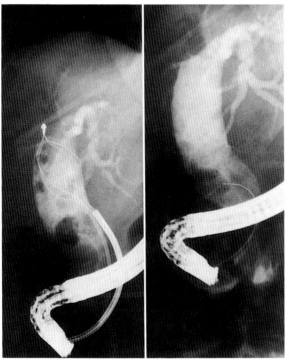

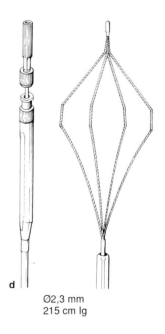

Ø2,3 mm
215 cm lg

However, clinical pancreatitis after diagnostic or therapeutic ERCP may also occur (1–3%) and is associated with significant morbidity (11). Subclinical hyperamylasemia (chemical pancreatitis) is frequent (25%) following routine ERCP/ES. Absolute amylase levels are elevated to a similar degree in chemical and clinical pancreatitis and are of no use in differentiating between these two conditions (13). A serum amylase should only be requested post ERCP if clinical pancreatitis is suggested. Mechanical injury of the am-

pulla or pancreatic duct at cannulation or at ES or over-injection of the pancreatic duct are all associated with post ERCP acute pancreatitis. Procedure-related pancreatitis becomes clinically manifest within hours of ERCP, and it is essential that the ward staff are familiar with the early symptoms and signs to ensure prompt diagnosis. When detected, early conservative treatment is usually sufficient. Early computed tomography to exclude rapidly advancing pancreatic necrosis is essential if the patient's condition worsens within 24 hours of the sphincterotomy. Sepsis may be a major problem and, once detected, a pancreatic abscess demands early radiological or surgical drainage. Appropriate antibiotic treatment may prevent the development of an abscess, but overenthusiastic use of inappropriate antibiotics may lead to other complications.

Cholangitis

On occasion, a dilated biliary tree is opacified with contrast demonstrating large stones that cannot be removed via ES. It is important to establish drainage of the bile duct to minimize the risk of cholangitis, which can occur despite pre- and postprocedure antibiotic therapy. In such instances, it is our practice to immediately insert a nasobiliary drain above the level of the obstruction and to clear the biliary tree of contrast by alternately aspirating and flushing the system with sterile saline (Fig. 9.5). The drain can be left in situ (on free drainage) and removed prior to a subsequent attempt to clear the duct endoscopically. Such later attempts are invariably successful due to a combination of resolved edema and/or bleeding (which may have attended the initial ES) and the mechanical degrading effect of the nasobiliary drain itself on the stone. Another advantage of the drain is to allow interval nasobilography to check the ductal caliber, stone position, and size. If available on site, ESWL may be employed to fragment large stones. A high degree of accuracy is attained in delivering the ESWL energies to stones targeted by nasobilography.

The nasobiliary drain may also be employed to deliver dissolving agents in an attempt to completely dissolve or reduce the size of the stone prior to subsequent mechanical extraction.

Rarely, ES is contraindicated due to the coagulopathy of disseminated intravascular coagulation (DIC) secondary to overwhelming stone-related ascending cholangitis with septicemia. This critical situation can be retrieved by instituting temporizing drainage with a nasobiliary tube. In our experience, once the pus is aspirated, the septicemia can be readily controlled with intravenous antibiotic therapy, and the DIC rapidly resolves. ES and stone extraction can be performed safely later.

Other techniques that are gaining increasing acceptance for patients in whom ES would be associated with an unacceptably high risk of complications are endoscopic balloon sphincteroplasty (5) followed by stone extraction, and endoprosthesis (stent) insertion (13) to facilitate drainage while leaving the stones in situ. Such procedures are not addressed here but should be within the interventional armamentarium of a therapeutic ERCPist.

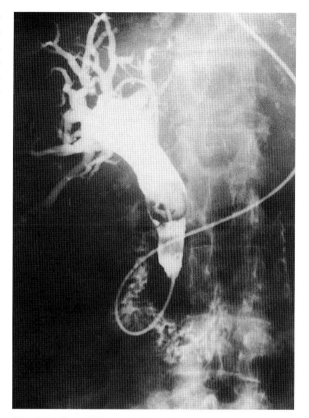

Fig. 9.**5** **Nasobiliary drainage for sepsis with bile duct stones**

Perforation

Retroperitoneal perforation after ES (4) is becoming rarer (1%) due to better technique and improved sphincterotomes with shorter wires. Early recognition of perforation is important because the institution of appropriate management reduces morbidity. If the incision is made with repeated short bursts of current in controlled increments of length it is unlikely that a rapid, uncontrolled ("zipper") cut will occur. Even if this happens, an additional precaution is to cut with only one-half of the wire inserted into the ampulla. This limited length will not cut beyond the intramural segment of the duct unless this is unusually short. A high degree of suspicion is advisable if the incision is uncontrolled. The opening to the retroperitoneum is not usually visible but can be confirmed if extravasation of contrast is seen or if air outlines the kidney and/or other structures. Leakage of air is associated with less subsequent morbidity than fluid, which is often infected bile and gastric contents. The correct management should include the immediate passage of a nasobiliary drain and a nasogastric tube. The patient is kept fasting and receives intravenous fluids, H_2-receptor antagonists or proton pump blockers (as an anti-secretory measure), broad spectrum antibiotic therapy, and appropriate analgesia. Depending on the size and nature of the leak, these measures can be withdrawn after a few days (usually) to a few weeks (rarely). Closure of the perforation can be demonstrated by the infusion of a water-soluble contrast medium down the nasobiliary drain or nasogastric tube. Fortunately, most patients recover with conservative treatment, though very rarely percutaneous and/or surgical drainage of a retroperitoneal collection (sometimes multiple and distant) is required.

Stenosis

If an adequate ES has been performed through all fibers of the sphincter of Oddi (as distinct from an endoscopic ampullotomy), functional stenosis is rather uncommon (less than 5%) (12). The sphincterotomy may narrow to a degree that remains functionally adequate in another 5% of cases. To evaluate the possibility of stenosis, an informed radiologist can easily demonstrate patency of the ES during a barium meal by tilting the patient's head down allowing barium to delineate the biliary tree. Patency can also be demonstrated at ERCP by trawling a balloon through the sphincterotomy. If stenosis has occurred it may be endoscopically treated by repeat ES, but caution is advised as there may be an increased incidence of bleeding. Balloon sphincteroplasty may be more appropriate in this instance. Vague or nonspecific abdominal symptoms usually point to another diagnosis rather than stenosis of a previous ES.

Summary

ES is an increasingly used and valuable minimally invasive technique that spares many patients the increased morbidity and mortality of open surgery. Com-plications are clearly defined, occur with an acceptably low frequency, and are readily recognized and treated in well-functioning units. Morbidity should not exceed 10%, mortality 1%, and surgical intervention 1%. Future refinements in equipment and technique will reduce these percentages further.

References

1. Cotton PB. Endoscopic management of bile duct stones (apples and oranges). Gut 1984; 25:587–97.
2. Cotton PB, Kozarek RA, Schapiro RH, et al. Endoscopic laser lithotripsy of large bile duct stones. Gastroenterology 1990; 99(4):1128–33.
3. Cotton PB, Williams CB. Practical Gastrointestinal Endoscopy. Oxford: Blackwell Scientific Publications, 1990.
4. Dunham F, Burgeois N, Gelin M, Jeanmart J, Toussaint J, Cremer M. Retroperitoneal perforations following endoscopic sphincterotomy, clinical course and management. Endoscopy 1982; 14:92–6.
5. Geenan JE, Derfus D, Welch JM. Biliary balloon dilatation. Endoscope Rev 1985; 2:10–6.
6. Hwang MH, Yang JC, Lin J. The treatment of retained intrahepatic stones with electrohydraulic and ultrasonic shock waves. Dig Dis Sci 1986; 31(Suppl): 10.
7. Lamber ME, Betts CD, Hill J, et al. Endoscopic sphincterotomy: the whole truth. Br J Surg 1991; 78:473–6.
8. Murray WR, LaFerla G, Fullarton GM. Choledocholithiasis: in vivo stone dissolution using methyl tertiary butyl ether (MTBE), GUT 1988; 29:143–5.
9. Neoptolemos JP, Carr-Locke DL, London NJ, et al. Controlled trial of urgent endoscopic retrograde cholangiopancreatography and endoscopic sphincterotomy versus conservative management for acute pancreatitis due to gallstones. Lancet 1988; 2:979–83.
10. Sauerbruch T, Stern M, Stzudy group for shockwave lithotripsy of bile duct stones. Fragmentation of bile duct stones by extracorporeal shock waves. Gastroenterology 1989; 961:146–52.
11. Siegel JH, Veerappan A. Complications of endoscopic sphincterotomy. In: Kozarek RA, ed. Clinics of gastrointestinal endoscopy. New York: WB Saunders, 1991.
12. Siegel JH. Endoscopic Sphincterotomy. In: Siegel JH, ed. Endoscopic retrograde cholangiopancreatography, technique, diagnosis and therapy. New York: Raven Press, 1992.
13. Soomers AJ, Nagengast FM, Yap SH. Endoscopic placement of biliary endoprostheses in patients with endoscopically unextractable common bile duct stones. A longterm follow-up study of 26 patients. Endoscopy 1990; 22:24–26.

10 Percutaneous Techniques for Bile Duct Stone Removal

Minimally invasive therapy of stone disease of the biliary tract is highly successful by endoscopic or percutaneous transtrack or transhepatic methods. Percutaneous and endoscopic therapy of biliary duct stone disease is widely practiced throughout the world by gastroenterologists, radiologists, and surgeons (1, 5, 6, 12, 14, 16, 20, 21, 24).

Endoscopic sphincterotomy and stone removal is the preferred technique in the elderly unless access to the bile ducts is present after cholecystectomy. Reoperation on bile duct stones in this age group has a high morbidity and mortality. However, endoscopic sphincterotomy has a complication rate as high as 10% and a mortality of 0.5% to 1.3%, so safer alternatives, such as percutaneous extraction through a T-tube track when it is present, are preferred (25). Long-term complications of sphincterotomy should still cause some concern (6, 22, 24, 25). In most patients, endoscopic sphincterotomy is an uneventful procedure when performed by experts.

When asymptomatic gallbladder stones coexist with common bile duct stones, the latter are removed endoscopically without treating the gallbladder stones until (if and when) they become symptomatic. This procedure is adopted in high-risk patients, while in patients younger than 50 years, surgery is probably preferable. In high-risk patients with combined gallbladder and ductal stones, a combination of techniques, such as endoscopic ductal stone removal plus ESWL of the gallbladder stones before dissolution with contact solvents following percutaneous transhepatic or endoscopic gallbladder catheterization (10), is recommended.

When ERCP and sphincterotomy fail because of previous gastrointestinal surgery, duodenal diverticulum, or other reasons, FN PTHC is necessary to demonstrate the biliary tract. The demonstration of stones in the biliary ducts (often associated with infected bile) is an indication for percutaneous transhepatic catheterization of the common bile duct for drainage. This may be accompanied by endoscopic sphincterotomy with guidance from above, by transhepatic sphincterotomy with or without endoscopic positioning of the sphincterotome, or by transhepatic balloon dilatation of the ampulla and evacuation of stones into the duodenum by Dormia basket or Fogarty-type balloon catheter (17, 18, 22, 23). Stones in the ducts, if larger than 1.5–2 cm, require other

methods of therapy such as ESWL, ISWL, laser lithotripsy, or dissolution with MTBE to reduce stone size to 3–5 mm for endoscopic or percutaneous extraction (7, 9, 11, 12, 13, 26).

Our experience using contact dissolution of common bile duct stones has been disappointing, although some stones can be reduced in size by this method.

Percutaneous Trans–T-Tube Track Biliary Stone Removal

This is the ideal, least harmful method of removing stones from the bile ducts in the patient after cholecystectomy and postoperative T-tube drainage. If the bile duct is explored at surgery, a T tube is placed in the common bile duct; this is used in the postoperative period to assess that the duct is free of stones.

It is usual at present to do routine operative cholangiography during laparoscopic cholecystectomy, and if a stone is present in the bile duct, the procedure is converted to open cholecystectomy and the stone removed. It is also possible to place a tube in the bile duct at laparoscopic cholecystectomy.

This method of external drainage is sufficient to provide bile diversion postoperatively, and in the young patient the fistula created may be used to dilate a passage into the common bile duct for stone removal.

Instrumentation is now available to remove an unsuspected biliary duct stone at laparoscopic cholecystectomy. Learning to succeed with this procedure in every patient is a difficult problem. Often it is stated that there are good reasons for immediate endoscopic stone removal in the immediate postoperative period because the presence of a T tube causes pain, the tube may fall out, cause intermittent fever or biliary colic, or jaundice may occur. This is not our experience when a stone is found at postoperative T-tube cholangiography, the T tube is clamped and fixed securely to the skin. All other drains are removed. It is known that internal fistulas develop between the T-tube track and subhepatic drains, which make track formation incomplete and cause leaks from the track during the procedure. The patient is told to report to the hospital if any symptoms are noted. Only one of our patients returned to the hospital when her T tube fell out. The tube was easily replaced by a new T tube. A 4-week delay was the average time in one large series for patients to come to endoscopic stone removal. We have treated patients referred for stone removal after a 6-month asymptomatic period with a T tube in situ. The 4-week delay necessary for track maturation is not a sufficient argument for immediate postoperative endoscopic stone therapy when the risks of complications of sphincterotomy are considerable, and its long-term effects are unknown. The development of postoperative jaundice due to an impacted stone at the ampulla is an indication for endoscopic stone removal to prevent cholangitis. An impacted stone is rare with a

T tube in situ. During the waiting period, the patient is not placed on antibiotics and leads as normal a life as possible. After 4 weeks the patient is admitted for stone removal the evening before the procedure, although this is not totally necessary, and the procedure may be carried out as a day case without admission to the hospital (Table 10.1).

Preparation of the Patient

The procedure is performed on the fasting patient without sedation. Pethidine (meperidine) analgesia may be given to relieve pain during the procedure or to produce euphoria in the nervous patient before beginning stone removal. Preprocedure blood chemistry is necessary to exclude pancreatic inflammation. If the serum amylase is elevated the procedure is postponed. Gentamicin (80 mg) is given intravenously 1 hour before stone removal and continued for 3 days. It is our practice to indicate to the patient our desire to complete the procedure in one visit and also to inform the patient of the necessity of a postprocedure cholangiogram at 24 or 48 hours after successful stone removal. Informed consent is obtained for the procedure. Because of the nature of our practice, most patients are referred from other hospitals often at a distance, and it is therefore more practical for the patient to seek hospital admission for 24–48 hours.

Contrast medium allergy is not a contraindication provided the procedure is undertaken without high-pressure contrast injections into the ductal system to prevent biliovenous or biliolymphatic reflux of contrast agent from the bile ducts. We use a nonionic contrast medium for bile duct opacification to reduce any risks of contrast medium reactions during stone removal.

Table 10.1 Trans–T-Tube track retained stone removal (1977–1992)

Total number of patients	172
Total number of stones removed	269
Number of failed stone removals	5
Reasons for failure	
Stone impacted duct–track junction	1
Stones within wall of CBD	1
T-tube track not complete	2
Acute angle entry of track into CBD	1
Complications of stone removal	17
Septic shock	1
Postprocedure cholangitis	2
Acute pancreatitis	1
Transient raised serum amylase	39
Postprocedure abdominal pain	10
Transient postprocedure fever	7
Procedure mortality	0
Total number of cases not treated	10
Reasons for refusing therapy	
T tube not in bile duct	1
T-tube track 7 Fr and large stone	1
T-tube track pus and incomplete track	4
T-tube angle with CBD acute	2
T-tube track-drain fistula	1
Maximum number of stones removed from one patient	12
Number of patients with one stone	92
Number of cases of intrahepatic stones	5
Number of cases with 2–4 stones	40
Number of cases with 5–8 stones	21
Number of cases with more than 8 stones	2
Number of cases requiring balloon dilatation of the ampulla	5
Number of cases requiring descending trans-track sphincterotomy	2

Preparation for Stone Removal

We carry out this procedure on a conventional fluoroscopy table with an undercouch tube and high-quality image television in the X-ray department. The lead protection is removed in order to give open access to instrumentation of the T-tube track on the right side of the abdomen. The technique is carried out as a sterile procedure using a gown and sterile gloves, preferably lead lined, to reduce exposure to the operators hands. Adequate lead-apron protection must be used by the radiologist, assistants, nursing staff, and technicians while in the X-ray room during the procedure. Since concentration by the radiologist and staff on the procedure at hand is essential for success, the procedure room should be quiet at all times and access to the room denied during the procedure. While many instruments are available for stone removal, we use only four. A guide wire, a steerable catheter, a Dormia basket, and a balloon catheter for dilatation of the ampulla when necessary (Table 10.2). An angiogra-

Table 10.**2**   Equipment for transtrack biliary stone removal

1. Steerable catheters	
Cook, Denmark	15 Fr
Medi-tech, Inc.	10 Fr and 13 Fr
(Watertown, Mass., USA)	
2. Sheathed Wire Baskets	Three sizes to fit
Cook	steerable cathe-
Medi-tech, Inc.	ters
Dormia	
3. Angioplasty Balloon Cathe-	
ters	
4. Fogarty balloon catheters	
Edwards Labs (La Jolla,	
Ca., USA)	
5. Straight rubber catheters	10 Fr, 12 Fr, 14 Fr,
(Davol Inc., Cranston, R.I.,	16 Fr
USA)	

phy guide wire with a short soft C tip is used to wire the ducts through the T tube before it is removed to prevent loss of the track (if the latter is stenosed, incomplete, or tortuous) and thus failure of the procedure. The steerable catheter used is the largest size that will enter the track and bile duct. When used frequently this catheter should be replaced often. The Dormia basket used should be of sufficient size to engage the stone in the duct for removal. Different sizes are available for different stone sizes. The basket must also fit the steerable catheter lumen. An angioplasty

catheter with an inflated balloon diameter of 10 mm or 15 mm is also used occasionally to dilate the ampulla in order to push a stone into the duodenum. Recently, a balloon on a guide wire has become available, which can be inserted through the steerable catheter directly to the ampulla without the need for passing a wire into the duodenum and an angioplasty catheter over the wire across the ampulla. Any Dormia basket that can engage the duct stone may be used for stone removal. Larger baskets are needed when the bile duct is dilated and also to trap large stones. Ideally the basket, when fully expanded, should rest on the wall of the bile duct. Small stones in a dilated bile duct are difficult to engage in the basket and are perhaps best treated by pushing individual stones into the duodenum using a Fogarty-type balloon after ampullary dilatation. A small basket is only useful for a small stone in a narrow bile duct, such as an intrahepatic duct or a fine caliber common bile duct.

Technique of Stone Removal (Fig. 10.**1**)

The procedure is performed on the fasting patient.

The patient is placed in the supine position on the X-ray fluoroscopy table and a T-tube cholangiogram is performed.

The position and number of stones in the duct are carefully observed, taking care to exclude air bubbles from the contrast medium system. The abdomen around the T-tube exit is cleaned with antiseptic and draped with sterile towels. Before any ligature around the T tube that is fastening it to the skin is severed, a guide wire is inserted into the bile duct through the exit hole of the T tube. Inspection of the skin around the T tube should show no evidence of pus. The latter suggests track infection and a poorly formed track. If only a single small stone is present, we continue the

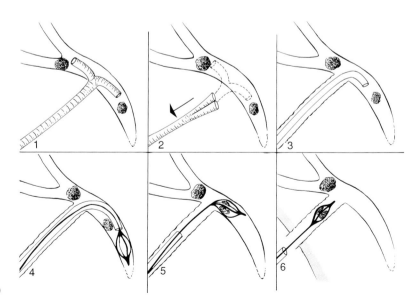

Fig. 10.**1   Percutaneous technique of bile duct stone removal**
(1–6: Maneuvers for stone removal)

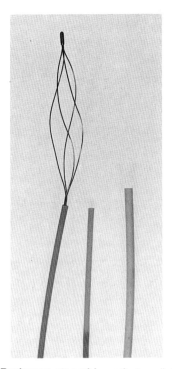

Fig. 10.**2** **Burhenne steerable catheter,** distal end with stone basket

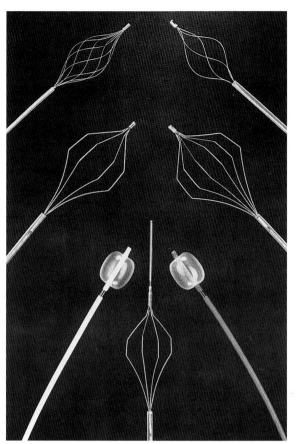

Fig. 10.**3** **Dormia baskets and Fogarty balloon catheters**

procedure. If multiple stones are present we defer the procedure in the presence of an infected track exit since a poorly formed track cannot be dilated and will not withstand multiple duct manipulations for stone removal.

The T tube is removed by a gentle but firm continuous pull on its external limb. We have never failed to remove a T tube from the bile duct during this procedure. Ease of T-tube removal suggests that a good track is present down to the bile duct. After removal, the intraduct ends of the T tube are inspected for adherent stones. On two occasions, inspection of the removed T tube showed an adherent stone. More contrast injection showed the duct to be free of a previous stone. If the T tube is cut across near the skin, care should be taken not to let it fall into the track since, even with a guide wire in situ, it may be difficult to retrieve the external limb of the tube. When the T tube is removed, bile and contrast flow from the track. The steerable catheter connected to a syringe of contrast medium is introduced into the external track orifice, and the track is outlined with contrast medium.

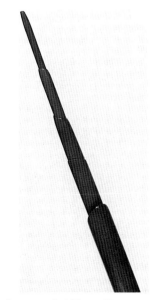

Fig. 10.**4** **Concentric biliary dilators** (Cook, Denmark)

The track is now studied by fluoroscopy. A search is made for track stenoses and acute bends with in the track to the bile duct. Any movement of the bile duct stones after T-tube removal is also noted and recorded. The ampullary region is also studied using contrast injection until the duodenum is clearly documented, and a search is made for abnormal entry of the bile duct into a duodenal diverticulum since the latter when incompletely outlined with contrast medium may present with a meniscus sign and mimic an impacted stone in the lower common bile duct (Fig. 10.5). Attempts at removal of this "stone" with a basket may cause perforation of the diverticulum. An air bubble–free duct is preferable and reduces procedure time.

If a track stenosis is demonstrated, it is dilated by a balloon catheter or concentric biliary dilators (Fig. 10.4) inserted over the in situ guide wire. If multiple angles are present in the length of the track, it is best at this stage to dilate the track and insert an Amplatz sheath. All manipulations are now carried out through this sheath which remains in situ down into the bile duct until all stones have been removed.

The steerable catheter (Figs. 10.2 and 10.3) is now inserted into the common bile duct and steered in the direction of the stones identified by further contrast medium injection if necessary.

The tip of the steerable catheter is placed just beyond the stone. The closed stone basket is then inserted through the steerable catheter and beyond the stone. The basket is opened and withdrawn until it lies

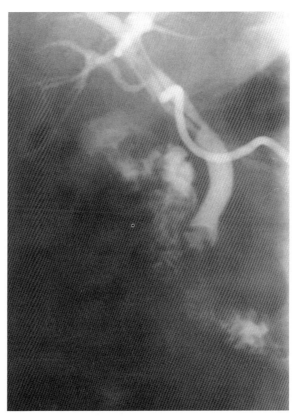

Fig. 10.**5** **Common bile duct entering duodenal diverticulum.** If the diverticulum is not outlined, the cholangiographic appearances may be mistaken for a duct stone

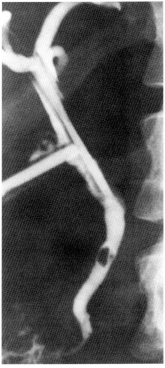
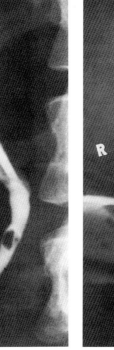
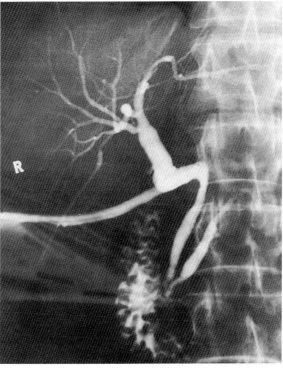

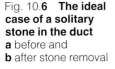
Fig. 10.**6** **The ideal case of a solitary stone in the duct**
a before and
b after stone removal

a   b

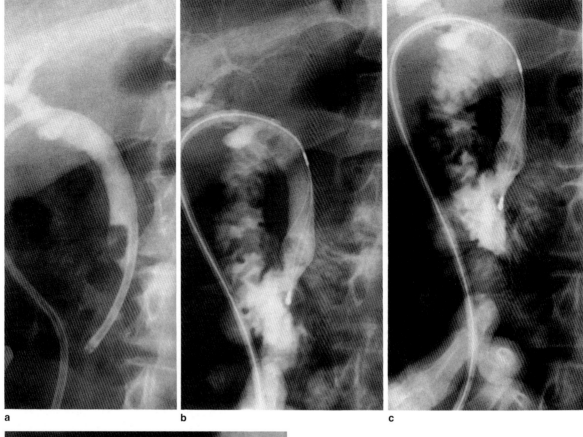

a   b   c

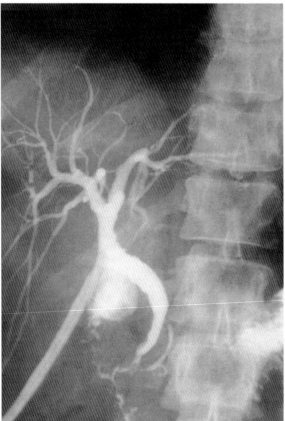

d

alongside the stone and gently rotated to engage the stone. When the stone is engaged, the steerable catheter basket and stone are withdrawn in one movement out through the track to the skin (Figs. 10.**6** and 10.**7**). When multiple stones are present, smaller stones are removed first and the largest stone is the last to be removed (Fig. 10.**8**). This prevents track injury during larger stone removals with other stones still in situ in the bile duct.

Track injury even with a guide wire in situ may make reentry into the bile duct very difficult and even prevent removal of other stones during the procedure or at a later date by preventing recatheterization of the bile duct and a failed examination.

When multiple stones are present, the procedure of catheterization, basketing of the stone, and removal is repeated until all the stones have been removed. When all stones have been removed or displaced into the duodenum, a final cholangiogram is performed via the sinus track. A rubber catheter is placed in the track for 24–48 hours, and a repeat cholangiogram is carried out to confirm a clear ductal system.

Fig. 10.**7 Single large stone successfully removed with large basket (a, b, c)** and **d** after stone removal

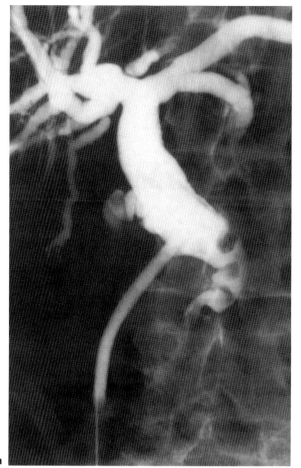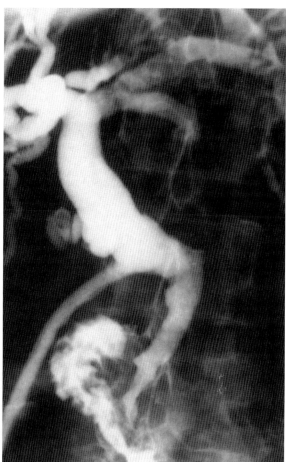

Fig. 10.**8** **Multiple stones a** before and **b** after removal

It is preferable to remove all the stones present during a first intervention via the T-tube track even when 10–12 stones are present, if there is a good track to the bile duct and the patient is cooperative. Manipulations within the bile ducts must be gentle at all times, but particularly when the Dormia basket is outside its sheath and engaging a calculus. Patient cooperation is increased if the physician advises him or her of the alternatives to a failed procedure due to noncooperation. The status of the interventional radiologist increases in the surgeon's or physician's estimation, and they will make other referrals. Physicians who perform procedures that compete with this technique try to achieve a once-only procedure, and therefore, radiologists must also try to achieve this goal.

Procedure Duration

With a single stone in a narrow duct below the T tube, this a 5-minute procedure for the experienced biliary stone remover. When a single stone is present in a dilated duct, it is a much more time-consuming procedure because it is difficult to engage the stone with the Dormia basket. In this event, after 15 minutes, we revert to dilating the ampulla and pushing the stone into the duodenum with the steerable catheter or Fogarty balloon catheter. Multiple small stones in a slightly dilated duct are also fairly easily removed. Large stones in a dilated duct and an adequate track to the skin are easily removed.

Multiple small stones in a dilated duct are difficult to remove and require great skill and tenacity for success. Many may be pushed into the duodenum by a balloon catheter after angioplasty by balloon dilatation or transtrack sphincterotomy of the ampulla.

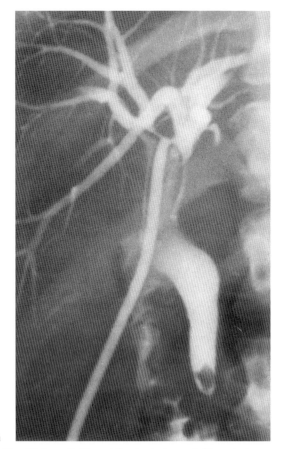
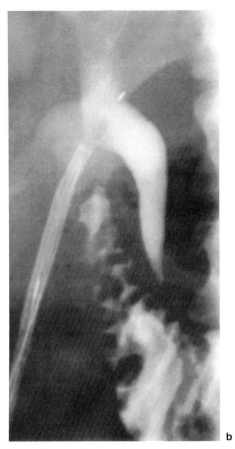

a

b

Fig. 10.**9   a Solitary bile duct stone. b** Stone being removed within dormia basket

Special Stone Sites

Stones in the main right or left hepatic duct are removed by the same method as common bile duct stones. More peripheral intrahepatic duct stones require segmental duct localization before inserting a catheter and basket into the duct site above the stone and proceeding as with common bile stones. Occasionally, after exact location of the ductal stones, saline may be used to wash the stones into the main bile ducts. If the stones are small they may be displaced into the duodenum. A cystic duct remnant stone may present a difficult problem if the stone cannot be dislodged into the bile duct. It is possible in some patients to catheterize the cystic duct with the steerable catheter. Attempts may be made to flush the stone from the cystic duct into the bile duct or retrieve the stone by basket into the bile duct and extract it. A stone impacted at the ampulla may be impossible to move but if a guide wire can be inserted into the duodenum, an attempt may be made to dilate the ampulla and retrieve the stone by basket or push it into the duodenum (Figs. 10.**10** – 10.**13**).

Complications of Stone Removal

When multiple stones are present in a dilated bile duct, infection is common, and instrumentation is likely to promote cholangitis. One patient with an infected track exit on the skin and a single stone in the common bile duct developed *septic shock* 30 minutes after successful removal of an 11-mm stone.

Two patients with multiple stones developed *ascending cholangitis*. One patient developed *acute pancreatitis*. All four patients recovered. Asymptomatic *elevation of serum amylase* occurred in 39 patients. Most were associated with manipulations at the lower end of the common bile duct without ampullary dilatation. *Fever* occurred in seven patients and lasted 24–48 hours. Ten patients experienced *abdominal pain,* which abated within 24 hours. It was not associated with paralytic ileus or altered liver function tests. In one case, *track rupture* was noted at removal of a large stone. This occurred at the site of a dilated track stenosis. The stone was removed, and the patient did not develop peritonitis. We considered that ten patients were not suitable for this form of treatment.

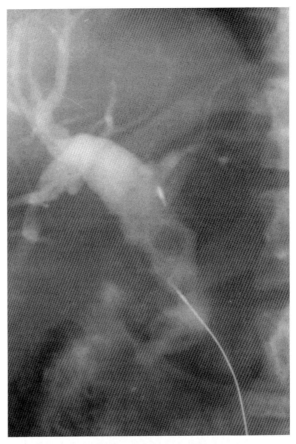

Fig. 10.**10**   **Stone impacted at the track–duct junction**

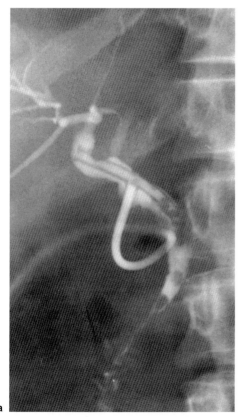

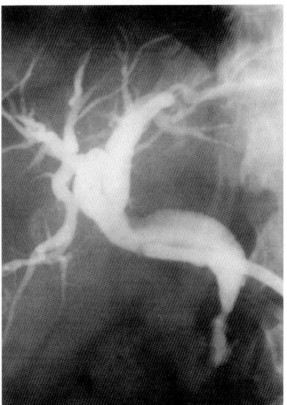

a

b

Fig. 10.**11**   **Multiple stones**   **a** before and **b** after removal

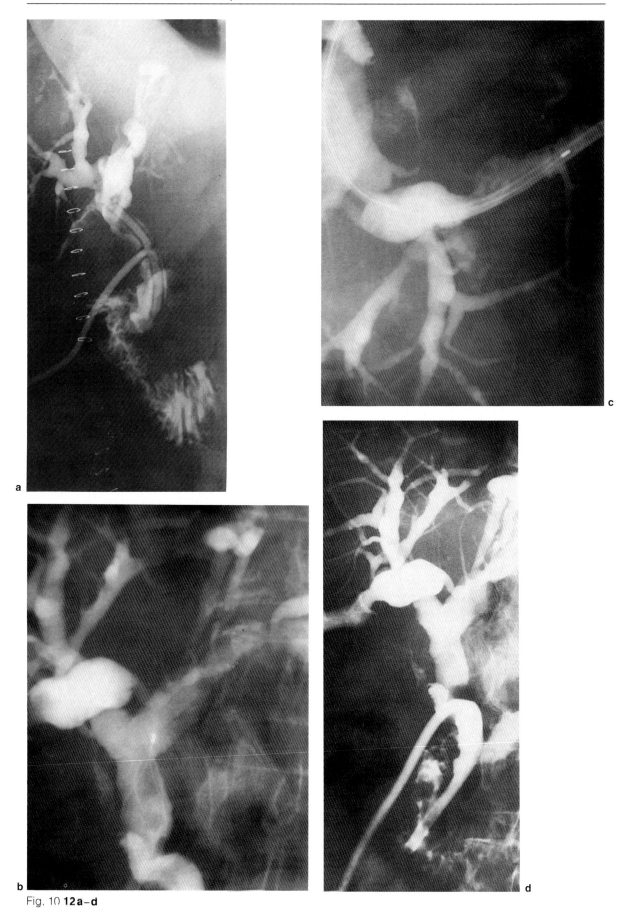

Fig. 10 **12a–d**

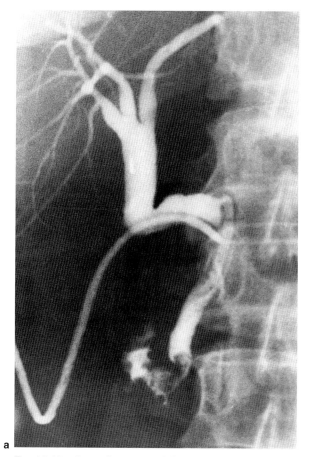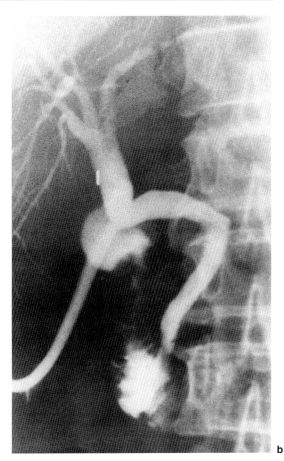

Fig. 10.**13**   **A small common bile duct stone**   **a** before and **b** after removal

These included cases of T tube not in the bile duct, small track and large stone, infected incomplete track, an acute-angle track–duct junction, and, in another case, a fistula was present from the track to a drain site in the subhepatic region. These are not included in the 172 cases reported.

Transtrack Failed Stone Removal
(Table 10.**3**)

This occurred in five patients. In one case the stone became impacted at the tract–duct junction and could not be fragmented by the wire basket. In another

◄ Fig. 10.**12**   **a Cholangiogram showing multiple stones 24 hours after emergency cholecystectomy** (no operative cholangiogram)
b Common bile duct stones in Dormia basket
c Right intrahepatic duct stones being engaged by basket after duct catheterization with steerable catheter
d Cholangiogram at 24 hours showing stone-free bile ducts

patient with a T tube in situ for 4 months, the stones were embedded in the wall of the duct. This patient had received infusions of monoctanoin (Fig. 10.**16**) in an attempt to dissolve the stones. In two patients, an incomplete track was present. These cases were associated with an infected track exit and failure to recatheterize the bile duct after one stone was removed. In one patient with a track exit in the right iliac fossa,

Table 10.**3**   Success rate of stone removal by extraction via a T-tube track

Author	Year	Number of cases
Mazzariello	1976	516 (97.5% success rate)
Burhenne	1980	661 (95.0% success rate)
Mason	1980	131 (70.0% success rate)
Caprini	1980	100 (96.0% success rate)
Taylor	1984	80 (80.0% success rate)
Geisinger	1989	189 (88.0% success rate)
Mc Nulty	1989	172 (96.0% success rate)

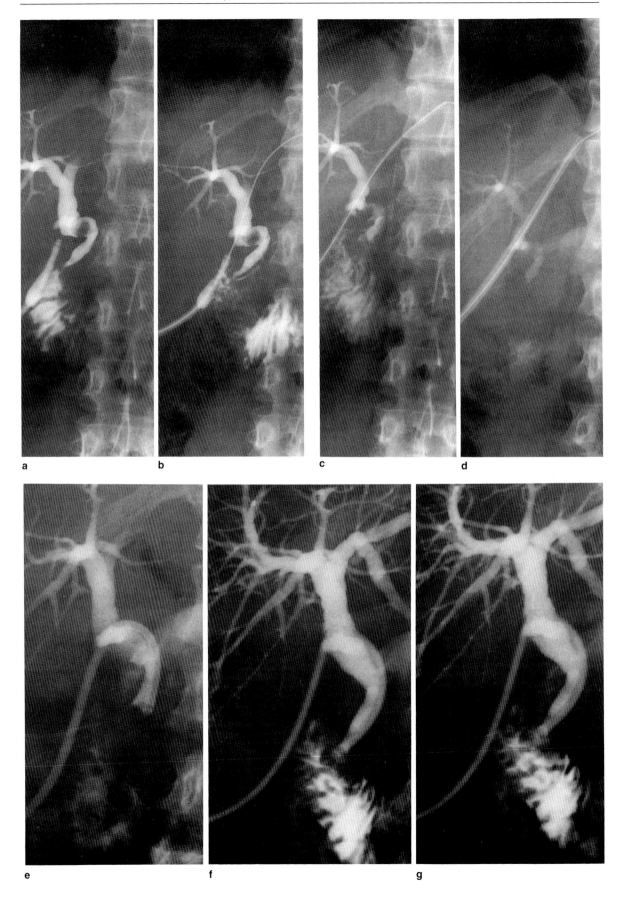

a

b

c

d

e

f

g

an acute-angle track–duct junction was present, and the steerable catheter could not be inserted into the bile duct.

Percutaneous Stone Removal after Laparoscopic Cholecystectomy
(Fig. 10.**14**)

Laparoscopic stone removal from the common bile duct following dilatation of the cystic duct is performed by Dormia-basket extraction and may be a very prolonged procedure as judged by satellite broadcasting from experts to the recent World Congress of Minimally Invasive Therapy.

A simple alternative for the laparoscopic surgeon is to insert a rubber catheter via the cystic duct into the common bile duct from a side port and complete the cholecystectomy.

Later, the mature track formed by the rubber catheter serves as a route to the bile duct for percutaneous stone extraction by endoscopic or Burhenne techniques after dilatation of the track to 14–15 Fr (Fig. 10.**14**) (36).

Balloon Dilatation of the Ampulla of Vater

We have used this technique in eight patients since the original description of the method (3). Balloon dilatation of the ampulla may be performed endoscopically (9), transhepatically (3, 4, 5, 6, 8), or via a T-tube track or fistula to the bile duct. We have used the method as an aid in bile duct stone removal and also in chronic pancreatitis with bile duct stricture formation in the head of the pancreas. However, the preferred treatment in stricture secondary to chronic pancreatitis is surgery. Endoscopic balloon dilatation is only limited by the channel diameter of the endoscope. Percutaneous transhepatic dilatation of the papilla is less safe than dilatation carried out through a T-tube track or external biliary fistula. When the gallbladder is in situ, percutaneous transcholecystic catheterization of the common bile duct and ampulla is a safer procedure than the transhepatic route.

◀ Fig. 10.**14 Retained stone after laparoscopic cholecystectomy without conversion to open cholecystectomy**
a Cholangiogram via catheter track to the bile duct showing retained stone
b Guide wire inserted into the left intrahepatic duct
c and **d** Track dilatation to the common bile duct using concentric teflon biliary dilators
e, **f**, and **g** Steerable catheter inserted into the duct and used to push the stone into the duodenum

1. Endoscopic Dilatation of the Papilla

After insertion of a side-viewing endoscope into the duodenum, and location and catheterization of the papilla, a guide wire is inserted via the catheter into the bile duct and up into an intrahepatic duct under fluoroscopic guidance. The catheter is removed ("wire in, catheter out") taking care not to dislodge the guide wire from its intrahepatic duct location. Next, an angioplasty balloon catheter (Blue Max) is inserted over the guide wire into the bile duct, and the guide wire is removed taking care not to dislodge the balloon catheter. The balloon is now positioned using the limit markers on the balloon catheter, and it is inflated using air or contrast medium in an attached syringe. The balloon is left positioned across the ampulla and used to opacify the duct system after the balloon is deflated. A Fogarty balloon or a wire basket may then be inserted for stone removal.

2. Percutaneous Transhepatic Dilatation of the Ampulla of Vater

Following "clean" FN PTHC and demonstration of the biliary tract, the common bile duct is catheterized, and a guide wire is inserted into the duodenum. A 7-Fr dilator is inserted over the wire into the common bile duct to dilate a track through the liver parenchyma. A 10-Fr sheath is now inserted into the common bile duct; this sheath is used to introduce an angioplasty balloon catheter over the guide wire into the duodenum.

The markers on the catheter are used to position the balloon across the ampulla. The balloon is inflated with air or contrast medium and kept inflated until the waist caused by the ampulla is no longer evident. The ampulla may be dilated up to 1.5 cm using successive diameter balloon catheters. If a stone is present in the bile duct, it is pushed into the duodenum by a Fogarty balloon catheter or Dormia basket.

The liver puncture site is sealed at the liver capsule following 24-hour drainage of the bile duct. The liver track may be occluded with a Gelfoam strip or a spring coil.

3. Percutaneous Transtrack Dilatation of the Ampulla (Figs. 10.**15** and 10.**16**)

When a T-tube track or external fistula is present, a steerable catheter is used to introduce a guide wire into the common bile duct and into the duodenum. An angioplasty balloon catheter is inserted into the duct over the wire, positioned across the ampulla, and inflated with air or contrast medium. The ampulla may be dilated by this method to 1.5 cm without complications. During laparoscopic cholecystectomy, if unsuggested bile duct stones are shown by cholangiography and a catheter is positioned in the bile duct through the

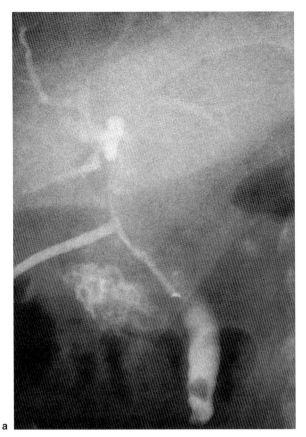

a

Fig. 10.**15   a A small retained stone is demonstrated in common bile duct** (arrow)
b c d e f The stone could not be engaged by the wire basket so the ampulla was dilated by balloon catheter and the stone was pushed into duodenum
g Cholangiogram at 24 hours showing a stone-free bile duct

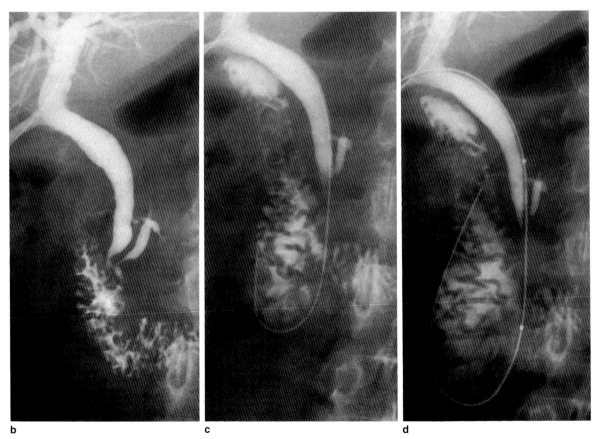

b   c   d

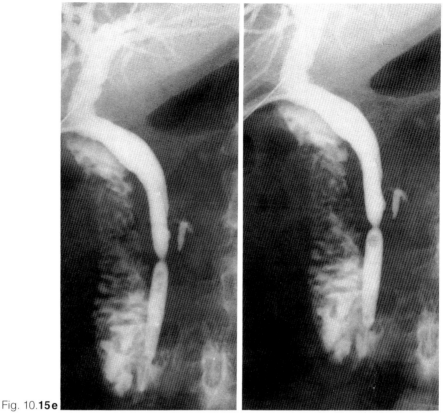

Fig. 10.**15e**   f

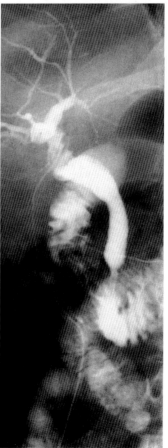

cystic duct, the track formed may be dilated to pass a balloon catheter over a guide wire into the common bile duct for dilatation of the ampulla. We prefer to use biliary dilators to enlarge this track to the bile duct from the skin and use great care to prevent loss of the track during manipulations. After dilatation of the ampulla, retained duct stones may be removed by basketing into the duodenum. During ampullary dilatations, pethidine (meperidine), 50–100 mg, is given i. v. to relieve pain.

Complications of Balloon Dilatation of the Ampulla

Complications following balloon dilatation of the ampulla are rare using the transtrack and endoscopic routes. The transcholecystic route is also safe. Major complications may follow the percutaneous route. These include hemorrhage (hemobilia or hemoperitoneum), bile leaks, and septicemia. One series reported complications in 21% of cases (4). Thirty-eight procedures were performed in 35 patients with jaundice, cholangitis, and biliary colic. A follow-up series by the same authors reported no complications in the last 17 cases of percutaneous transhepatic dilatation of the ampulla (10). Pancreatitis is always a possible complication in manipulations involving the papilla.

Fig. 10.**15g**

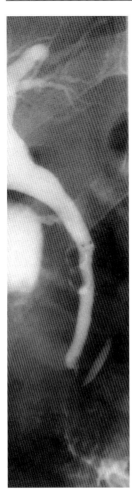

Fig. 10.**16** **Catheter cholangiogram showing two
stones embedded in the
wall of the bile duct.** These
could not be displaced into
the duct lumen or extracted

We have used this technique in eight patients (including one patient via the transcholecystic route) without
any evidence of liver trauma, bleeding, or pancreatitis, and we believe that it is a very useful technique for preventing failure of bile duct stone removal.

Percutaneous Sphincterotomy

Percutaneous sphincterotomy may be carried out by
the transhepatic route after FN PTHC or via a T-tube
track or external fistula after laparoscopic cholecystectomy (2, 4, 5, 7).

The latter two routes are obviously safer than the
transhepatic route. The technique is used for stone removal when ERCP fails for any reason, such as
duodenal diverticulum, previous gastric surgery, or
ampullary stricture.

Following FN PTHC and opacification of the common bile duct and intrahepatic ducts, and in the absence of overt cholangitis, a suitable duct is chosen for
catheterization of the common bile duct. A 9-Fr catheter is inserted into the common bile duct over a guide
wire. If there is clean puncture of the biliary tract,

we prefer to proceed directly with sphincterotomy.
Others prefer to wait for 7 days to allow a track to
form around the transhepatic catheter (9).

Coagulation screen should be normal; i. v. antibiotic is given immediately before the procedure. A
guide wire is inserted into the duodenum through the
9-Fr catheter. The catheter is exchanged for a 9-Fr
Teflon dilator. A standard Classen-type endoscopic
papillotome is passed down the sheath into the
duodenum beyond the papilla. The papillotome wire
is positioned fluoroscopically between 11 o'clock and
1 o'clock and checked with an end-viewing, duodenoscope, and sphincterotomy is performed. Carefully
performed, this procedure is as useful as the endoscopic technique and has similar complications. Morbidity is minimal if the sphincterotome loop wire is
correctly positioned and checked endoscopically.
Using a mature T-tube track the procedure is easier,
and the complications of liver catheterization are absent. An external fistula from the bile duct following
laparoscopic cholecystectomy may also be used to
catheterize the bile duct and a track established to the
common bile duct using biliary dilators. A sheath may
be introduced into the common bile duct and sphincterotomy carried out as above.

Other alternatives to standard sphincterotomy
have been reported, but their overall success rates and
morbidity figures are far from optimal (6, 9). If perforation into the peritoneum occurs, the risk of severe
infection is less than that with endoscopic sphincterotomy with perforation since drainage is already established by the transhepatic catheter (9). The most serious complication of the technique is bleeding. If endoscopic visualization of the papilla is performed to
position the papillotome, the risk is reduced and it is
similar to endoscopic sphincterotomy (1, 6). Since balloon sphincterotomy is a much safer technique, we
only use percutaneous sphincterotomy when the balloon dilatation fails.

Percutaneous Transhepatic
Removal of Bile Duct Stones

(Table 10.**4**)

When external drainage of the bile duct is absent there
are four alternatives for treating bile duct stones.
When ERCP fails or is not possible, percutaneous removal is an attractive alternative. In these circumstances, the diagnosis of bile duct stones is often made
by FN PTHC. The usual precautions for FN PTHC are
observed. The bile ducts are outlined with contrast medium, and the number and size of the ductal stones are
observed and recorded. A transhepatic catheter is now
introduced into the common bile duct using the same
technique used for stent insertion.

The right intercostal or left xiphisternal route is
used to catheterize the right or left hepatic duct and

Table 10.**4**   Percutaneous   transhepatic   stone   removal

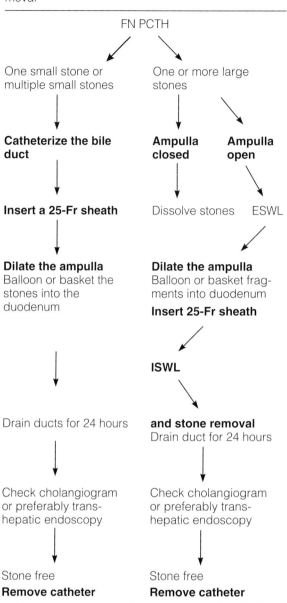

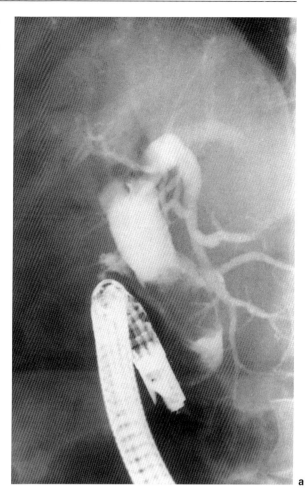

a

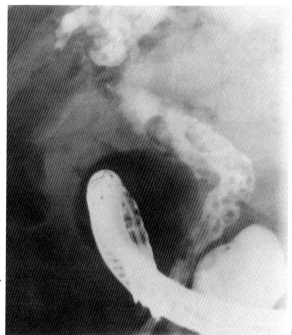

b

Fig. 10.**17   a ERCP showing large stone in common ▶ bile duct**
b Repeat ERCP 24 hours after sphincterotomy and ESWL of the common bile duct stone showing multiple stone fragments. These were easily removed by balloon catheter

the common bile duct. Presence or absence of contrast flow through the ampulla into the duodenum is observed. The technique of stone removal depends on the number and size of the calculi demonstrated and on whether the ampulla is draining (Fig. 10.**18**). If one small stone is present, preparations are made to remove it. If multiple small stones are present, these can also be removed. If one or more large stones are present and the ampulla is not draining contrast medium, an attempt is made to dissolve the stones or reduce their size before removal (see following section for technique of MTBE dissolution of ductal stones). If the ampulla is not occluded, we prefer to dilate the ampulla with a balloon and use fluoroscopy-guided ESWL to fragment the stones before removal. If this fails, consultation with our urologist follows, and intracorporeal shock wave lithotripsy (ISWL) is performed to fragment and remove the stones (see below). If this fails, transhepatic sphincterotomy is performed and a 10-Fr stent is inserted through the ampulla for duct drainage and to prevent stone impaction.

Removal of One or More Small Stones from the Common Bile Duct

Success with removal of one or several small stones from the bile duct after demonstration by FN PTHC depends on the catheterization of the bile duct via the liver in an atraumatic manner in order to prevent bleeding. A guide wire is passed into the duodenum, and a balloon catheter is inserted over the wire after dilating the liver track to take a 25-Fr sheath, which is inserted as far as its length allows into the common bile duct. All procedures are carried out through this sheath in order to protect the liver during stone manipulations.

Using successive balloon catheters, the ampulla may be dilated to 1–1.5 cm. This allows passage of stones up to 1–1.5 cm in diameter. These may be pushed into the duodenum by a Fogarty balloon catheter or by basketing one or more stones at a time through the ampulla, depending on stone size. The only contraindication to this procedure is the presence of infection in the bile ducts. After removal of all stones, the bile duct is drained externally for 24 hours, and a check cholangiogram or, preferably, fiberoptic endoscopy is carried out. If the duct is clear of stones the catheter is removed.

Removal of One or More Large Stones from the Bile Duct (Fig. 10.**18**)

Following demonstration of the stones by FN PTHC or ERCP with failed bile duct catheterization, if facilities are available and *the ampulla is closed on contrast injection,* an attempt may be made to reduce stone size with MTBE infusions after bile duct catheterization with a 5-Fr pigtail catheter containing multiple side holes (see below). The procedure is labor intensive and requires a special room with ventilation facilities and an automatic pump system.

Following reduction in stone size, a guide wire is inserted into the duodenum and, via transhepatic sheath, successive balloon catheters are inserted across the ampulla to dilate it to 1–1.5 cm. This is followed by stone removal as above. If *the ampulla is open* a catheter is inserted across the ampulla and the patient is referred for ESWL using contrast opacification of the bile duct to target the stones.

If stone fragmentation is successful, the stones are removed by basket or balloon into the duodenum as above.

If fragmentation with ESWL is unsuccessful, consultation with our urologists follows, and a track is dilated through the liver to 25 Fr to allow ISWL to be performed. This is a high-risk procedure that we try to avoid if possible. The stones are fragmented by this method and removed via the Amplatz sheath. After completion of the procedure, a large rubber catheter is inserted into the bile duct, and 24–48 hours later, a cholangiogram is performed to check for residual stones. If the duct is stone free and there is free drainage into the duodenum, the catheter is removed within 1 week. This allows a track to form to the skin and prevents leakage into the peritoneum.

If ISWL fails and the patient is unfit for surgery, transhepatic sphincterotomy may be performed and a 10-Fr stent inserted through the ampulla to prevent stone impaction.

Removal of Large Stones from the Bile Ducts

Most patients with large stones in the common bile duct are elderly. Large stones that prevent endoscopic bile duct catheterization are difficult to treat, even at choledochotomy. Even wide sphincterotomy may be insufficient for stone removal, so it is often necessary to fragment the stones or attempt to reduce their size before endoscopic removal. This may be performed by (1) mechanical lithotripsy, (2) ESWL, (3) ICSWL, EHL, ultrasound or laser techniques, (4) stone dissolution, or size reduction by MTBE. Mechanical lithotripsy by endoscopic, transtrack, percutaneous transhepatic, or transcholecystic catheterization of the bile duct is the simplest procedure. Laser lithotripsy is very expensive to establish initially but may be performed through a relatively small access route. Intracorporeal shock wave lithotripsy requires a larger access route to the bile duct and therefore has a higher incidence of complications. ESWL of bile duct stones is a less invasive form of therapy but requires additional sphincterotomy or dilatation of the ampulla for removal of fragments.

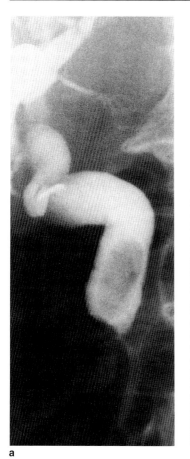

a

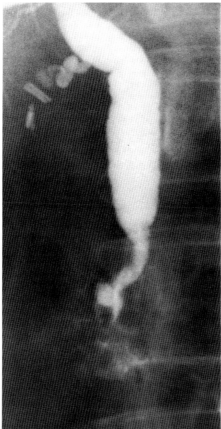

b

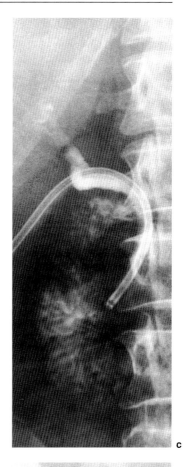

c

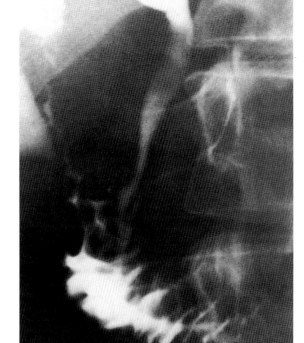

d

Fig. 10.**18 a Cholangiogram showing solitary common bile duct stone.** The papilla is closed
b Stone size reduction by contact dissolution with MTBE
c The stone fragment was pushed into the duodenum
d A cholangiogram at 24 hours shows changes in the lower common bile duct and pancreatic duct consistant with acute pancreatic swelling due to pancreatitis caused by stone manipulation. The patient recovered on conservative therapy

1. Mechanical Lithotripsy

Preprocedure i. v. antibiotics and sedation are given. After standard catheterization of the common bile duct through the liver or the gallbladder, if the latter is present, a track to the bile duct is dilated to take a 12- or 14-Fr catheter or sheath. After external drainage (after PTHC) for 2–3 days, or immediately after percutaneous transcholecystic drainage, or via a mature T-tube track, a Dormia basket–type mechanical lithotripter is inserted into the bile duct (BML3Q Olympus Corp, Lake Success, New York) contained within a Teflon sheath, and with an outer metal coil for stone crushing. A stone is engaged in the basket and a weight force of 80 lb may be applied to crush the stone. Stones up to 3 cm in diameter may be trapped in the basket. Any stone engaged by the basket may be crushed. Limitations on this form of therapy are due mainly to inability to trap the stone within the basket because of the size or position of the stone. The stone fragments are next removed by conventional Dormia-type basket. Percutaneous endoscopic inspection of the bile duct is used to confirm stone clearance from the ducts. The bile duct is drained for 24 hours after stone clearance. The patency of the ampulla and absence of stones are recorded by cholangiography and the external catheter removed.

This technique fails if multiple large stones occupy the entire duct system. External removal of the stone fragments avoids the risk of pancreatitis since there is no risk of trauma to the papilla.

2. Extracorporeal Shock Wave Lithotripsy
(Table 10.5)

Preparation

Preparation for ESWL includes normal coagulation, absence of anticoagulant therapy for 10 days before the procedure, absence of pregnancy, aortic aneurysm, and cardiac pacemakers. Endoscopic or percutaneous catheterization of the bile duct is necessary for contrast opacification of the stone(s) in the bile duct. I. v. antibiotic is given to limit or prevent cholangitis.

Technique

Radiological stone location using a renal lithotripter and biplane screening is best for therapy. The aim is to fragment the stones to 2–5-mm-diameter size. These can be removed without difficulty following sphincterotomy or by the Burhenne technique after dilatation of the ampulla by balloon catheter to 1–1.5 cm.

ESWL of bile duct stones is often an emergency procedure in obstructive jaundice. If cholangitis is present, nasobiliary or external catheter drainage is instituted until infection subsides.

Treatment success requires accurate demonstra-

Table 10.**5**   Indications for ESWL of bile duct stones

Large stones (3 cm or larger)
Hard stones
Failure to engage stones in Dormia basket
Intrahepatic stones inaccessible by PTHC
  or ERC routes
Stones above biliary stricture

tion of the stones. Ultrasound does not achieve this in the presence of an intraduct catheter. Air bubbles may be mistaken for stones.

Duct clearance is rarely achieved without a drainage procedure such as endoscopic sphincterotomy or balloon dilatation of the sphincter of Oddi. Electrohydraulic lithotripsy, with its greater power of fragmentation, gives the best results in the shortest time. Over 33% of patients may require a second treatment. Second or third treatment sessions are performed at intervals of 48 hours. Treatment success depends on accurate localization of the stones with X-ray imaging. The average duration of treatment with EHL is 30 minutes, and bile duct stones are fragmented in 95% of patients with extrahepatic biliary stones and in 55% of patients with intrahepatic stones.

Complications of ESWL of Bile Duct Stones

After ESWL of ductal stones, bacteremia occurs frequently because of the high incidence of infected bile in choledocholithiasis. Liver hematoma may occur and hemobilia has been reported. Lung tissue must be excluded from the shock wave area. Fragmentation of the stones by ESWL is followed by stone fragment removal. Other complications include those of endoscopic sphincterotomy in the elderly. The time-consuming extraction of fragments of large fragmented stone volumes by basket or balloon catheter may be difficult.

Discussion

Electromagnetic and piezoelectric lithotripsy units are less powerful but adequate for ESWL of ductal stones. The smaller the stone fragments and the wider the sphincterotomy or dilatation of the papilla, the earlier the stone fragments are cleared from the bile duct. Multiple stones larger than 3 cm in diameter still pose a difficult therapeutic problem without intracorporeal laser or lithotripsy therapy.

3. Percutaneous Biliary Endoscopy for Stone Lithotripsy

Percutaneous transhepatic, trans-T-tube track or transcholecystic endoscopic examination of the bile ducts and gallbladder is a valuable addition to the interventional procedures available for therapy of biliary stone disease. Radiation is avoided or minimal during the procedure, and areas not accessible by other methods, including the mother/daughter scope, may be reached. The procedure is valuable in the therapy of intrahepatic and common bile duct stone disease including intrahepatic stones in Caroli disease (5) and for tumor endoluminal forceps or brush biopsy (6, 9, 11).

Indications

The indications for percutaneous endoscopy of the biliary tract include both gallbladder and bile duct disease. The demonstration of stone disease, particularly of the intrahepatic ducts, which cannot be removed by conventional methods such as the Burhenne technique or peroral endoscopy, or the presence of *large ductal stones* requiring lithotripsy for fragmentation before removal are all indications for this procedure. ESWL requires a previous wide sphincterotomy to allow stone passage prior to therapy. Undiagnosed duct filling defects, tissue diagnosis of biliodigestive stenotic lesions after surgery, and endoluminal tumor radiation are other indications. Endoscopic inspection of the gallbladder or bile ducts after stone removal or after ESWL, plus MTBE fragment dissolution or cholecystolithotomy are also indications (1, 6, 7).

Preparation of the Patient

The patient is prepared as for any percutaneous transhepatic procedure including i. v. antibiotics, normal coagulation, hematology screening and, fasting for 8 hours.

Technique

Following FN PTHC and catheterization of the bile duct and duodenum or via a mature T-tube track, a 15-Fr sheath is inserted into the bile duct. Guide wires are placed via the sheath into the duodenum or an intrahepatic duct. The left duct is used for endoscopy of right duct area lesions and vice versa. We use a 15-Fr (6.6-Fr channel) nonrigid endoscope inserted into the bile duct through *a 5-day mature track through the liver* or inserted the same day into the gallbladder. The delay for track maturation, which is very important if serious complications are to be avoided, is poorly tolerated in modern hospital practice (2, 8, 10). The endoscope is irrigated by normal saline, which distends the ducts and aids lesion visualization.

The endoscope is particularly valuable for directing a flushing catheter or Dormia basket into a peripheral duct for stone removal. Common bile duct stones may be fragmented by basket crushing or intracorporeal lithotripsy with an electrohydraulic probe under direct vision and flushing during fragmentation

with N/6 saline to improve shock wave conduction for stone fragmentation. Picus et al. (1989) performed intracorporeal shock wave lithotripsy via Teflon sheath after acute track dilatation without complications. Nimura (1984) carried out 239 percutaneous transhepatic cholangioscopy procedures without any serious complications following track dilatation over 3 weeks. Bonnell et al. (1991) performed intracorporeal shock wave lithotripsy of intrahepatic and common bile duct stones in 50 patients following percutaneous transhepatic duct catheterization via the right lobe (22 cases), left lobe (5 cases), via two tracks, one in the right and one in the left lobe (11 cases), or multiple tracks (3 cases). They recommended formation of a track in two sessions. On day one, a track was dilated to 14 Fr and drained by catheter for 48 hours. At that time, the track was dilated to 20 Fr and drained by an 18-Fr catheter. Next, endoscopic or transhepatic sphincterotomy or balloon dilatation of the ampulla was performed to allow easy passage of stone fragments into the intestine. Stones above a biliary–intestinal anastomosis were treated by balloon dilatation of the anastomotic stricture prior to lithotripsy. Cholangioendoscopy was performed using a flexible endoscope, 5 mm in diameter, with a 2-mm working channel, 6 days after track preparation. Endoscopic irrigation was performed with saline 60–100 mL/min. Stones were fragmented by a 3-Fr lithotripsy probe under direct viewing. Pulses of 2 seconds duration and 40 impulses per second at 0.26 joules per impulse energy were used for stone fragmentation and fragments pushed or washed into the duodenum. After stone clearance, the ducts were drained externally for 3 days by a 14-Fr catheter, which was removed after final contrast cholangiography. Severe complications occurred in 11 cases (22%), and four patients died (8%). Bleeding caused two deaths. Hemobilia was massive in six cases. Hemorrhage occurred during track formation or during cholangioscopy. Intrahepatic duct perforation occurred in three cases; septic shock caused death in one of these. Fatal pulmonary edema from intestinal irrigation fluid absorption occurred in one patient with cardiac failure. Minor ductal hemorrhage was common secondary to lithotripsy injury. Small peripheral intrahepatic calculi were left untreated. Nishioka et al. (1987), Dawson et al. (1991), Ponchon et al. (1991), Sullivan et al. (1991), and Berci et al. (1990) used a pulsed tunable dye laser to fragment intrahepatic and common bile duct stones by transhepatic track, T-tube track, or endoscopically using a mother/daughter scope with an 85–92% fragmentation rate and a 75% to 95% clearance of all stones from the bile ducts without complications. The laser fiber is small (0.2–0.4 mm) and may be inserted transhepatically into the bile duct via a 4-Fr sheath, thus avoiding the known risks of large tracks through the liver (1, 3, 4, 7, 10, 11).

Complications

Hemorrhage is the most serious complication of percutaneous transhepatic endoscopic procedures. It is created by the initial bile duct puncture and may be minimized by slow needle insertion through the liver parenchyma under fluoroscopic vision. Larger tracks are more commonly associated with bleeding than tracks of 10 Fr or less. Track maturation before instrumentation also reduces the incidence of bleeding. Intrahepatic manipulation of the endoscope during endoscopy should only be performed by direct vision, and never blindly, to prevent duct injury or rupture.

4. Dissolution of Large Bile Duct Stones with MTBE

MTBE is an effective agent for dissolving cholesterol gallstones in the gallbladder following percutaneous or endoscopic gallbladder catheterization. The drug may be used to treat bile duct stones via a percutaneous or T-tube track or an endoscopically inserted nasobiliary catheter. It is difficult to control this technique and to prevent spill of MTBE into the duodenum.

MTBE only dissolves cholesterol stones that show minimal or absent rim calcification on computed tomography. Treatment time for stone lysis depends on stone position as well as stone size and composition. It is essential to occlude the bile duct below to prevent MTBE entering the duodenum. *This is a dangerous technique if the ampulla is not occluded.* Bile diversion during treatment enhances the effect of MTBE on the ductal stone(s). *Mechanical obstruction of the ampulla should not be used without bile diversion.* The technique may be used to reduce stone size or dissolve cholesterol stones completely.

Ductal Stone Dissolution with MTBE

a. Via a T-tube Track

Provided the track to the bile duct from the skin is adequate, this is the safest method of attempted stone dissolution. Two occlusion balloon catheters and a 5-Fr pigtail catheter are inserted into the bile duct. I. v. antibiotics are given, and the T tube is removed. A guide wire is inserted into the lower bile duct. A second guide wire is inserted into an intrahepatic duct. Balloon catheters resistant to MTBE (Blue Max, Meditech) are inserted over the guide wires into (a) the duct above the stone(s) and (b) the duct at the ampulla below the stone(s). A 5-Fr catheter (Thistle, Cook, Denmark) with a pigtail containing 32 side holes is now inserted into the bile duct preferably around the stone(s). Contrast medium is now injected into the 5-Fr pigtail catheter to determine the isolated bile duct volume and confirm occlusion of the duct above and below the stone(s). Duct distension with contrast agent is avoided.

The isolated bile duct volume is the maximum volume of MTBE that may be injected into the closed system for dissolution. The aspirate must be carefully monitored to prevent MTBE loss and to clinically confirm stone dissolution. Stone dissolution times vary from 2 to 12 hours. A small intrahepatic stone may dissolve within 30 minutes if the stone is bathed in MTBE by the catheter positioned at the stone. MTBE is infused by glass syringe only. Successful lysis requires that the pigtail catheter lie around the stone(s) and that the exclusion of bile from the stone-containing area of duct accelerate the action of the solvent on the stone(s). Most results of this technique report a reduction in stone size in 50% of cases and complete dissolution of small intrahepatic stones. Large ductal stones are completely dissolved in 33–60% of patients.

b. Via Percutaneous Transhepatic Catheterization

FN PTHC is performed, and the bile duct is catheterized. A track to the common bile duct is dilated to 20 Fr and a 20-Fr sheath is inserted into the bile duct. A balloon catheter, 5–7 Fr, (Blue Max resistant to MTBE) is inserted over a guide wire into the duct and across the ampulla. A 5-Fr pigtail catheter with 32 side holes in the loop of the pigtail is then inserted over a guide wire and positioned using the guide wire around the stone(s). A second 10-Fr pigtail catheter is inserted and positioned in the duct above the stone(s). Bile diversion by this route is performed by continued intermittent bile aspiration during MTBE syringe changes. A bile-free ductal area containing the stones cannot be achieved by the percutaneous route.

Occlusion of the lower end of the common bile duct is vital with this technique. The catheter is fixed to the skin with a suture and its position observed carefully at routine intervals during stone lysis. Its position is checked regularly before intervals of lysis therapy are commenced, and again at the end of all treatment sessions. The isolated bile duct volume is determined by contrast medium injection into the 5-Fr pigtail catheter as above. Stone lysis is performed in 3-hour sessions as with gallbladder stone MTBE therapy. Contrast injections are used to monitor stone size and pigtail catheter position at regular intervals. Stone dissolution is carried out in a special room with adequate ventilation and extraction facilities as described for gallbladder stones.

Complications of Bile Duct Stone Lysis with MTBE

As with cholesterol stone dissolution in the gallbladder, absorption of MTBE must not be permitted. The ideal route for this therapy is via a T-tube track. Bile duct stone dissolution may be performed via a nasobiliary catheter, but catheter positioning around the stone(s) for dissolution is more difficult and less successful than the T-tube track route. Keeping MTBE from reaching the duodenum prevents excessive sedation or coma, abdominal pain, nausea, hemolysis, and renal failure. Transhepatic bile duct stone dissolution is more difficult because of the problem of bile diversion from the stone-containing area of bile duct.

Infusion pumps, when available commercially, will provide decreased dissolution time for MTBE therapy.

Results of MTBE Therapy of Bile Duct Stones

In general, results of this therapy in ductal stones are poor even when combined with other dissolution agents. The lower cholesterol content of ductal stones, the difficulty of excluding bile from the stone dissolution area after endoscopic or percutaneous duct catheterization (which results in poor solvent contact), and difficulties in excluding MTBE from the duodenum when dissolution is performed by nasobiliary catheter all reduce success.

In 10 patients with common bile duct stones who we treated with MTBE infusions via a carefully positioned nasobiliary catheter, there was no significant stone dissolution after up to 10 hours of solvent treatment, and excessive sedation occurred following loss of MTBE into the duodenum. Others have reported limited successes with this therapy.

The Formation of Tracks from the Biliary Tract to the Skin

Dissolution of cholesterol gallstones with MTBE requires insertion of a percutaneous transhepatic catheter from the skin to the gallbladder lumen. A track from the gallbladder through the liver to the skin of the abdominal wall forms around a percutaneously inserted 5-Fr catheter within 6 days or less (4), and a track from the gallbladder mucosa to the liver capsule is present after 4 days of MTBE therapy. The catheter in the gallbladder is made from material such as polyethylene, polyurethane, or Teflon. These materials resist dissolution with MTBE (2). T tubes for postoperative biliary drainage are made from silastic rubber, which causes a foreign body reaction around the tube with fibrous tissue and a stronger track within 7–10 days than other T-tube materials. From experience of incomplete T-tube tracks, we believe that track formation around an indwelling T tube begins from the bile duct and continues laterally to the abdominal wall. Infection around the exit of the T tube at the skin of the abdominal wall often results in the track being incomplete laterally for 3–4 cm. In such cases, if the T tube is removed without inserting a guide wire into the bile duct, the track is lost from the skin and the procedure fails. A mature T-tube track (4–5 weeks dura-

tion) may be dilated from 7 Fr to 14–16 Fr without loss of or injury to the channel to the bile duct. A straight rubber catheter inserted into the bile duct at laparoscopic cholecystectomy also provides a track suitable for stone removal when it has matured. All other drains are removed from the liver and subhepatic areas to prevent formation of internal fistulas and an incomplete track for transtrack removal of retained bile duct stones.

Our experience with percutaneous transhepatic cholecystostomy catheter drainage shows that with a 5-Fr pigtail catheter in situ for 7 days, there is always an intact track present through the liver from the gallbladder to the skin (4).

D'Agostino et al. (1991) studied the track to the skin from the gallbladder by contrast injection. They used larger catheters to drain the gallbladder (7 Fr) or an 18-Fr track reduced to a 7-Fr catheter for drainage after stone removal. These authors considered that a 20-day period was necessary to develop a well-formed track in the absence of track infection or tumor or biliary tract obstruction. When the gallbladder is emptied completely after percutaneous drainage for stone dissolution, or stent insertion via the cystic duct, and extrahepatic obstruction is absent, no significant leakage occurs from the gallbladder. In 13 of 39 cases that we treated, without plugging the percutaneous track with Gelfoam, there were no cases of bile spill into the peritoneum. One patient developed nausea that lasted 24 hours. No fluid collections were detected by ultrasound in the perihepatic or pericholecystic areas.

Tissue from the track wall, perhaps formed by local intratrack bleeding during catheter insertion into the gallbladder, may adhere to the catheter and cause disruption of the track when the catheter is removed from the bile duct or gallbladder. Large cholecystostomy tracks used for stone removal are drained for 14 days by Foley catheter, and the catheter is removed only when there is free flow of contrast agent into the cystic duct, common bile duct, and duodenum. This 14-day period allows adhesions to develop from the gallbladder to the abdominal wall. Surgical cholecystostomy catheters may be removed in 6–7 days (5). Defective T-tube tracks are found in association with diabetes mellitus, steroid therapy, malnutrition, infection, and chronic renal failure (1, 2, 3).

References

Percutaneous Trans–T-tube track Stone Removal

1. Bean WJ, Smith SL, Calan JE. Percutaneous removal of residual biliary tract stones. Radiology 1974; 113:1–9.
2. Burhenne HJ. The technique of bile duct stone extraction. Radiology 1974; 113:567–572.
3. Burhenne HJ. Complications of non-operative extraction of retained common bile duct stones. Am J Surg 1976; 131:260–262.

4. Burhenne HJ. Percutaneous extraction of retained biliary tract stones; 661 cases. AJR 1980; 134:888–898.
5. Braun MA, Collins MB. A simple method for reducing air bubble artifacts during percutaneous extraction of biliary stones. AJR 1992; 158:309–310.
6. Caprini JA, Crampton AR, Swan VM. Nonoperative extraction of retained common duct stones. Arch Surg 1976; 111:445–451.
7. Clarsen M, Ossenberg FW. Non surgical removal of common bile duct stones. Gut 1977; 18:760–769.
8. Dahnert W, Gunter R, Schmidt HD, et al. Entfernen zurückgelassener Gallengangskonkremente durch den T-drainkanal. Rofo 1984; 141:63–66.
9. Fennessy JJ, You KD. A method for the expulsion of stones retained in the common bile duct. AJR 1970; 110:256–259.
10. Ferrucci JT, Mueller PR. Postoperative instrumentation of the biliary tract. In: Ferrucci JT, Mueller PR, eds. Interventional radiology of the abdomen. Baltimore: Williams and Wilkins, 1981; 11–52.
11. Galloway SJ, Casarella WJ, Seaman WB. The non-operative treatment of retained stones in the common bile duct. Surg Gynecol Obstet 1973; 137:55–58.
12. Garrow DG. The removal of retained common bile duct stones. Report of 105 cases. Br J Radiol 1977; 50:777–782.
13. Gunther R, Schmidt HD, Braun B. Perkutane transhepatische Gallensteinextraktion. Deutsche Med Wschr 1981; 106:615–617.
14. Hare WSC. Treatment of retained stones in common bile duct. Austral NZ J Med 1978; 8:563–568.
15. Ho CS. Non-operative removal of retained common bile duct stones. Canad J Surg 1978; 21:244–247.
16. Hublitz UF, Cogliano FD, Arean PJ. Early extraction of residual biliary tract stones: a two guide wire technique. AJR 1984; 143:1090–1092.
17. Kadir S, Kaufman SL, Barth KH, White R. Selected techniques in interventional radiology. Philadelphia: Saunders, 1982; 128–138.
18. Kadir S, Gadacz TR. Adjuncts and modifications to basket retrieval of retained biliary calculi. Cardiovasc Intervent Radiol 1987; 10:295–300.
19. Lagrave G, Plessis JL, Pougeard-Dulimbert G, et al. Lithiase biliaire residuelle: extraction a la sonde de dormia par la drain de Kehr. Mem Acad Chir (Paris) 1969; 95:431–455.
20. Lams A, Letton AH, Wilson JP. Retained common bile duct stones, a new nonoperative technique for treatment. Surgery 1969; 66:291–296.
21. Light W. Extraction of retained biliary calculi in the X-ray department. Can Ass Radiol J 1974; 24:209–214.
22. Leary JB, Parshall WA. Percutaneous common duct stone extraction. Radiology 1972; 105:452–454.
23. Mack E, Patzer EM, Crummy AE, et al. Retained biliary tract stones. Arch Surg 1981; 116:341–344.
24. Magarey CJ. Non-surgical removal of retained biliary calculi. Lancet 1971; 1:1044–1046.
25. Magill HL, Baker CRF Jr. A simple catheter suction technique for nonoperative retrieval of a retained common bile duct stone. Radiology 1982; 142:788–789.
26. Mc Nulty J, Collins PG, Lane BE. Non-operative removal of retained common bile duct stones. Irish Med J 1984; 77:318–321.
27. Mason R. Percutaneous extraction of retained gallstones. Clin Gastroenterol 1985; 14:403–419.
28. Mazzariello RM. A Fourteen year experience with non operative instrument extraction of retained bile duct stones. World J Surg 1978; 2:447–455.
29. Mondet A. Tecnica de la extraccion incruenta de los calculos on la lithiasis residual del coledoco. Bol Soc Cir B Aires 1962; 46:278–290.
30. Meranze SG, Stein EJ, Burke DR, et al. Removal of retained common bile duct stones with angiographic occlusion balloons. AJR 1986; 146:383–386.
31. Nussinson E, Cairns SR, Vaira D, et al. A 10 year single centre experience of percutaneous and endoscopic extraction of bile duct stones with T tube in situ. Gut 1991; 32:1040–1043.
32. Polack EP, Fainsinger MH, Bonnano SV. A death following complications of roentgenologic non-operative manipulation of common bile duct calculi. Radiology 1977; 123:585–586.
33. Schwartz W, Long WB, Ring EJ, Rosato EF. Biliary stone removal: the interventional radiologist's role. Europ J Radiol 1983; 3:341–347.
34. Taylor BR, Ho CS. Non-surgical treatment of common bile duct stones. Can J Surg 1984; 27:28–32.
35. Geisinger MA, Owens DB, Meaney TF. Radiological methods of bile duct stone extraction. Am J Surg 1989; 158:222–227.
36. World congress of minimally invasive therapy. Dublin, Ireland, November 1992.

Balloon Dilatation of the Papilla

1. Berkman WA, Bishop AF, Palagallo GL, Cashman MD. Transhepatic balloon dilatation of the distal common bile duct and ampulla of Vater for removal of calculi. Radiology 1988; 167:453–455.
2. Bret PM. Les techniques d'abord direct ottes invatives: opacification directe, prelevements traitements par voie Percutanée. In: Doyon D, Amiel M, eds. Voies biliaries: aspects diagnostiques et therapeutiques. Paris: Masson, 1984: 67–99.
3. Centola CAP, Jander HP, Stauffer A, Russinovich NAE. Balloon dilatation of the papilla of vater to allow biliary stone passage. AJR 1981; 136:613–614.
4. Clouse ME, Stokes KR, Lee RGL, Falchuk KR. Bile duct stones: percutaneous transhepatic removal. Radiology 1986; 160:525–529.
5. Fataar S, Bassiony H, Abou-Neema H. The percutaneous stretch and push technique for removing retained bile duct stones. Br J Radiol 1982; 55:456–459.
6. Graciani L, Fabrizzi G, Manfrini E, Galeazzi R, Freddara U. Percutaneous transhepatic Oddi sphincter dilatation for bile duct stone removal. AJR 1989; 152:73–75.
7. Meranze SG, Stein EJ, Burke DR, et al. Removal of retained common bile duct stones with angiographic occlusion balloons. AJR 1986; 146:383–384.
8. Saeed M, Newman GE, Dunnick NR. Use of angioplasty balloons in the percutaneous management of biliary calculi: Tandem balloon method. AJR 1987; 148:745–746.
9. Staritz M, Ewe K, Meyer-zum Buschenfelde KH. Endoscopic papillary dilation (EPD) for the treatment of common bile duct stones and papillary stenosis. Endoscopy 1983; 15:197–198.
10. Stokes KR, Falchuk K, Clouse ME. Biliary duct stones; update of 54 cases after percutaneous transhepatic removal. Radiology 1989; 170:999–1001.

Percutaneous Sphincterotomy

1. Bonnel D, Liguory C, Cornud F, Lefebvre JF. Percutaneous transhepatic sphincterotomy (PTS): early experience in 7 patients. Proceedings of the Third Annual meeting of the International Society of Biliary Radiology Chicago: International Society of Biliary Radiology, 1991.
2. Burhenne HJ, Scudmore CH. Antegrade transcholecystic sphincterotomy; canine study of a new interventional technique. Gastrointest Radiol 1986; 11:73–76.
3. Cobourn CL, Makowka L, Chia Sing Ho B, et al. Percutaneous transhepatic sphincterotomy in the management of biliary tract disease. Gastrointest Radiol 11:273–277.
4. Gunther RW, Klose KJ, Storkel S. Percutaneous antegrade electropapillotomy: study in dogs. Cardiovasc. Intervent Radiol 1984; 7:270–276.
5. Passi RB, Rankin RN. The transhepatic approach to a failed endoscopic sphincterotomy. Gastrointest Endoscopy 1986; 32:211–2225.
6. Ponchon TPJ, Valette R, et al. Evaluation of combined percutaneous endoscopic procedure for the treatment of choledocholithiasis and benign papillary stenosis. Endoscopy 1987; 19:194.
7. Staritz M, Poralla T, et al. Endoscopic removal of common bile duct stones through the intact papilla after medical sphincter dilation. Gastroenterology 1985; 88:1807–1811
8. Wurbs D, Hagenmuller F, Classen M. Descending sphincterotomy of the papilla of Vater through a choledochoduodenostomy under endoscopic view. Endoscopy 1980; 12:38–40.

9. Wurbs D, Dammermann R, Ossenberg FW, Classen M. Descending sphincterotomy of the papilla of Vater through the T drain under endoscopic view. Endoscopy 1978; 10:199–203.
10. Zanon E, Righi D, Maisano U, Regge D, Ferrari A, Recchia S, Gandini G. Percutaneous transhepatic sphincterotomy. Endoscopy 1991; 23:25–28.

Percutaneous Transhepatic Removal of Bile Duct Stones

1. Berci G, Hamlin JA, Dayhofsky L, PazPartlow M. Common bile duct laser lithotripsy. Gastrointest Endosc 1990; 36:137–138.
2. Bonnel DH, Liguory CE, Cornud FE, Lefebvre JFP. Common bile duct and intrahepatic stones: Results of transhepatic electrohydraulic lithotripsy in 50 patients. Radiology 1991; 180:345–348.
3. Dawson SL, Mueller PR, Lee MJ, et al. Treatment of bile duct stones by laser lithotripsy. AJR 1992; 158:1007–1009.
4. Feldman RK, Freeny PC, Kozarek RA. Pancreatic and biliary calculi: percutaneous treatment with tunable dye laser lithotripsy. Radiology 1990; 174:793–795.
5. King J, Orrison WW, Davis M, Kleinman R. Percutaneous choledochoscopic choledocholithotomy in Caroli's disease. Gastrointest Radiol 1990; 15:137–138.
6. Liguory CL, Lefebvre JF, Bonnel D, et al. Indications for cholangioscopy. Endoscopy 1989; 21:341–343.
7. Nimura Y. Percutaneous transhepatic cholangioscopy (PTCS). Stomach Intestire 1980; 16:681–689.
8. Nishioka NS, Levins PC, Murray SC, et al. Fragmentation of biliary calculi with tunable dye lasers. Gastroenterology 1987; 93:250–255.
9. Picus D, Weyman PJ, Marx MV. Role of percutaneous intracorporeal electrohydraulic lithotripsy in the treatment of biliary tract calculi, Work in progress. Radiology 1989; 170:989–993.
10. Ponchon T, Gagnon P, Valette PJ, et al. Pulsed dye laser lithotripsy of bile duct stones. Gastroenterology 1991; 100:1730–1736.
11. Sullivan KL, Bagley DH, Gordon SJ, et al. Transhepatic laser lithotripsy of choledocholithiasis: initial clinical experience. J. Vasc. Intervent Radiol 1991; 2:387–391.

The Formation of Tracks from the Biliary Tract to the Skin

1. Andersson R, Tramberg KG, Bengmark S. Isolated intraperitoneal accumulations of bile after surgical or diagnostic procedures. Acta Chir Scand 1988; 154:375–377.
2. D'Agostino HB, van Sonnenberg E, Sanchez RB. Imaging of the percutaneous cholecystostomy tract: observations and utility. Radiology 1991; 181:675–678.
3. Gillatt DA, May RE, Kennedy R, Longstaff AJ. Complications of T-tube drainage of the common bile duct. Ann R Coll Surg Eng 1985; 67:370–371.
4. Mc Nulty JG. Interventional radiology of the gallbladder. Berlin: Springer, 1990:47–48.
5. Troidl H. Surgical alternatives in the treatment of cholelithiasis, cholecystostomy. In: Kremer K, Lierse W, Platzer W, et al., eds. Atlas of operative surgery-Gallbladder bile ducts and pancreas. Stuttgart: Thieme, 1992:145–148.

11   Benign Bile Duct Stricture and Postsurgical Bile Duct Trauma

Minimally invasive therapy in benign bile duct diseases has as its aim complete cure of the disease process. In order to compete with other forms of therapy, the treatment should, if possible, be completed during a single visit to the interventional unit. In these times of accountable hospital procedure costs, it benefits all concerned that treatment procedures are performed as rapidly and carefully as possible with minimal morbidity and no procedure-related mortality.

Etiology

Most benign bile duct strictures are caused by surgeons during surgery on the biliary tract including laparoscopic cholecystectomy. A few are the result of chronic pancreatitis, sclerosing cholangitis, blunt abdominal trauma; anastomotic strictures occur in liver transplant. Surgical cure is rare, and a stricture may recur even after 20 years (3, 5, 7, 10, 22, 23, 33). If bile duct injury is recognized at cholecystectomy, direct end-to-end anastomosis over a T tube should be performed. If this is not possible, immediate choledochojejunostomy and Roux-en-Y anastomosis are carried out.

Most strictures are not recognized at the time of the initial surgery, and while immediate jaundice may occur postoperatively, symptoms may be delayed or intermittent for months or years (33). Bouts of cholangitis, pain, and jaundice are the characteristic clinical manifestations of benign bile duct stricture. Eventually, secondary biliary cirrhosis develops with portal hypertension (5). The latter and sepsis are the major causes of death in such patients.

Stricture recurrence is common after biliointestinal anastomosis performed for benign stricture. Intermittent cholangitis is the best index of restenosis with or without calculi (5). Reoperation has a mortality rate of 15% (18, 20, 33), and it may reach 25% when portal hypertension is present (26).

Four alternatives are presently available for interventional therapy of benign bile duct stricture. These are:

1. Percutaneous dilatation by balloon catheter
2. Percutaneous trans–T-tube track balloon dilatation
3. Endoscopic balloon dilatation
4. Stent insertion

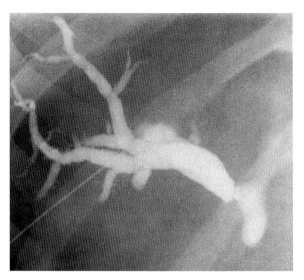

Fig. 11.**1**   **FN PTHC showing ligated bile duct not suitable for minimally invasive therapy**

Before any form of therapy is instituted, a firm diagnosis of benign stricture of the bile duct must be established by biopsy if necessary. This particularly applies to endoscopic diagnosis of biliary stricture.

Percutaneous and endoscopic methods of therapy of benign bile duct stricture are equally effective. Endoscopic methods cannot be used once a biliary intestinal anastomosis has been performed. **Both methods of therapy are contraindicated when the bile duct is ligated accidently by the surgeon** (Fig. 11.1).

Incomplete primary duct trauma may be treated initially by endoscopic or percutaneous duct dilata-

Fig. 11.**2**   **a ERCP showing questionable duct narrow-** ▶
ing in the common hepatic duct
b After 24 months the patient returned with cholangitis, and ERCP shows a stricture with multiple hepatic duct stones
c Endoscopic balloon dilatation was performed
d Repeat ERCP after 6 months shows a stone-free ductal system and minimal stricture, which was dilated by balloon catheter

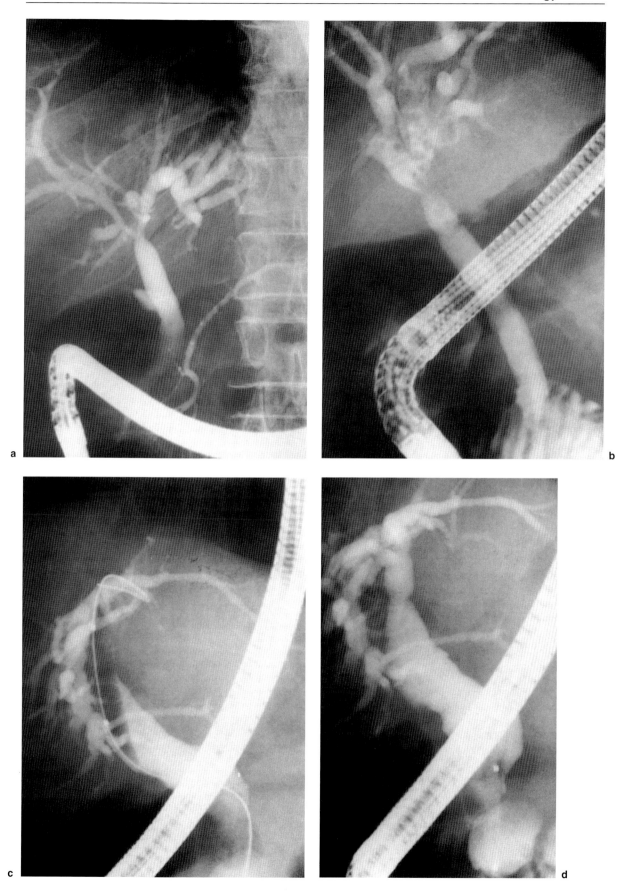

tion by balloon catheter when a firm diagnosis has been established. However, a severed bile duct or ligated bile duct must be treated initially by surgical mucosal-to-mucosal anastomosis of the duct above the injury to the jejunum with a Roux-en-Y anastomosis for drainage.

A track to the duct from the skin (formed by a tube inserted at laparoscopic cholecystectomy or a T-tube track) is safer for balloon dilatation of a stricture than a transhepatic track route after FN PTHC.

Pathology of Benign Bile Duct Stricture

The pathological changes found after bile duct injury vary in extent depending on the cause of injury and the duration of partial or complete biliary obstruction. In the bile duct wall at the site of injury, inflammatory changes and fibrosis cause the stricture. Local bile extravasation may cause the inflammatory response. The ducts proximal to the obstruction become dilated and fibrotic with mucosal atrophy, necrosis, and squamous metaplasia. In the submucosa there is an inflammatory cell infiltrate with fibrosis. The same changes cause obliteration of the duct distally. Duct wall ischemia may be responsible. Proximal to the stricture the bile is almost always infected. *Surgical treatment by mucosal-to-mucosal anastomosis is the best primary form of treatment,* but fibrosis almost always develops eventually at the ductal jejunal anastomosis.

Both external and internal fistulas may occur in association with ductal stricture. Jaundice is absent when there is an external fistula, and there is intermittent jaundice when an internal fistula is present. This usually occurs to the duodenum and is associated with recurrent cholangitis. Periportal fibrosis and biliary cirrhosis occur in the untreated patient. Portal hypertension with bleeding varices occurs in 20% of patients, associated with inadequate stricture treatment that causes biliary cirrhosis.

In chronic pancreatitis, a long narrow stricture occurs in the retropancreatic part of the common bile duct. This type of stricture is more common in alcoholic pancreatitis. Bile duct dilatation above the stricture may be moderate or marked. This stricture should be treated by surgery. Less commonly, there is papillary fibrosis or a short stricture above the papilla.

Strictures in sclerosing cholangitis are usually multiple and involve the entire ductal system. Histology shows mucosal atrophy, necrosis, submucosal inflammatory changes, and fibrosis. Multifocal strictures occur and eventually biliary cirrhosis.

Diagnosis of Benign Bile Duct Stricture

The diagnosis of postsurgical stricture is usually made during investigation of postoperative jaundice by FN PTHC or ERCP. In incomplete stricture, the upper and lower limits of the stricture may be demonstrated by both techniques. When the duct is severed

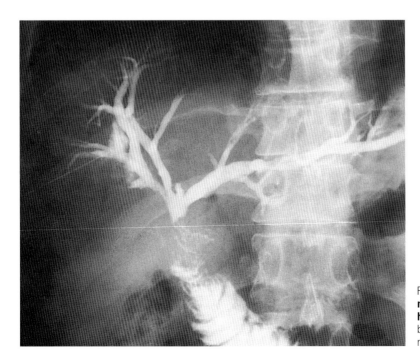

Fig. 11.**3 FN PTHC showing a normal anastomosis and slight right hepatic duct narrowing.** Forceps biopsy revealed cholangiocarcinoma.

or ligated, the proximal bile ducts are only demonstrated by FN PTHC. Similarly, after biliointestinal anastomosis, the stricture is only demonstrated by FN PTHC. Minimal ductal narrowing or irregularity shown by FN PTHC or ERCP may be difficult to confirm as a benign stricture without brush or forceps biopsy of the site.

Benign stricture occurs mostly at the junction of the main right and left hepatic ducts and in the upper common hepatic duct. Jaundice is present when advanced strictures occur in sclerosing cholangitis, although deep jaundice may be present with marked ductal changes without any dominant strictures being visible at cholangiography. Traumatic strictures after blunt abdominal trauma usually sever the common bile duct above the pancreas.

The long narrow stricture of chronic pancreatitis is characteristically located in the lower third of the common bile duct.

Shorter strictures involving the duct at and above the ampulla also occur in pancreatitis, and there may be associated stricturing of the distal pancreatic duct.

1. Percutaneous Transhepatic Stricture Dilatation

Indications

The main indication for this procedure is the demonstration of a benign bile duct stricture in which there is continuity of the extrahepatic ducts with a local stricture in the common hepatic duct or in the main right hepatic duct, or less commonly, in the left hepatic duct. Short strictures at the lower end of the common bile duct in chronic pancreatitis, or papillary stenosis in chronic pancreatitis are also suitable for percutaneous dilatation. Long strictures in chronic pancreatitis are not an indication. These require bypass surgery. Stricture at the site of a biliointestinal anastomosis is an important indication for balloon dilatation (Fig. 11.4). Strictures in sclerosing cholangitis may be dilated by percutaneous catheterization or by endoscopic balloon dilatation. The technique is usually not possible in most primary duct strictures or in duct ligation because of absence of duct continuity. Stricture diagnosis may be made by FN PTHC, sinography, or ERCP. In the absence of pus in the bile, minimally invasive therapy is instituted immediately on discovery of the lesion. If there is evidence of cholangitis, external drainage is performed by percutaneous catheter or endoscopically by nasobiliary drain. Drainage is continued until biliary infection resolves.

Technique

Preparation

Precautions for FN PTHC are observed. I.v. antibiotics are given. Success with this technique depends on "clean" bile duct catheterization without extravasation into the liver parenchyma or perihepatic area.

Technique of Stricture Dilatation (Fig. 11.5)

A bile duct in the right or left lobe of the liver is catheterized, and a guide wire is inserted into the intestine through the stricture. Analgesia (i.v.) and sedation are given, and a series of Teflon dilators are inserted into the bile duct to form a track for the balloon dilators. We prefer to complete the dilatation in one session using high-pressure angioplasty balloons with inflated balloon diameters up to the size of the normal bile duct in the individual patient. Balloon inflation is maintained with each catheter size until the waist on the balloon caused by the stricture is no longer visible. When calculi are located above an anastomotic stricture, balloon dilatation may be sufficient to allow the stones to pass into the intestine or to flush or push the stones into the jejunum.

Successful therapy of a tight stricture is accompanied by some bleeding, but this should not be sufficient to require transfusions of blood. After stricture dilatation we do not use external drainage except when the stricture is located at the papilla.

Complications

This is a painful procedure requiring i.v. pethidine (meperidine) during dilatations. Some authors use general anesthesia (16).

The morbidity of this procedure is related to biliary catheterization and drainage and not to balloon dilatation of the stricture (29). Septic cholangitis has been reported in 5% to 25% of treated cases (5, 23). Hemorrhage may occur and require transfusion. Pancreatitis may follow dilatations of the papilla.

No deaths have been reported from this procedure.

In a personal series of 11 cases, there were no serious complications. One patient with an anastomotic stricture and intrahepatic stones developed cholangitis following stricture dilatation and stone removal. This resolved on conservative therapy with external drainage. Since it is more difficult to catheterize the bile ducts in the absence of dilated ducts, some surgeons create a jejunal loop, which provides easy access to the bile ducts for repeated stricture dilatation with less morbidity (29).

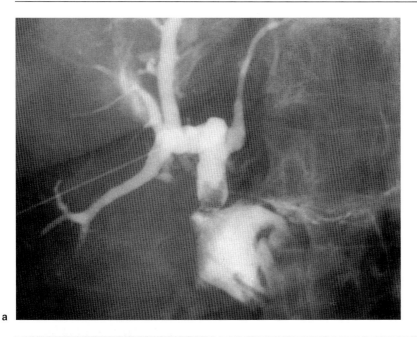

a

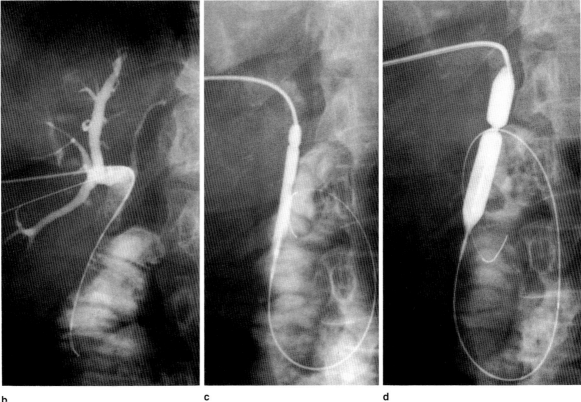

b   c   d

Fig. 11.**4   a FN PTHC showing stones above a biliointestinal anastomosis and stricture formation**
b The bile duct was catheterized
c A balloon catheter was inserted to dilate the stricture
d The stones were washed into the duodenum

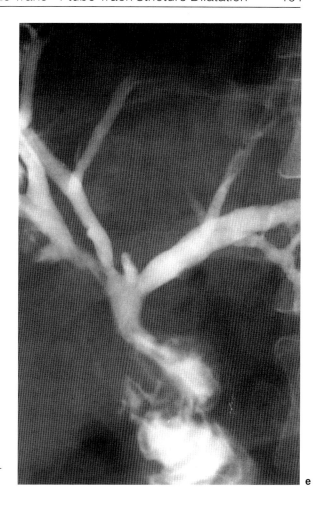

e Poststricture angioplasty shows a good result and absence of calculi. The patient remains well at 24 months

e

Results

The long-term results of this procedure are unknown. Stricture patency for 2.5 years has been reported. Biliary surgeons would not consider this a good result (10, 33). We have not used stents in the treatment of benign bile duct stricture, although others have used metal stents that cannot be removed from the stricture once inserted (6, 8, 28). Long stents should be used to avoid difficulties in stent placement (28).

2. Percutaneous Trans–T-tube Track Stricture Dilatation

The main indication for this procedure is the demonstration of a benign bile duct stricture by T-tube cholangiography or a "tubogram" at 7 days after laparoscopic cholangiography. At 3–5 weeks after surgery, cholangiography is repeated via the in situ tube.

Technique

Analgesia and i.v. antibiotics are given, and the tube is removed from the bile duct over a guide wire. A steerable catheter or angiographic curved catheter is now inserted into the duct system in the direction of the stricture, and a guide wire is directed across the stricture into the duodenum or into an intrahepatic duct. A series of angioplasty balloon catheters are now inserted over the guide wire across the stricture and balloon inflation maintained until the stricture waist is no longer visible on the dilated balloon. When the normal duct width is achieved, the balloon is removed and a catheter inserted for ampullary drainage in periampullary strictures for 24–48 hours, and serum amylase levels are recorded. If these are normal, the catheter is removed and the patient discharged.

This is the safest technique of stricture dilatation since the complications of transhepatic catheterization are absent. However, in most bile duct strictures the T-tube track is also absent.

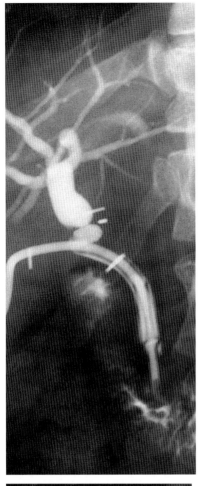

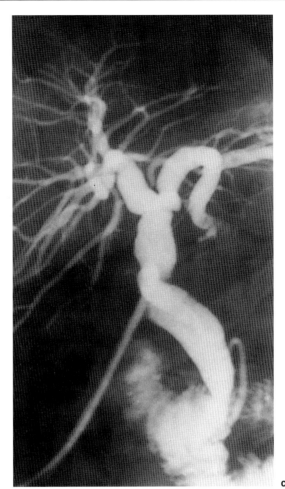

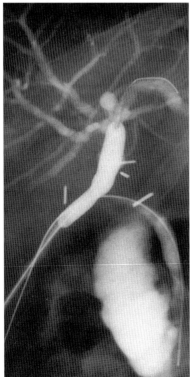

Fig. 11.**5 Postlaparoscopic cholecystectomy stricture(s)?**
a Catheter cholangiogram
b Balloon catheter stricture dilatation
c Postdilatation cholangiogram. The patient remains symptom free at 18 months

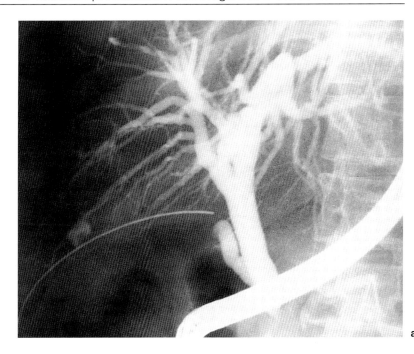

Fig. 11.**6   a Postcholecys-
tectomy biliary leak from a right
hepatic duct** is opacified by ERCP
b A straight stent was inserted into
the right hepatic duct. The leak
closed within 4 days

a

3. Endoscopic Dilatation of Benign Bile Duct Strictures

Indications

The main indication is the demonstration of a benign
bile duct stricture during endoscopic cholangiography in the symptomatic patient with a history of
cholecystectomy and pain, jaundice, or cholangitis.
This method cannot be used to treat biliointestinal
anastomoses since the route to the bile duct is no
longer available after surgery. In papillary fibrosis or
short peripapillary strictures associated with pancreatitis or passage of a bile duct stone, this is the ideal
method of therapy. It is contraindicated in long strictures of the lower common bile duct due to chronic
pancreatitis, which are best treated by bypass surgery.

Technique

When ERCP demonstrates a ductal stricture, the absence of malignancy must be confirmed by biopsy.
After diagnostic ERCP it is necessary to perform a
sphincterotomy to allow the insertion of a balloon
catheter into the bile duct. After duct catheterization a
guide wire is inserted into the bile duct and its tip positioned in an intrahepatic duct above the stricture.
Next, a balloon angioplasty catheter is inserted across
the stricture over the wire and inflated until the stricture waist is no longer visible.

This is repeated until the stricture is dilated to the
size of the bile duct. Strictures involving both the right
and left hepatic ducts are dilated individually at the
same session.

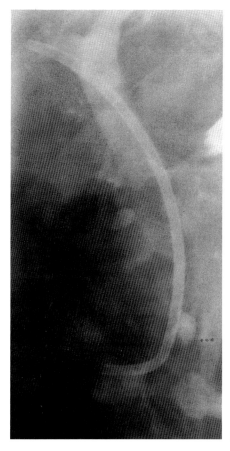

b

Complications

Complications are rare after endoscopic stricture dilatation. Complications of sphincterotomy may occur. Ascending cholangitis occurs in the presence of infected bile. Nasobiliary drainage should be performed if pus is encountered.

4. Stent Insertion in Benign Stricture or Postsurgical Leakage from the Bile Ducts

Endoscopic stent insertion may only be used in primary duct strictures and not in biliointestinal anastomoses as the route is no longer available. Recent indications for endoscopic stenting after laparoscopic cholecystectomy include bile leakage from an anomalous duct in the right lobe of the liver or from the cystic duct stump, or from a choledochotomy without T-tube drainage after open cholecystectomy and bile duct exploration.

Technique

The diagnosis is established by diagnostic ERCP. This may show:

1. A hilar stricture
2. Leakage of contrast medium from a duct in the gallbladder fossa
3. Leakage from the cystic duct
4. Leakage from a choledochotomy site

1. *Benign duct stricture*
After stricture dilatation, a 10- or 12-Fr stent is inserted across the stricture, and the stricture is reviewed in 3 months.

2. *Anomalous duct leakage*
When this is demonstrated, a stent is inserted into the right hepatic duct (Fig. 11.**6**). This allows healing of the injured duct by draining bile away from the site of leakage across the papilla into the duodenum.

3. *Cystic duct or choledochotomy leakage*
This is treated by inserting a stent that extends from the ducts above the leakage into the duodenum to divert bile away from the lesion and overcome papillary obstruction, which is thought to prolong biliary leakage. Sphincterotomy may be used for the same purpose. When FN PTHC demonstrates a postsurgical stricture and there is continuity of the bile duct to the duodenum and minimal or no leakage of contrast medium from the stricture site, the patient should be referred to a competent and experienced biliary surgeon since the best hope of a successful outcome lies in early surgery by biliointestinal anastomosis. A minor stricture (diaphragm) in the duct at the site may be treated by balloon angioplasty and a 10-Fr teflon stent inserted across the stricture and its lower end positioned in the duodenum. The patient is reviewed at 3 months; the stent is removed with a snare by endoscopy or fluoroscopy. A decision is now made whether or not to recommend surgical stricture correction. Surgery in bile duct stricture must not be delayed in order to avoid the development of cholangitis, liver abscess formation, or biliary cirrhosis.

References

1. Browder IW, Dowling JB. Early management of operative injuries of the extrahepatic biliary tract. Ann Surg 1987; 205:649–658.
2. Bezzi M, Salvatori FM, Maccioni J, et al. Biliary metal stents in benign strictures. Semin Intervent Radiol 1991; 8:321–330.
3. Burhenne JH. Dilatation of biliary tract strictures. Radiol Clin North Am 1975; 14:153–159.
3. Christenson RA, van Sonnenberg E, Nemcek AA, et al. Inadvertant ligation of the aberrant right hepatic duct at cholecystectomy: Radiological diagnosis and therapy. Radiology 1992; 183:549–554.
4. Citron SJ, Martin LG. Benign bile duct strictures: Treatment with percutaneous cholangioplasty. Radiology 1991; 178:339–341.
5. Collins PG, Gorey TF. Iatrogenic biliary stricture: presentation and management. Br J Surg 1984; 71:980–982.
6. Crist DW, Kadir S, Cameron JL. The value of preoperatively placed percutaneous catheters in reconstruction of the proximal part of the biliary tract. Surg Gynec Obstet 1987; 165:421–424.
7. Dick R, Gillams A, Dooley J, et al. Stainless steel mesh stents for biliary strictures. J Intervent Radiol 1989; 4:95–98.
8. Gallagher DJ, Kadir S, Kaufman SL, et al. Nonoperative management of benign postoperative biliary strictures. Radiology 1985; 156:625 –629.
9. Gillams A, Dick R, Dooley J, et al. Self expandable stainless steel braided endoprosthesis for biliary strictures. Radiology 1990; 174:137–140.
10. Goldin E, Katz E, Wengrower D, et al. Treatment of fistulas of the biliary tract by endoscopic insertion of endoprostheses. Surg Gynecol Obstet 1990; 170:418–423.
11. Gya D, Sali A, Hennessey O, Kune GA. Balloon dilatation of biliary strictures: Experience and review of the literature. Aust NZ J Surg 1990; 60:361–364.
12. Huibregtse K. Endoscopic biliary and pancreatic drainage. Stuttgart: Thieme, 1988:59–86.
13. Irving JD, Adam A, Dick R, et al. Gianturco expandable metal stents: results of a European clinical trial. Radiology 1989; 170:199–206.
14. Kaufman SL, Kadir S, Mitchell SE, et al. Percutaneous transhepatic biliary drainage for leaks and fistulas. AJR 1985; 144:1055–1058.
15. Kaufman SL. Interventional procedures for the treatment of benign diseases of the biliary tract. Radiology Reviews 1992; 1:122 –133.
16. Lee MJ, Mueller PR, Saini S. Percutaneous dilatation of benign biliary strictures: single session therapy with general anaesthesia. AJR 1991; 157:1263–1266.
17. Lee Y, Lee BH, Park, et al. Balloon dilatation of intrahepatic biliary strictures for percutaneous extraction of residual intrahepatic stones. Cardiovasc Intervent Radiol 1991; 14:102–105.
18. Lillimoe KD, Pitt HA, Cameron JL. Postoperative bile duct strictures. Surg Clin North Am 1990; 70:1355–1380.
19. May GR, Bender CE, LaRusso NJ, et al. Nonoperative dilatation of dominant strictures in primary sclerosing cholangitis. AJR 1985; 145:1061 –1065.
20. Molner W, Stockton AE. Transhepatic dilatation of choledochoenterostomy strictures. Radiology 1978; 129:59–64.
21. Moore, AV Jr, Illescas FF, Mills SR, et al. Percutaneous dilatation of benign biliary strictures. Radiology 1987; 163:625–628.

22. Morrison MC, Lee MJ, Saini S, et al. Percutaneous dilatation of benign biliary strictures. Rad Clin North Am 1990; 28:1191–1201.
23. Mueller PR, van Sonnenberg E. Ferrucci JT Jr, et al. Biliary stricture dilatation; Multicenter review of clinical management in 73 patients. Radiology 1986; 160:17–22.
24. Nilsson U, Ekelund L: Balloon dilatation of stenotic common bile duct anastomoses in the pig. Acta Radiol 1987; 28:115–120.
25. Ponchon T, Gallez JDF, Valette PJ, et al. Endoscopic treatment of biliary tract fistula. Gastrointest Endosc 1989; 35:490–498.
26. Pitt HA, Kaufmann SL, Coleman J, et al. Benign post operative biliary strictures: operate or dilate? Ann Surg 1989; 210:417–427.
27. Rao KJM, Blake H, Thoedossi A. Use of a modified angioplasty balloon catheter in the dilatation of tight biliary strictures. Gut 1990; 31:565–567.
28. Rossi P, Bezzi M, Salvatori F, et al. Recurrent benign biliary strictures: Management with self expanding metal stents. Radiology 1990; 175:661–665.
29. Russell E, Yrizarry JM, Huber JS, Guerra JJ Jr, et al. Percutaneous transjejunal biliary dilatation: alternative management for benign strictures. Radiology 1986; 159:209–214.
30. Salmonowitz E, Casteneda-Zuniga WR, Lund G, et al. Balloon dilatation of benign biliary strictures. Radiology 1984; 151:513–616.
31. Sauerbruch T, Weinzierl M. Treatment of postoperative biliary fistulae by internal endoscopic biliary drainage. Gastroenterology 1986; 90:1998–2002.
32. Skolkin MD, Alspaugh JP, Caseralla WP, et al. Sclerosing cholangitis: Palliation with percutaneous cholangioplasty. Radiology 1989; 170:199–206.
33. Smith RE. Obstruction of the bile duct. Br J Surg 1979; 66:79–84.
34. Stringer R. Catheter a Ballonets d'angioplastie de Grunzig dans le traitment des stenoses de la voie biliare. Ann Radiol 1984; 27:125–129.
35. Trambert JJ, Bron KM, Zaiko AB, et al. Percutaneous transhepatic balloon dilatation of benign biliary strictures. AJR 1987; 149:945–948.
36. Vogel SB, Howard RJ. Evaluation of percutaneous transhepatic balloon dilatation of benign biliary structures in high risk patients. Am J Surg 1985; 149:73–79.
37. Weyman PJ, Balf DM. Percutaneous dilatation of biliary strictures. Semin Intervent Radiol 1985; 2:50–59.
38. Williams HJ, Bender CE, May GR. Benign postoperative biliary strictures: Dilatation with fluoroscopic guidance. Radiology 1987; 163:629–634.
39. Yee ACN, Ho CS. Complications of percutaneous biliary drainage. Benign vs malignant disease. AJR 1987; 148:1207–1209.
40. Zuidema GD, Cameron JL, Sitzmann JV, et al. Percutaneous transhepatic management of complex biliary problems. Ann Surg 1983; 197:584–593.

12 Drainage Procedures in Biliary Infection and Liver Abscess

Infected bile is common in patients with cholelithiasis and biliary obstruction. Infection is always present in the patient with an external biliary fistula. Infection is less common in tumoral biliary obstruction. Manipulations within the bile duct in the presence of infection may lead to severe ascending cholangitis. Cholangitis is common after second attempts at endoscopic biliary catheterization or percutaneous transhepatic catheterization after endoscopic cholangiography, and failed endoscopic catheterization of the bile duct. It is a recognized complication of endoscopic and percutaneous stent insertion.

Suppurative cholangitis may follow ascending cholangitis and it carries a high mortality. Stent occlusion or dislodgement and failure to drain an obstructed segment of the liver are important causes of cholangitis. When biliary obstruction is demonstrated, it is essential to provide immediate emergency drainage by endoscopic or transhepatic catheter. There are three alternative methods of therapy of acute obstructive suppurative cholangitis:

1. Surgical decompression
2. Endoscopic drainage
3. Percutaneous transhepatic external drainage

Surgical decompression is now much less commonly used in clinical practice. If pus is encountered during exploration of the bile duct, the bile duct is drained by T tube and surgery deferred. Most clinicians would consider endoscopic drainage the procedure of choice in suppurative cholangitis. If ERCP fails or access cannot be gained to the obstructing lesion, percutaneous drainage may be lifesaving. This may be performed by transhepatic or transcholecystic drainage after percutaneous cholecystostomy.

Endoscopic Drainage by Nasobiliary Catheter

Indications for Nasobillary Drainage

When infected bile (pus) is seen during ERCP or following endoscopic sphincterotomy, it is essential to drain the biliary tract as an emergency procedure. Demonstration of intrahepatic abscesses communicating with the bile ducts during diagnostic ERCP is also an indication for drainage.

Technique of Insertion of Nasobiliary Catheter

Following ERCP and demonstration of infected bile and stone or tumor obstruction, a guide wire is introduced into the bile duct above the obstruction. The nasobiliary catheter is now introduced over the wire and positioned in the bile duct above the obstruction, and the endoscope is slowly withdrawn under fluoroscopic control while the nasobiliary catheter is advanced down the scope until the latter is outside the mouth leaving the catheter in place. The nasobiliary tube is now rerouted through the nasal cavity by inserting a tube through the nasal cavity into the mouth and pushing the nasobiliary catheter through the nasal catheter from the mouth to the external nares. Positioning of loops of the tube in the duodenum prevents its dislodgement from the bile duct.

A 7-Fr nasobiliary tube can often be inserted without sphincterotomy. A 9-Fr or larger nasobiliary catheter requires endoscopic sphincterotomy before tube insertion. The nasobiliary catheter may be used to drain the bile externally, or saline or antibiotic solutions may be infused. Drug infusions may be used in the therapy of sclerosing cholangitis. We use the nasobiliary catheter developed by Wurbs (Wilson Cook) for endoscopic external drainage, and we have found that if the tube is correctly positioned in the bile duct above the obstruction and looped in the duodenum, it rarely becomes dislodged. A 2.8-mm endoscope channel is sufficient for insertion of the 7-Fr tube. Larger endoscope channels are needed for the 9- or 10-Fr nasobiliary drains (Fig. 12.**1**).

Nasobiliary drainage is also valuable for:

1. Decompression of an obstructed bile duct as an immediate alternative to stenting in the presence of overtly infected bile
2. Prevention of stone impaction after endoscopic sphincterotomy
3. Treatment of an external biliary fistula
4. Aspiration of bile for cytology, chemical, or bacterial analysis
5. Temporary drainage of a malignant biliary stricture following failure of stent insertion
6. Attempted dissolution of bile duct stones with or without ESWL
7. Opacification of the duct system for ESWL of bile duct calculi

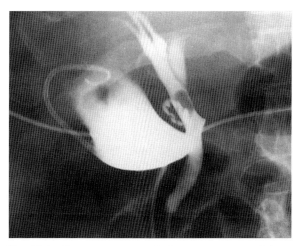

Fig. 12.**1 Percutaneous cholecystomy combined with endoscopic nasobiliary drainage in cholangitis associated with stone disease**

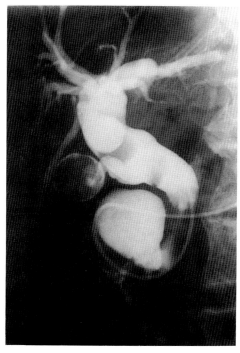

Fig. 12.**2   Nasobiliary drainage in choledocholithiasis with cholangitis and sepsis**

1. Decompression of Biliary Obstruction

It is our policy to insert a nasobiliary tube into the bile duct and position it above the obstructing lesion as a primary treatment in acute obstruction with cholangitis (Figs. 12.**2** and 12.**3**). Further endoscopic stenting is delayed until the infection has resolved.

2. Prevention of Stone Impaction

After sphincterotomy for stone removal it may be impossible to remove large stone(s). While treatment by ESWL is awaited, a nasobiliary catheter is inserted into the bile duct to prevent stone impaction.

It may be used later to opacify the duct with contrast medium to demonstrate stone position for ESWL therapy.

3. Treatment of an External Biliary Fistula

External biliary fistulas are rare, and most are caused during surgery or follow abdominal trauma or rarely, acute cholecystitis. Formerly, surgery was the only treatment. Endoscopic drainage of the bile duct is curative in most cases after removing any obstructing lesion such as a stone in the bile duct or stenting of a stricture below the site of the fistula. Stenting alone is sufficient in most cases, but drainage by nasobiliary catheter may be used as a primary treatment if biliary infection is evident. This is followed by delayed stenting.

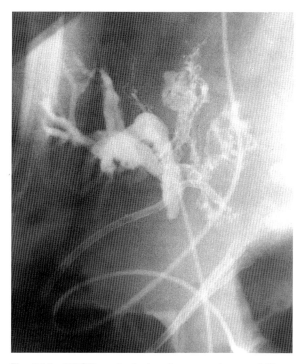

Fig. 12.**3 ERCP and cholangiogram via nasobiliary catheter showing abscess cavity in benign bile duct stricture communication with the bile ducts in the right lobe of the liver.** The external drainage catheter is extruded partly from the abscess cavity. The patient died from septicemia

4. Aspiration of Bile for Chemistry, Bacteriology, or Cytology

To demonstrate bacterial colonization, the first 10 mL of aspirated bile is discarded. Aspiration may be used to study concentrations of antibiotic in bile during systemic chemotherapy. Bile composition may be studied over several days under differing conditions.

5. Temporary Drainage of Malignant Biliary Stricture

Most bile duct tumors are not removable by surgery and are treated by endoscopically or transhepatically placed stents across the obstruction. If a stent cannot be inserted through the tumor, drainage may be possible by nasobiliary catheter as a temporary measure to relieve pruritus prior to surgery.

6. Dissolution of Biliary Calculi with MTBE

Our experience of 10 cases using MTBE via a nasobiliary drain for stone dissolution showed 50% success in assisting stone clearance by mechanical methods. The procedure was only successful in reducing stone size if it was possible to insert the catheter into the bile duct without sphincterotomy. Otherwise, leakage of MTBE into the duodenum caused sedation and cessation of stone dissolution.

Percutaneous Transhepatic Biliary Drainage in Acute Cholangitis

Percutaneous transhepatic biliary drainage was one of the first forms of biliary interventional radiology. Following FN PTHC a catheter is inserted into the bile duct for external drainage. This was formerly used as a preparation for surgery in obstructive jaundice and later as a form of internal/external biliary drainage. Today we use it only when there is evidence of biliary infection at FN PTHC or as a temporary measure during percutaneous transhepatic stent insertion.

Percutaneous biliary drainage is often carried out as an emergency treatment following failed endoscopic drainage in the presence of known or documented biliary sepsis.

Technique of Percutaneous Biliary Drainage (Figs. 12.4–12.6)

Under local anesthesia and antibiotic cover, FN PTHC is performed from the right axilla or the left xiphisternal area. "Clean" cholangiography without intraparenchymal contrast deposition is preferred.

Preferably a duct is chosen that is a secondary branch of the right or left hepatic duct. The ducts in the liver are opacified as is the proximal common bile duct. Next a 0.16 guide wire is introduced through the Chiba needle into the hepatic duct and into the bile

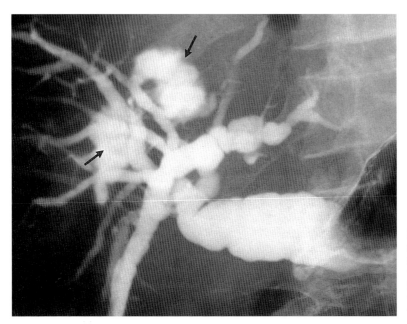

Fig. 12.**4** **Abscess cavities** (arrows) **communicating with the bile ducts in the right lobe of liver treated by external drainage after insertion of a transhepatic catheter.** There is complete tumor obstruction of the common bile duct

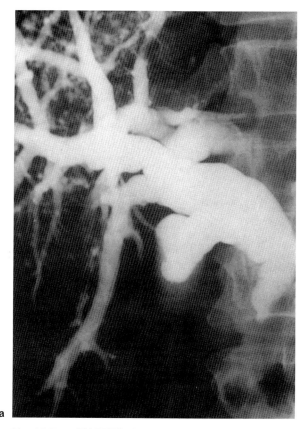
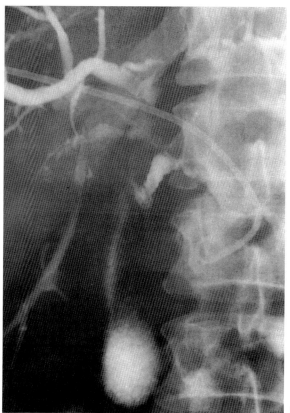

Fig. 12.**5   a FN PTHC showing carcinoma of the head of the pancreas and intrahepatic abscesses communicating with the bile ducts.**
b Percutaneous external drainage cholangiogram at 72 hours; the abscesses have resolved

duct. The double catheter of the Accustick set (Meditech) is inserted over the wire into the bile duct. The fine wire is removed with the inner sheath of the Accustick, and a Lunderquist Ring Torque guide wire is inserted down the sheath into the common bile duct. The sheath is removed and 5-, 7-, and 9-Fr dilators are inserted over the wire to make a track through the liver. Finally a 9-Fr catheter with a retaining pigtail containing multiple side holes is inserted over the wire into the duct and fixed at the skin to prevent dislodgement. This technique, puncturing a more peripheral intrahepatic duct, is less likely to cause arterial injury within the liver than using an 18-gauge sheathed needle for duct catheterization.

The drainage catheter is connected to a closed drainage system to prevent introduction of further sepsis. All of the side holes in the drainage catheter must lie within the bile duct.

External drainage is continued, and i.v. fluids and antibiotics are given until sepsis resolves. This usually occurs within 3 days.

When sepsis is no longer present, external drainage is converted to internal drainage by percutaneous stent insertion.

External Drainage in Biliary Fistula
(Figs. 12. **8** and 12.**9**)

Demonstration of an external biliary fistula is usually made by sinography. The latter does not show the communication to the bile duct in the acute situation; then, FN PTHC is necessary to outline the bile ducts. Since the ducts are not dilated this may be a difficult procedure in the immediately postoperative and probably uncooperative patient. A chronic external fistula is easily demonstrated by sinography. If there is no injury to the extrahepatic biliary tract, external drainage lowers biliary pressure, and the cause of the fistula is determined by contrast cholangiography. Leakage from an injured anomalous bile duct or cystic duct stump after gallbladder removal, choledochotomy without drainage, and benign bile duct stricture are

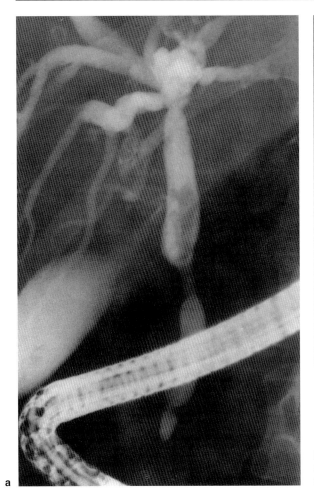

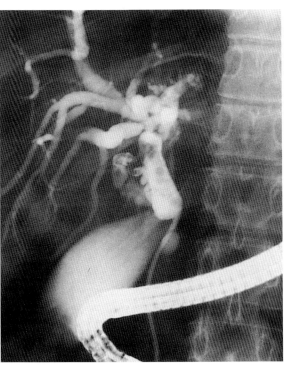

Fig. 12.**6 a ERCP showing fungus ball in the bile duct in immunosuppressed patient. b** A nasobiliary catheter was inserted for drainage

the common causes of fistula. A subhepatic or perihepatic bile collection occurs and continues to accumulate until the biliary tract is drained to reduce biliary pressure by sphincterotomy, nasobiliary drainage, stent insertion, or percutaneous drainage via a transhepatic catheter inserted into the common bile duct and across the papilla into the duodenum. Drainage allows the site of leakage of bile from the injured duct or cystic duct stump to heal. An external fistula in association with a postsurgical bile duct stricture usually requires excision and choledochojejunostomy for treatment but occasionally in an incomplete stricture, drainage may be used to allow stricture healing. The lesion may then be dilated by an angioplasty balloon catheter. Internal biliary fistulas require surgery for therapy.

Percutaneous Drainage of Liver Abscess

Pyogenic liver abscess is a serious disorder, and multiple pyogenic liver abscesses are usually fatal. Prompt diagnosis and therapy are essential. Percutaneous drainage is now considered the ideal procedure for therapy of most intra-abdominal fluid collections and abscesses, and it is the treatment of choice for liver abscess. Careful insertion and positioning of the drainage catheter is essential for successful treatment. Ultrasound and CT sectional imaging assist in correct catheter positioning. Pyogenic abscess is most common in the right lobe of the liver.

Multiple liver abscesses have a poor prognosis and respond poorly to multiple percutaneously inserted drainage catheters. Only a mature abscess that shows

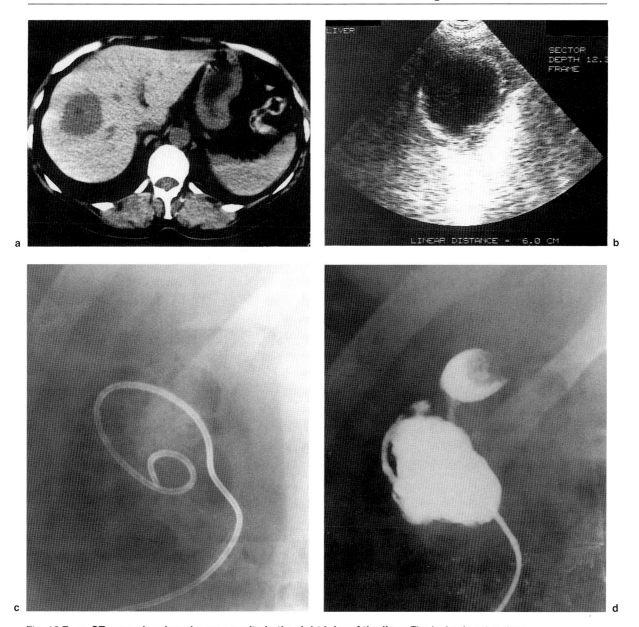

Fig. 12.**7   a CT scan showing abscess cavity in the right lobe of the liver.** The lesion is not mature.
b Ultrasound 5 days later showing a mature thick-walled abscess in the right lobe.
c Percutaneous external drainage by pigtail catheter.
d Abscess opacification via the drainage catheter at 7 days shows communication with the gallbladder fundus.
The lesion resolved after 5 days drainage and did not recur

a fluid collection within it on ultrasound responds to percutaneous drainage. Multilocular abscess responds less well to percutaneous drainage even though the loculations may intercommunicate. Most amebic abscesses are diagnosed by clinical methods with the assistance of serological tests and resolve with drug therapy alone without percutaneous drainage. The latter is, however, beneficial in some patients including those with large abscess collections that may rupture if not drained, failed response to drug therapy, ruptured abscess, or suggested bacterial infection.

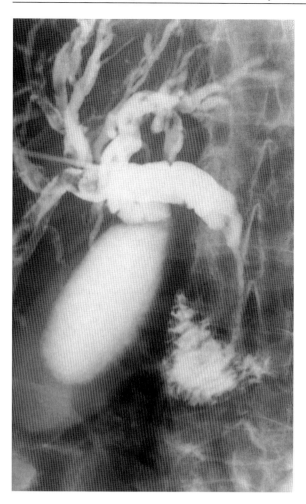

Fig. 12.**8 Percutaneous biliary external drainage in cholangitis** associated with choledocholithiasis and cholangitis

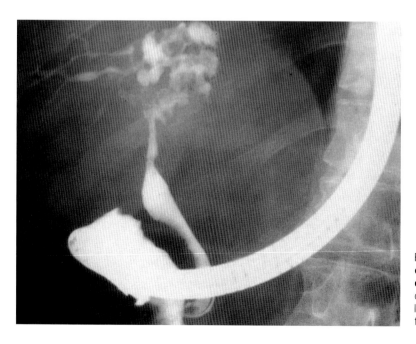

Fig. 12.**9 Abscess in the left lobe of liver in liver transplant with early duct stricture.** Nasobiliary endoscopic drainage failed to heal the lesion, which was related to infarction of the left lobe

Indications for Percutaneous Drainage

The major indication is the presence of a fluid collection within the liver in a septic patient.

Contraindications to Percutaneous Drainage

The procedure is contraindicated in the presence of coagulation disorders that cannot be corrected. An uncooperative patient is a contraindication. The procedure is performed only after consultation with an experienced surgeon.

Technique of Abscess Drainage

Preparation of the Patient

The procedure is discussed with the patient or the responsible person in case of a very ill patient. The benefits of the procedure, including avoiding surgery, are outlined, and the possible risks including hemorrhage, bowel injury, septic shock, additional infection, pneumothorax, or pleural infections are discussed. *The likelihood of long-term catheter drainage is emphasized.* Anticoagulant and aspirin therapy are suspended, and coagulation studies should be normal. The platelet count should be more than 50 000.

Antibiotic therapy is given i.v. immediately before drainage. This reduces the effects of bacteremia and sepsis related to the procedure.

Sedation and analgesia are given, and vital signs are monitored during the drainage procedure.

Technique of Drainage and Equipment
(Figs. 12.**7**, 12.**9**, and 12.**10**)

We use drainage catheters including an 18-gauge sheathed needle for initial entry into the cavity, and for guide wire insertion (Surgimed, Denmark), pigtail catheters, 5 Fr to 10 Fr for clear fluid contents, and 12- to 16-Fr pigtail catheters for purulent collections.

Puncture of the abscess cavity may be performed using CT, ultrasound, fluoroscopy, or a combination of these. Location of the abscess cavity and its relations with the surface of the abdomen is most accurately demonstrated and measured by contrast CT of the liver using 10-mm contiguous slices. Contrast CT also helps to avoid major vessels near the needle/catheter pathway during initial liver puncture. With the aid of skin markers and CT calipers, the exact path to the center of the abscess may be calculated with precision. Drainage is performed as a sterile procedure. We prefer to do this in the interventional suite after abscess localization by CT. The skin is prepared with antiseptic and suitably draped. The area is infiltrated with local anesthetic. An incision is made in the skin with a scalpel, and using mosquito forceps, the soft tissues are separated for the catheter needle track to the

liver capsule. The catheter needle is now inserted to the predetermined depth into the center of the abscess, and a small (5–10 mL) sample of fluid or pus is aspirated. A guide wire is inserted and coiled in the abscess cavity. The catheter sheath is removed, leaving the wire coiled within the cavity. Dilators are now inserted over the guide wire up to the size next to the pigtail catheter caliber to be used for drainage. The pigtail catheter is now inserted over the wire and coiled within the abscess. The abscess contents are aspirated by syringe and the volume recorded. The catheter is connected to a closed drainage system and secured to the skin by sutures to prevent displacement. An abscess in the left lobe of the liver is drained using an anterior approach. An abscess in the right lobe is drained from the axilla if located superiorly, or from the right hypochondrium if located inferiorly.

A repeat CT scan may be used to confirm the correct position of the catheter within the cavity prior to the patient's return to the ward. Adequate drainage and antibiotic therapy (based on organisms and sensitivity) are the two essentials of success of percutaneous abscess drainage therapy.

We perform a contrast study of the abscess cavity under sterile conditions within 3–4 days or earlier if there is copious drainage from the abscess to demonstrate or exclude a communication with the bile ducts in the liver. Correct positioning and maintaining of the catheter's position within the abscess cavity is the most important factor for the success of this therapy. The pigtail catheter is secured to the skin and connected to a drainage bag. Drainage from the catheter is by gravity at the patient's bedside. The volume of the contents of drainage bags is recorded daily.

Sudden cessation of drainage without catheter displacement at the skin indicates a blocked catheter, which is unblocked by sterile saline. The catheter is kept in place until the abscess is "dry." In 23 of our patients, pyogenic liver abscess treatment was successful for mature abscess cavities in 20 patients. Three patients developed pyogenic abscess secondary to inadequate surgical and endoscopic therapy of benign bile duct stricture and their abscesses proved fatal (Fig. 12.**3**). In these patients, percutaneous drainage was not effective because of continued communication with the biliary tract during drainage, and drainage was instituted too late to be effective. This therapy is less useful in the presence of a multilocular abscess. If a discrete abscess cavity is not demonstrated by ultrasound or CT, percutaneous drainage fails as a procedure. Infected metastatic tumors, if multiple, are not suitable for this form of treatment. An infected hematoma is suitable for this therapy only if it is completely intrahepatic, and the liver capsule is intact. Imaging techniques may show an apparently multilocular abscess cavity, but it is often possible to drain this type of cavity using a correctly positioned single pigtail catheter.

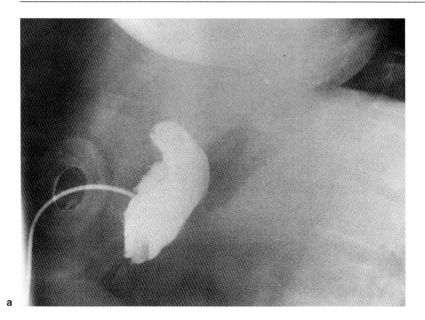

a

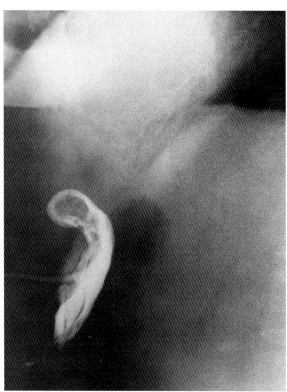

b

Fig. 12.**10 a Percutaneous catheter drainage four weeks after insertion into an abscess in the left lobe of the liver**
b Abscess cavity at 6 weeks: only a potential space remains

An abscess cavity smaller than 4 cm in diameter is best treated by aspiration, repeated if necessary, rather than catheter drainage. Prolonged drainage is required in some patients. In our experience, drainage times have varied from 2 to 30 days. The most frequent duration of drainage was 2 to 5 days. Communication with the biliary tree delays abscess resolution. Contrast radiology by sinogram or ERCP readily demonstrates the biliary–abscess fistula (Fig. 12.**6**). A nasobiliary catheter inserted into an intrahepatic duct on the side of the abscess (right intrahepatic duct for right lobe and visa versa) diverts bile away from the abscess cavity by overcoming the effect of an intact ampulla.

Fine-needle diagnostic aspiration may be used to diagnose **amebic abscess** by demonstrating an "anchovy-sauce" fluid aspirate only present in 50% of cases in one series (18). It is more important to demonstrate the absence of bacteria from the abscess cavity. It is disputed whether or not percutaneous drainage is necessary for therapy (18, 25). When there is failure to respond to drug therapy (chloroquine or metronidazole), percutaneous drainage may be used to drain an amebic abscess by the same method as that described for pyogenic abscess. **Fungal abscesses** (Fig. 12.**11**) are usually small and disseminated throughout the liver, and percutaneous drainage is contraindicated in the usual immunosuppressed patient in whom these infections occur. Fine-needle aspiration of one of the hepatic abscesses usually has a low positive culture yield.

Complications

A 10% complication rate is reported for drainage of abdominal fluid collections and abscesses. Drainage failure, sepsis, or bowel perforation occurred in 2.8% of cases. Minor complications included hemorrhage, pleural lesions, bacteremia, and local infection. Careful attention to contraindications, proper drainage catheter selection, insertion, positioning, localization, aftercare, and effective antibiotic therapy greatly aid abscess cure and reduce complications to a minimum.

Percutaneous Drainage of Simple Liver Cyst

Congenital cysts have a characteristic appearance at ultrasound and CT scanning. Most are small and asymptomatic and do not require treatment. Large cysts cause pain because of their size and position.

Needle aspiration is of no value because the cyst recurs.

Percutaneous endothelial sclerosis of the lining of the inner wall may be performed by injecting sterile alcohol after cyst aspiration. Cyst fluid is sent to the laboratory for cytology and culture. Bean and Roden (1985) used an amount of alcohol equal to 25% of the cyst volume. The alcohol was removed after 15–20 minutes, and the cysts did not recur (7, 31). The technique is not useful in giant cysts, which may be removed successfully by laparoscopy. Complications of cyst puncture include transient pain, cyst hemorrhage and a rise in body temperature.

Percutaneous Drainage of Hydatid Cyst

The treatment of choice for *hydatid cyst of the liver* is surgical (31, 36) or percutaneous drainage (1, 7, 9, 10, 19, 32, 36). The latter is now considered safe, while formerly it was considered to be contraindicated.

Percutaneous drainage of hydatid cyst is now a recognized form of treatment for selected hydatid cysts of the liver (Fig. 12.**12**).

Contraindications to Percutaneous Drainage

Excluded from this form of treatment are cysts with a hyperechoic solid pattern without posterior wall echoes on ultrasound, infected cysts, and cysts that have ruptured into the biliary tract, peritoneum, or pleura.

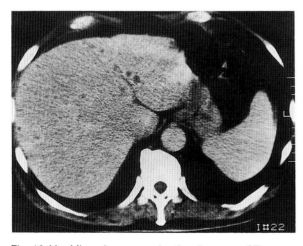

Fig. 12.**11** Microabscesses in the liver on CT scan. Drainage is not possible

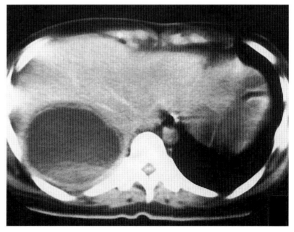

Fig. 12.**12** **CT scan in hydatid cyst.** Sand is visible in the dependent part of the cavity. Percutaneous drainage was successful in obliterating the cyst cavity with alcohol

Technique of Drainage

Two types of percutaneous therapy have been described. Both are performed under local anesthesia. The first type of therapy involves cyst puncture insertion of a scolicidal agent and drainage of the cyst (1, 7, 9, 10, 19, 32). The second type of percutaneous therapy described by Saremi (1992) is much more elaborate. It involves drainage, injection of a scolicidal agent, and removal of the cyst contents and the endocyst lining after fragmentation and endoscopic inspection of the inner lining of the cyst. This is followed by external drainage until the cyst is "dry". This method would seem to provide ideal percutaneous therapy without any recurrences (37). *The cyst is punctured through an area of thick normal liver tissue via a right intercostal approach* using an aseptic technique and under local anesthesia.

Percutaneous drainage of hydatid cysts is best performed through the nondependent aspect of the hydatid cyst. This minimizes the risk of fluid leaks. Anterior cysts are drained in the supine position and posterior cysts in the prone position. Drainage is carried out using fluoroscopy after determining the cyst position and puncture site by CT. In the technique described by Saremi (1992) designed to remove the endocyst and daughter cysts, the cyst is punctured by a 7-Fr teflon multiple–side hole catheter containing a stylet, and its contents aspirated and replaced by 20% saline or 0.5% silver nitrate (32) for 10–15 minutes. A Lunderquist torque wire is now inserted and a 12-Fr dilator is inserted over the 7-Fr catheter. He described a metal cutting device for fragmentation and removal of the separated endocyst wall and daughter cysts. This cutting device incorporates an endoscope for inspection and complete removal of fragments. After fragment removal a 10-Fr pigtail catheter is inserted into the cyst and remains within the cavity until the cavity is no longer visible. This may take several weeks.

Bret et al. (1988) treated three patients with percutaneous aspiration and injected various scolicidal agents without complications or recurrence in the 6–12 months after treatment. Georgio et al. (1992) used a technique of cyst puncture, aspiration, alcohol injection, and aspiration using a fine needle or an 18-gauge or 20-gauge needle in large cysts. Three days later a second injection of alcohol was made and left in situ. They did not employ catheter drainage, and the endocyst or any daughter cysts were not removed.

Acunas et al. (1992) treated 15 patients with needle (20-gauge) aspiration under CT control and used hypertonic saline as a scolicidal agent combined with chemotherapy (mebendazalone daily for 1 month).

Filice et al. (1992) treated 32 patients by cyst aspiration and injection of alcohol without recurrence at follow-up, which for some patients exceeded 4 years.

Complications of Hydatid Cyst Drainage

Conventional therapy for hydatid cysts in the liver is surgical. This involves aspiration of the contents of the cyst, injection of a scolicidal agent to destroy the parasite, and removal of the cyst by resection. The mortality is 3.9% after surgery. Postoperative morbidity is 8–16% and increases to 89% in infected cysts (32). Percutaneous aspiration has produced no serious complications in the cases reported to date. Complex cysts were not aspirated. Infection and communication with the biliary tract are contraindications to this therapy. There is no reported mortality from percutaneous therapy of hydatid cyst of the liver.

References

1. Acunas B, Rozanes I, Celik L, et al. Purely cystic hydatid disease of the liver: treatment with percutaneous aspiration and injection of hypertonic saline. Radiology 1992; 182:541–543.
2. Altemeir WA, Schowengerdt CG, Whitley DH. Abscess of the liver: surgical considerations. Arch Surg 1982; 101:258–263.
3. Bean WJ, Rodan BA. Hepatic cysts: Treatment with alcohol. AJR 1985; 144:237–240.
4. Beggs I. The radiological appearances of hydatid disease of the liver. Clin Radiol 1983; 34:555–560.
5. Bernadino ME, Berkman WA, Plemmons M, et al. Percutaneous drainage of multiseptated hepatic abscesses. J Comput Assist Tomogr 1984; 8:38–42.
6. Boey JH, Way LW. Acute cholangitis Ann Surg 1980; 191:264–270.
7. Bret PA, Fond A, Bretagnolle M. et al. Percutaneous aspiration and drainage of hydatid cysts in the liver. Radiology 1988; 168:617–620.
8. Deviere J. Endoscopic management of a post-operative traumatic biliary fistula. Endoscopy 1987; 19:136–139.
9. Filice C. Strosselli M, Brunetti E, et al. Percutaneous drainage of hydatid liver cysts. Radiology 1992; 184:579–580.
10. Giorgio A, Tarantino L, Francia G, et al. Unilocular hydatid liver cysts: Treatment with US guided double percutaneous aspiration and alcohol injection. Radiology 1992; 184:705–710.
11. Gogel HK, Runyon BA, Volpicelle, Palmer RC. Acute suppurative obstructive cholangitis due to stones: treatment by urgent endoscopic sphincterotomy. Gastrointest Endosc 1987; 33:210–213.
12. Himal HS, Lindsay T. Ascending cholangitis: surgery versus endoscopic or percutaneous drainage. JVIR 1991; 2:299–303.
13. Ikeda S, Tanaka M, Itoh H, et al. Emergency decompression of the bile duct in acute obstructive suppurative cholangitis by duodenoscopic cannulation: a life saving procedure. World J Surg 1981; 5:587–589.
14. Johnson RD, Mueller PR, Ferrucci JT Jr, et al. Percutaneous drainage of pyogenic liver abscess. AJR 1985; 144:483–487.
15. Kadir S, Baassiri A, Barth KH, et al. Percutaneous biliary drainage in the management of biliary sepsis. AJR 1982; 138:25–29.
16. Kairaluoma MII, Leinonen A, Stahlberg M, et al. Percutaneous aspiration and alcohol sclerotherapy for symptomatic hepatic cysts. Ann Surg 1988; 210:208–211.
17. Kaufman SL, Kadir S, Mitchell SE, et al. Percutaneous transhepatic drainage for leaks and fistulas. AJR 1985; 144:1055–1058.
18. Ken JG, van Sonnenberg E, Casola G, et al. Perforated amoebic liver abscesses successful percutaneous treatment. Radiology 1989; 170:195–198.
19. Khuros MS, Zargar SA, Mahajan R. Echinococcal granulosis cysts in the liver: management with percutaneous drainage. Radiology 1991; 180:141–145.

20. Kiil J, Kruse A, Rokkjaer M. Large bile duct stones treated by endoscopic biliary drainage. Surgery 1989; 105:51–56.
21. Kuligowska E, Conners SK, Shapiro JN. Liver abscess: sonography in diagnosis and treatment. AJR 1982; 138:353–356.
22. Lai ECS, Paterson JA, Tam PC, et al. Severe acute cholangitis: the role of emergency biliary drainage. Surgery 1990; 107:268–272.
23. Lai ECS, Tam PC, Paterson JA, et al. Emergency surgery for severe acute cholangitis: the high risk patients. Ann Surg 1990; 211:55–59.
24. Lai ECS, Mok FPT, Tan ESY, et al. Endoscopic biliary drainage for severe acute cholangitis. N Eng J Med 1992; 326:1582–1586.
25. Lambiase RE, Doyoe L. Cronan J, Dorfman GS. Percutaneous drainage of 335 consecutive abscesses: results of primary drainage with 1 year follow up. Radiology 1992; 184:167–169.
26. Leese T, Neoptolemos JP, Baker AR, Carr-Locke DL. Management of acute cholangitis and the impact of endoscopic sphincterotomy. Br J Surg 1986; 73:988–992.
27. Leung JWC. Endoscopic management of postoperative biliary fistula. Surg Endosc 1988; 2:190–193.
28. Leung JWC, Chung SCS, Sung JJY. Urgent endoscopic drainage for acute suppurative cholangitis. Lancet 1989; 1:1307–1309.
29. MacErlean DP, Gibney RG. Radiological management of abdominal abscess. J Roy Soc Med 1983; 76:254–257.
30. Mc Fadzean AJS, Chang KPS, Wong CC. Solitary pyogenic abscess of the liver treated by closed aspiration and antibiotics: a report of 14 consecutive cases with recovery. Br J Surg 1954; 41:141–144.
31. Morris DL, Richards KS. Hydatid disease: current medical and surgical management. Oxford: Butterworth-Heinmann, 1992.
32. Mueller PR, Dawson SL, Ferrucci JT Jr, Nardi GL. Hepatic echinococcal cyst: successful percutaneous drainage. Radiology 1985; 155:627–628.
33. Mueller PR, van Sonnenberg E, Ferrucci JT Jr. Percutaneous drainage of 250 abdominal abscesses and fluid collections part. 2. Current procedural concepts. Radiology 1984; 151:343–347.
34. Nunez D Jr, Guerra JJ, Al-Sheikh WA, et al. Percutaneous biliary drainage in acute suppurative cholangitis. Gastrointest Radiol 1986; 11:85–89.
35. Pessa ME, Hawkins IF, Vogel SB. The treatment of acute cholangitis: percutaneous transhepatic biliary drainage before definitive therapy. Ann Surg 1987; 205:389–392.
36. Saidi F. Hydatid cysts of the liver: In: Saidi F. Surgery of hydatid disease 1st ed. Philadelphia: Saunders, 1976.
37. Saremi F. Percutaneous drainage of hydatid cysts. Use of a new cutting device to avoid leakage. AJR 1992; 158:83–85.
38. Sones PJ. Percutaneous drainage of abdominal abscesses. AJR 1984; 142:35–40.
39. Vaccaro JP, Dorfman GS, Lambiase RE. Treatment of biliary leaks and fistulas by simultaneous percutaneous drainage and diversion. Cardiovasc Intervent Radiol 1991; 14:109–112.
40. Van Sonnenberg ED, D'Agnostino HB, Casola G. et al. Percutaneous abscess drainage: current concepts. Radiology 1992; 181:617–626.
41. Van Sonnenberg ED, D'Agostino HB, Sanchez RB, Casola G. Percutaneous abscess drainage: Editorial Comments. Radiology 1992; 184:27–29.
42. Worthley CS, Toouli J. Endoscopic decompression for acute cholangitis due to stones. Aust NZ J Surg 1990; 60:355–359.
43. Wurbs D. Results of bilionasal drainage. In: Classen M, Geelen J, Kawai K, eds. Nonsurgical biliary drainage. Berlin: Springer 1984:75–80.

13 Radiology, the Liver, and the Biliary Tract in AIDS

J. Keating and B. G. Gazzard

Background

The acquired immune deficiency syndrome (AIDS) was first described simultaneously in New York and San Francisco in the latter part of 1981 (6, 22). In 1983 the causative virus, the human immunodeficiency virus (HIV), was discovered in Paris, and these findings were amplified in America during 1984 (2, 14). Antibody tests to detect infection rapidly became available following the discovery of the virus, and we now recognize that HIV infection typically follows four phases.

Up to 50% of individuals who develop HIV infection have a seroconversion illness about 3 months after exposure. This is a fairly nonspecific flu-like illness, rather like glandular fever, associated with a rash, lymphadenopathy, and various neurological complaints, including occasionally encephalitis and transverse myelitis (34). Severe immunosuppression may develop and opportunistic infections, particularly *Pneumocystis carinii* pneumonia (Fig. 13.1) or esophageal candidiasis (Fig. 13.2), can occur. Gastrointestinal manifestations are common during this period. Abnormal liver function tests are well described, and these may be sufficiently severe for a diagnosis of hepatitis to be suggested.

Seroconversion is followed by an asymptomatic phase that typically lasts for a number of years. During this period there is a pronounced humoral and cell-mediated immune response directed against HIV. One of the conundrums as to the pathogenesis of AIDS is why this pronounced immune response gradually wanes. The onset of symptomatic disease is usually associated with a reduction in antibodies directed toward core components of the virus (27). A number

Fig. 13.**1 Chest radiograph showing typical features of *Pneumocystitis carinii* pneumonia.** Infiltrate more marked in right lung

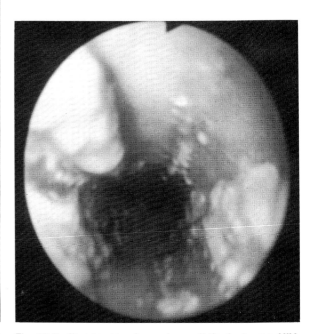

Fig. 13.**2 Dense esophageal candidiasis in an HIV-positive patient**

of groups have now established that approximately 50–60% of HIV-seropositive individuals will develop AIDS over a period of 10 years following seroconversion (29, 37).

Symptomatic Disease

The pre-AIDS constitutional symptoms associated with HIV disease are variable, but lethargy frequently predominates and a number of skin conditions occur. During this phase, temperature and diarrhea are relatively common. Two conditions of the mouth, buccal candidiasis and hairy leucoplakia, are both common and predict the development of full-blown AIDS within a short period.

AIDS-defining Illnesses

A variety of opportunistic infections are sufficiently predictive of an underlying immunodeficiency state for the diagnosis of AIDS to be made (31).

Opportunistic Infections in AIDS

Fungi

The most common opportunistic fungal infection in HIV-seropositive individuals is with *Candida albicans*. The presence of buccal candidiasis coupled with esophageal symptoms is sufficient to make a diagnosis of AIDS.

Pneumocystis carinii is now thought to be a fungus that may present as a flu-like illness with prominent shortness of breath. Hypoxia is a sign of advanced disease and chest X-ray appearances in such individuals are of pulmonary edema (30). *Pneumocystis carinii*, particularly with very severe immunosuppression, does disseminate, and infection has been documented in the liver and in other sites, including the eye.

The other fungus that commonly infects HIV-positive individuals is *Cryptococcus neoformans*, which is thought to be ubiquitous within the environment. The organism is probably inhaled and disseminates widely in the body, but the most common presentation is meningitis. Infection has been found in the liver, lungs, and gut.

A wide variety of other fungi have occasionally been reported in AIDS, causing disseminated infection that may involve the liver. These include histoplasmosis, coccidioidomycosis and paracoccidioidomycosis, all of which are common in Central and South America. Occasional reports, particularly of histoplasmosis, have occurred in patients who have not travelled to an endemic area. It is likely that with increasing immune suppression, a whole variety of other fungi previously regarded as pure saprophytes will produce symptoms in HIV-seropositive patients and may spread to the liver or biliary tract. Aspergillosis appears to be extremely uncommon in HIV-seropositive individuals, but may present with deranged liver function tests (11).

Protozoal

The most common protozoal infections of AIDS involve the gastrointestinal tract. Cryptosporidiosis is responsible for large volume diarrhea in severely immunosuppressed individuals. Biliary infection with cryptosporidiosis is probably an important cause of AIDS-related sclerosing cholangitis, and certainly biliary infection may provide a reservoir for infection of the gut. There is no known successful treatment.

Microsporidia are usually protozoa with a unique spiral filament that extrudes from the spore and penetrates epithelial cells. The contents of the spore are then extruded through the filament to cause an intracellular infection. Following the first description of microsporidia infection of the gut in 1985, it was shown that this is a common cause of diarrhea in advanced immune suppression. Microsporidiosis infection of the biliary tree may be important and was shown to be particularly frequent in a recent French study as a cause for AIDS-related sclerosing cholangitis.

Toxoplasmosis has a strong predilection for the brain, although disseminated disease does occur (35). About three-quarters of all cases are recrudescences of latent infection, and early in disease, such patients will have had positive toxoplasma serology. However, in up to a third of cases, infection may be due to newly acquired disease. Occasional toxoplasma infections of the liver are to be expected as the epidemic progresses.

Viruses

T-cell deficiencies appear to predispose to a variety of infections with herpes virus. The most important in AIDS-related immunosuppression is cytomegalovirus (CMV) infection. The most serious manifestation is infection of the eye, producing an ischemic retinitis, which will rapidly lead to blindness if not treated. Infection of the upper gut produces either a diffuse distal esophagitis or perhaps more commonly a discrete local esophageal ulceration (38). Infection of the stomach and small intestine is common, but the symptoms are nonspecific, and infection of the large bowel produces a colitis, which may be diffuse or limited to the right or left side of the colon. CMV colitis is associated with bloody diarrhea and abdominal pain (12). At postmortem, CMV infection of the liver appears common, but this is rarely symptomatic during life.

Bacteria

As the humoral immune system and B-cell function remains relatively intact until the late stages of AIDS, bacterial infection is not common and is mainly limited to organisms that grow intracellularly and are normally eradicated by the cell-mediated immune system. The most common of these is *Mycobacterium avium intracellulare* (MAI), which in late disease is a common cause of fever, diarrhea, and recurrent episodes of anemia (19). The diagnosis is most commonly made by a positive blood culture, but this may take from 4 to 6 weeks. Infection of the gut is common, producing an appearance similar to Whipple disease in the small intestine with associated thickening

of peritoneum and lymphadenopathy (Fig. 13.**3**); granuloma in the liver are also seen (Fig. 13.**4**).

Recurrent salmonellosis is also diagnostic of AIDS. Salmonella infection is frequent, noticeably from poorly cooked meals. A wide variety of species are found, some of which produce septicemia and recurrent infection (3).

Tumors

Two tumors, Kaposi sarcoma and non-Hodgkin lymphoma, are also diagnostic of AIDS. A major epidemic of Kaposi sarcoma has occurred following the introduction of HIV into the human population.

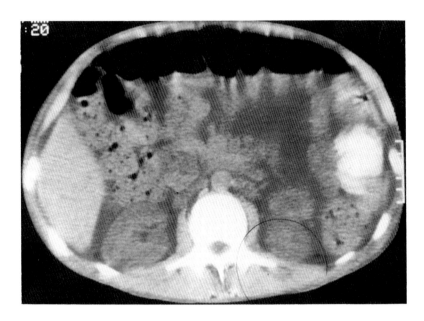

Fig. 13.**3   CT scan of abdomen showing thickening of peritoneum and lymphadenopathy** characteristic of disseminated *Mycobacterium avium intracellulare* (MAI) infection

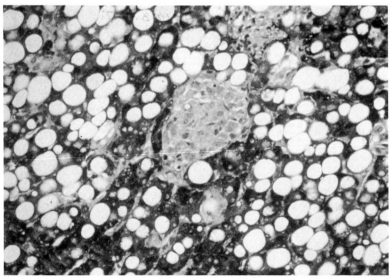

Fig. 13.**4   Histology of liver showing fatty change and a centrally located granuloma in a patient with MAI infection**

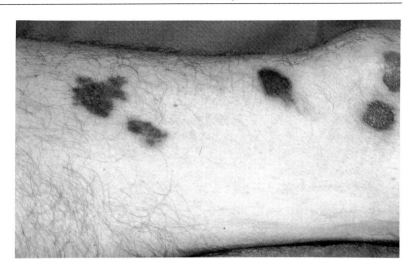

Fig. 13.**5** **Kaposi sarcoma of skin,** which are elevated and pale pink or brown

Kaposi sarcoma is most frequent among seropositive homosexual males, and there is also a raised incidence of the condition in homosexual individuals who are HIV negative. It has therefore been postulated that a second virus, which may also be venereally acquired, is important in the genesis of Kaposi sarcoma lesions. Although most noticeably a tumor of the skin (Fig. 13.**5**), involvement of the gut and liver is also common (18). Such spread is usually asymptomatic, although at postmortem, heavy tumor load is sometimes present within the abdominal cavity, indicating that death was probably related to the tumor itself. Involvement of the liver is common, producing a "mass" appearance on CT scan, but patients are rarely jaundiced or have markedly abnormal liver function tests.

The cause of the marked increase in incidence of non-Hodgkin lymphoma in HIV-seropositive individuals is unclear. In HIV-seropositive patients, non-Hodgkin lymphoma is commonly found in non-nodal sites and appears to have a particular predilection for the gut; liver involvement is common.

Liver Involvement in HIV-seropositive Individuals

Liver function tests are abnormal in more than 50% of individuals with HIV disease prior to death, and in 80% of postmortems there are histological abnormalities in the liver, most commonly fatty infiltration, similar to that seen in other groups of severely emaciated people (5). In a significant proportion of individuals there are poorly formed granulomas, which might be associated with a drug hypersensitivity reaction (15).

Invasive and noninvasive radiology is likely to assist in four groups of patients:

1. Those with a pyrexia of unknown origin
2. Those with abnormal liver function tests suggestive of hepatitis
3. Those with focal abnormalities on ultrasound or CT scanning
4. In the diagnosis of AIDS-related sclerosing cholangitis

Pyrexia of Unknown Origin

As the symptoms of HIV infection are protean and as such a wide variety of organisms may produce symptoms, a pyrexia of unknown origin with nonspecific symptomatology is common. A proportion of patients have *Pneumocystis carinii* infection without prominent respiratory symptoms, and thus all individuals should be screened with an arterial blood gas and chest X-ray. Other patients have symptoms or signs that clearly localize disease to a particular organ, such as meningitis associated with cryptococcal infection. A temperature without specific symptoms is a common presenting feature of MAI infections, less common of cytomegalovirus infection, and a frequent feature of non-Hodgkin lymphoma. A careful search of the retina for cytomegalovirus infection and gut biopsies help to exclude cytomegalovirus infection as a cause. Occasionally, liver biopsy shows cytomegalovirus inclusions. Such individuals usually have only mildly abnormal liver function tests.

The most common way of diagnosing MAI is by blood culture, but even with PCR probes this may take several weeks to give a positive answer. Liver biopsy has the advantage that in such individuals, poorly formed granuloma with acid-fast bacilli in the center can be seen. Guided-needle liver biopsy is particularly helpful in diagnosing non-Hodgkin lymphoma, which frequently causes multiple filling defects, either on ultrasound or CT scanning of the liver.

Liver biopsy also has a role in the diagnosis of a variety of exotic organisms that would not commonly

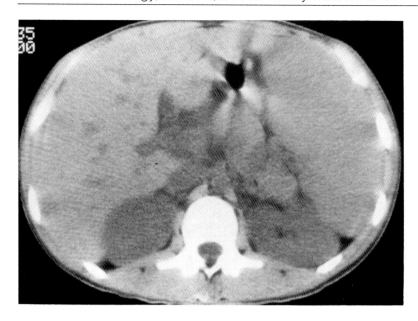

Fig. 13.**6** **CT of abdomen showing gross hepato-splenomegaly of disseminated lymphoma**

be considered, even in the HIV context, unless changes on liver biopsy were seen. Such organisms include *Leishmania donovani.*

Focal Lesions

As with the rest of gastroenterology, liver biopsy is most useful in the diagnosis of focal lesions. Guided liver biopsy may provide a diagnosis of lymphoma, liver abscesses, and tumors, noticeably Kaposi sarcoma, which, despite its vascularity, is probably safe to biopsy. Ileoscopy and abdominal CT (Fig. 13.**6**) can also aid in the diagnosis of lymphoma. ERCP combined with CT of the abdomen will define the tumor location (Figs. 13.**7**, 13.**8**).

Hepatitis

Liver biopsy is also of value in the diagnosis of apparent hepatitis. A wide range of drugs may be responsible for hepatitis, but important interactions also occur between HIV and a number of viruses.

Hepatitis C infection is more severe in HIV-seropositive people. Hepatitis C infection is not a major problem in homosexuals, but many intravenous drug users are infected with both HIV and hepatitis C (26, 1). Such co-infection appears to worsen the prognosis considerably. Asymptomatic individuals with HIV disease and hepatitis C are as likely to die of liver failure as of AIDS. Hepatitis D is cytopathic like hepatitis C, and co-infection of hepatitis D with HIV is thought to worsen the course of liver disease (13, 25).

Thus, although liver biopsy is usually unrewarding as a diagnostic tool in HIV-seropositive patients with abnormal liver function tests, it may have a role in providing a diagnosis and a prognosis in some cases of viral hepatitis.

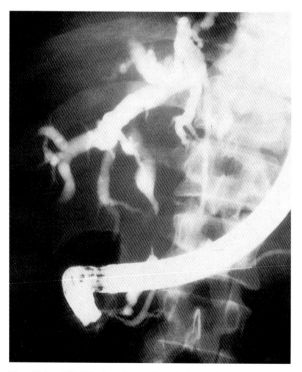

Fig. 13.**7** **ERCP showing dilated right biliary tree with compression of common bile duct by lymphoma**

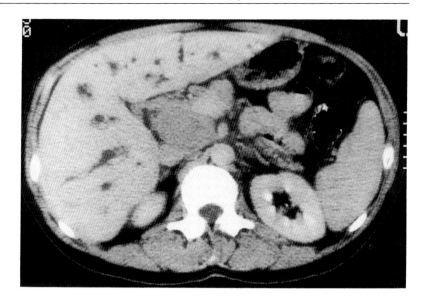

Fig. 13.**8   CT of abdomen showing mass (lymphoma) in head of pancreas and dilated intrahepatic ducts**

AIDS Cholangiography

Cholangiography is important in the diagnosis of AIDS-related sclerosing cholangitis (7, 8). The prevalence of this condition in HIV-infected patients is unclear. Most patients have been diagnosed on endoscopic retrograde cannulation, performed because of abdominal pain. For obvious reasons cholangiography in asymptomatic patients is rarely performed, but it is quite possible that asymptomatic cases are common in cases of gut infection. Similar criteria for the diagnosis of AIDS-related sclerosing cholangitis are used as in making a diagnosis of idiopathic sclerosing cholangitis. Although the changes are often less pronounced and some strictures are longer, overall types at cholangiography are similar. An ampullary stricture may be the cause of duct dilatation (Fig. 13.**9**) although biliary manometry has not been performed. Stricture may be coupled with beading and irregularity of the intra- or extrahepatic ducts, which are both more typical features of sclerosing cholangitis. Occasionally, long intraduct strictures occur without changes of cholangitis. Filling defects in the common bile duct are sometimes prominent, thought to be due to sloughing off of inflammatory material. Preliminary liver imaging will reveal dilated bile ducts in about a third to a half of cases, and all such patients who go on to have cholangiography have appearances that fit with sclerosing cholangitis (33).

In perhaps a third of individuals with abnormal cholangiograms, the pancreatic duct is also abnormal with beading and dilatation (Fig. 13. **9**). In cases of ampullary stenosis, it has been suggested that sphincterotomy may relieve pain (28). It has also been suggested that isolated strictures of the ampulla may be associated with cytomegalovirus infection. The natural history of AIDS-related sclerosing cholangitis is not clearly understood, but in our experience, pain commonly resolves spontaneously over a course of a few months. Thus, the likely role for sphincterotomy is small.

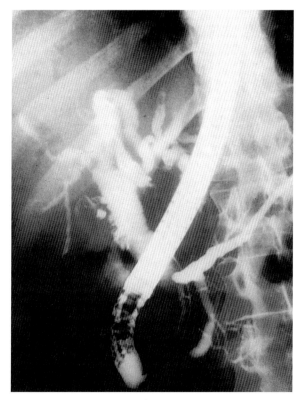

Fig. 13.**9   ERCP showing pancreatic and bile duct dilatation** due to AIDS-related sclerosing cholangitis (ARSC)

The etiology of AIDS-related sclerosing cholangitis is unclear, but most believe that these appearances are likely to be secondary to a variety of infections. In about half to two-thirds of cases, cryptosporidiosis is found elsewhere in the gut and occasionally can be demonstrated in aspirated bile or on ampullary biopsies or biopsies within the duct itself. Cytomegalovirus infection can be found in the ampulla within the bile duct or elsewhere in the gut. A proportion of patients have microsporidial infection.

Health and Safety Issues Related to Invasive Radiology in HIV-seropositive Patients

Risk to Health Care Worker

The transmission of HIV is relatively inefficient, partially because the lipid envelope of the virus is fragile. It is thus susceptible to a variety of detergents, which makes cleaning surfaces and equipment straightforward. However, HIV in dried blood samples stored at room temperature for some days can infect tissue cultures, but whether it would be capable of infecting humans is less certain. The total number of health care workers infected with HIV as a result of occupational exposure is small. Most of the documented seroconversions have been as the result of direct blood to blood contact following needlestick injury.

Thus, radiologists carrying out invasive procedures like other health care workers, are mainly at risk of HIV infection as a result of needlestick injuries. Using automatically resheathing needles and wearing gloves may reduce these risks.

If a needlestick injury does not occur, the overall risks of infection are very slight (less than 0.4% in all the published, prospective studies) (28). The amount of blood transmitted by a needlestick injury is highly likely to be important. All but one of the present reported seroconversions have involved a microtransfusion of blood.

If a needlestick injury does occur in a patient of unknown HIV status, it may create a great deal of anxiety. Our policy is to request a physician from another team to discuss with such an individual whether he would allow his blood to be tested for HIV and whether he would wish to know the result. So far all such patients have readily agreed.

If a needlestick injury involving known HIV-positive blood occurs, the question of the use of prophylactic AZT arises. There is no data that this is effective. A number of seroconversions have occurred despite the use of AZT early after needlestick injury, but it is not clear how many more may have been prevented. There is limited animal data, using retroviruses with similarities to HIV, to suggest that AZT given prior to or concurrently with an inoculum may reduce the degree of viranemia (36, 9, 23, 24). If this data is interpreted as a reason for the use of AZT in human needlestick injuries, it is clear that speed is important and that drug therapy should begin as soon as possible after the incident (perhaps even with intravenous AZT) and should be continued for 1 or 2 weeks thereafter. There are a number of potential side effects of AZT, particularly in big doses (10, 32, 21). Most of these are reversible on stopping therapy—however, the possibility of long-term oncogenesis and teratogenesis (although slight) remains. These potential disadvantages have to be weighed against no clear data for benefit, and this equation may well be different for people with a trivial needlestick injury, where no blood was drawn from either party, compared with a more serious incident (20).

Risk to Patient

Perhaps more important than the risk of HIV transmission from patients to health care workers is the risk of HIV infection being transmitted from one individual to another in the context of invasive radiology. This is most likely to occur during endoscopy, as other procedures use mainly disposable equipment. The presence of HIV has been detected by polymerase chain reaction on endoscopes immediately following procedures on HIV-seropositive patients. Such HIV did not infect tissue cultures and was removed by thorough washing of the endoscope (18, 17). Nevertheless, the potential for transmission remains and emphasizes the need for thorough washing of endoscopes prior to reuse. All such endoscopes must be "sterilized" as well; 2% of glutaraldehyde in contact with HIV for 4 minutes has been shown to be an effective virucidal agent. The percentage of glutaraldehyde in solution following reuse falls rapidly and may be below an effective level within a week of reuse. This emphasizes the importance of frequent reconstitution of fresh glutaraldehyde, taking adequate precautions including ventilation and closed systems to protect staff members (39).

In some units dealing with large numbers of HIV-seropositive patients, the situation arises in which one immunosuppressed patient who may carry opportunistic infections is endoscoped prior to a second patient with equally severe immunosuppression. Thus, there is potential for transmission of cryptosporidiosis, *Mycobacterium avium intracellulare* (MAI), and microsporidiosis. It is clear that spores of *Mycobacterium avium intracellulare* are relatively resistant to glutaraldehyde, and the infectivity of such organisms only decreases slowly following immersion. *Mycobacterium tuberculosis* is also relatively resistant but is inhibited more rapidly by glutaraldehyde, and thus standard advice is to immerse bronchoscopes or gastroscopes for one hour in glutaraldehyde if contamination is suspected. With MAI infection, thorough washing to reduce the number of organisms prior to immersion in glutaraldehyde is the most important step in avoiding cross contamination. The sensitivities of cryptosporidiosis and microsporidiosis to glutaraldehyde are unknown, but it is possible that spores will be resistant (16). Cryptosporidiosis spores are sensitive to hydrogen peroxide, which most manufacturers now agree would not be damaging to endoscopes. Nevertheless, for both infections, thorough washing is again the mainstay of prevention of transmission.

An enormous amount has been learned over the last 12 years about the etiology and pathogenesis of AIDS. However, many new syndromes remain to be described. It is therefore not surprising that the precise role of various investigations, including invasive radiology, are presently ill-defined. With such a common disease, it is imperative that all doctors continue to keep abreast of this important area.

References

1. Alter HJ, Purcell RH, Shih JW, et al. Detection of antibody to hepatitis C virus in prospectively followed transfusion of recipients with acute and chronic non-A, non-B hepatitis. N Eng J Med 1989; 321:1494–1500.
2. Barre-Sinoussi F, Cherman J-C, Rey F, et al. Isolation of a T-lymphotropic retrovirus from a patient at risk for acquired immune deficiency syndrome (AIDS). Science 1984; 224:500–503.
3. Bodey GP, Fainstein V, Guerrant R. Infections of the gastrointestinal tract in the immunocompromised patient: Annu Rev Med 1986; 37:271–281.
4. Canning EU, Hollister WS. Enterocytozoon bieneusi (microspora): prevalence and pathogenicity in AIDS patients. Trans R Soc Trop Med Hyg 1990; 84:181–186.
5. Cappell MS. Hepatobiliary manifestations of the acquired immunodeficiency syndrome. Am J Gastroenterol 1991; 86:1–15.
6. Centers for Disease Control. Pneumocystis pneumonia – Los Angeles. MMWR 1981; 30:250–252.
7. Cello JP. Acquired immunodeficiency syndrome cholangiography: Spectrum of disease. Am J Med 1989; 86:539–546.
8. Cello JP. Human immunodeficiency virus-associated biliary tract disease. Seminars in Liver Disease 1992; 12:213–218.
9. Centers for Disease Control. Public health service statement on management of occupational exposure to human immunodeficiency virus, including considerations regarding zidovudine post exposure. MMWR 1990; 39:RR-1.
10. Darnond DE, Le-Jeunne C, Hugues FC. Failure of prophylactic zidovudine after a suicidal seft-inoculation of HIV infected blood. N Eng J Med 1991; 323:1062.
11. Denning DW, Follansbee SE, Scolaro M, et al. Pulmonary aspergillosis in the acquired immunodeficiency syndrome. N Eng J Med 1991; 10;324:654–662.
12. Dietrich DT, Rahmin M. Cytomegalovirus colitis in AIDS: Presentation of 44 patients and a review of the literature. J Acquir Immune Defic Syndr 1991; 4 (suppl 1):S29–S35.
13. Farci P, Croxson TS, Taylor MB, et al. Effect of human immunodeficiency virus on the increased severity of liver disease associated with delta hepatitis (Abstract). Gastroenterol 1988; 94:A578.
14. Gallo RC, Salahuddin SZ, Popovic M, et al. Frequent detection and isolation of cytopathic retroviruses (HTLV-III) from patients with AIDS and at risk for AIDS. Science 1984; 224:500–503.
15. Grunfeld C, Kotler, DP. Wasting in the acquired immunodeficiency syndrome. Seminars in Liver Disease 1992; 12:175–187.
16. Hanson PJV, Gor D, Chadwick MV, et al: Endoscopy and AIDS – an evaluation of the risk of cross infection. Gut 1989; V40 N5:742.
17. Hanson PJV, Gor D, Clarke JR, et al. Contamination of fibreoptic endoscopes in AIDS. Lancet 1989a; 2:86–88.
17. Hanson PJV, Gor D, Jeffries D, et al. Chemical inactivation of HIV on surfaces. Br Med J 1989b; 298:862–864.
18. Herndier BG, Friedman SL: Neoplasms of the gastrointestinal tract and hepatobiliary system in acquired immunodeficiency syndrome. Seminars in Liver Disease 1992; 12:128–141.
19. Horsburgh CR Jr, Mason UG III, Farhi DC, et al. Disseminated infection with mycobacterium avium intracellulare – a report of 13 cases and a review of the literature. Medicine (Baltimore) 1983; 64:36–48.
20. Jeffries DJ. Zidovudine after occupational exposure to HIV. BMJ 1991; 302:1349–1351.
21. Jones PD. HIV transmission by stabbing in spite of zidovudine prophylaxis. Lancet 1991; 338:884.
22. Kaposi's sarcoma and pneumocystis pneumonia among homosexual men – New York City and California. MMWR 1981; 30:305–308.
23. Lange JMA, Boucher CAB, Hollak CEM, et al. Failure of zidovudine prophylaxis after accidental exposure to HIV-1. N Eng J Med 1990; 322:1375–1377.
24. Looke DFM, Grove DI. Failed prophylactic zidovudine after a needlestick injury. Lancet 1990; 335:1280.
25. Morante AL, De La Cruz F, De Lope CR, et al. Hepatitis B virus replication in hepatitis B and D coinfection. Liver 1989; 9:65–70.
26. McNair ANB, Main J, Thomas HC. Interactions of the human immunodeficiency virus and the hepatotropic viruses. Semin Liver Dis 1992; 12:188–196.
27. Pavlakis GN. Structure and function of the Human Immunodeficiency Virus Type 1. Semin Liver Dis 1992; 12:103–107.
28. Risks to surgeons and patients from HIV and hepatitis: guidelines on precautions and management of exposure to blood and body fluids. BMJ 1992; 305:1327–1343.
29. Rutherford GW, Lifson AR, Hessol NA, et al. Course of HIV-1 infection in a cohort of homosexual and bisexual men: An 11-year follow-up study. Br Med J 1990; 301:1183–1188.
30. Sattler FR, Feinberg J. New developments in the treatment of pneumocystis carinii pneumonia. Chest 1992; 101(2):451–457.
31. Selik RM, Starcher ET, Currn JW. Opportunistic infections reported in AIDS patients: Frequencies, association and trends. AIDS 1987; 1:175–182.
32. Tait DR, Pudifin DJ, Gathiram V, et al. Zidovudine after occupational exposure to HIV. BMJ 1991; 303:581.
33. Thuluvath PJ, Connolly GM, Forbes A, Gazzard BG. Abdominal pain in HIV infection. QJ Med 1991; V78:275–285.
34. Tindall B, Barker S, Donovan B, et al. Characterization of the acute clinical illness associated with human immunodelficiency virus infection. Arch Intern Med 1988; 148:945–949.
35. Tschirhart D, Klatt EC. Disseminated toxoplasmosis in the acquired immunodeficiency syndrome. Arch Pathol Lab Med 1988; 112:1237–1241.
36. United Kingdom Department of Health. Occupational exposure to HIV and the use of zidovudine. A statement from the expert advisory group on AIDS. Lancashire: Health Publications Unit, 1992.
37. Ward JW, Bush TJ, Perskin HA, et al. The natural history of transfusion-associated HIV infection: Factors influencing progression to disease. N Eng J Med 321:947–952.
38. Wilcox CM, Diehl DL, Cello JP, et al. Cytomegalovirus esophagitis in patients with AIDS – a clinical, endoscopic and pathologic correlation. Ann Intern Med 1990; 113:589–593.
39. A Working Party of the British Society of Gastroenterology. Cleaning and disinfection of equipment for gastrointestinal flexible endoscopy: interim recommendations. Gut 1988; 29:1134–1151.

Interventions for Tumor Disease of the Liver and Biliary Tract

14 Minimally Invasive Therapy of Liver Tumors

Malignant liver tumors may be treated by hepatic resection, systemic injection of chemotherapeutic agents, implanted programmable infusion pumps, or local intervention such as intra-arterial chemotherapy, endovascular embolization, or in small tumors, intratumoral alcohol administered percutaneously. Over the past 10 years it has been shown that examination of patients with cirrhosis or chronic hepatitis by ultrasound and ultrasonically guided fine-needle biopsy has lead to detection of increasing numbers of small asymptomatic hepatocellular carcinomas. Follow-up of patients with known primary cancer by ultrasound has increased the early detection of asymptomatic liver metastases. Small secondary liver tumors and precancerous nodules such as adenomatous hyperplasia in known liver disease may be diagnosed early by high-resolution ultrasound and fine-needle biopsy (3, 4, 5, 12).

Malignant hepatoma is one of the most common malignant tumors in the world. Modern imaging techniques combined with measurement of serum levels of alpha-fetoprotein are widely used in the screening of high-risk patients, such as hepatitis B carriers and patients with chronic liver disease (5, 6, 7, 11). Recently, repeated screening of high-risk patients has resulted in the detection of such tumors at an early stage (1, 4, 7). Alpha-fetoprotein levels are usually normal in small asymptomatic hepatocellular carcinomas.

The prognosis of the patient with hepatoma is poor, and surgery is the only hope of cure if the tumor is small, detected early, and concomitant liver disease allows major liver surgery.

In inoperable cases, transcatheter embolization and chemotherapy have been used, and in recent years, percutaneous transhepatic injection of alcohol has been used to obliterate small tumors (6, 8, 9, 13). The goal of percutaneous transhepatic alcohol injection is to destroy the lesion or lesions in the liver completely. This applies to one to three lesions all of less than 3.5 cm in diameter. Larger tumors over 4.0 cm in diameter may be treated to reduce tumor size.

Percutaneous alcohol injection is not successful in obliterating these or larger tumors. Studies have shown that alcohol causes coagulation necrosis after diffusion into tumor cells, and thrombosis of small tumor vessels follows. Cellular dehydration and protein denaturation may be the cause of tumor shrinkage after treatment. Because alcohol is confined to the lesion, healthy tissue is not damaged or destroyed as it is after surgical resections or endovascular embolizations. Most tumors occur in diseased livers with poor functional reserves. Any therapy that destroys tumor tissue without reducing the liver's functional reserve helps to delay the onset of terminal liver failure (13, 14, 17).

Pathology of Liver Tumors

Hepatocellular Carcinoma

This tumor arises from the hepatocytes. It is the most common primary malignant tumor of the liver, and it is most common in patients with cirrhosis. The presence of cirrhosis often delays diagnosis and often limits therapy of the neoplasm.

Ultrasound surveys of the liver in cases of chronic liver disease at regular intervals help to discover early tumors (14, 21, 28). This is a highly vascular tumor supplied by the hepatic artery. It grows into the portal and hepatic veins and may invade the bile ducts. Hepatoma (HCC) in cirrhosis is well differentiated, while HCC in noncirrhotics is poorly differentiated. Three varieties are described by gross appearances:

1. An *expanding lesion* with a fibrous capsule. This tumor is the common form found in Europe.
2. An *infiltrating tumor* composed of tumor nodules of various sizes within the liver parenchyma and tumor arteries within the lesions.
3. A *multifocal tumor* that causes small masses of equal size scattered throughout the liver. It has an extremely poor prognosis.

Other forms of HCC include:

4. *Small HCC,* a tumor with a 2-cm diameter or less. It is mostly found in advanced cirrhosis.
5. *Fibrolamellar hepatoma* is a rare tumor composed of eosinophilic neoplastic hepatocytes and fibrous tissue arranged in lamellar fashion. It is a well-demarcated tumor with fibrous septa. It occurs in the normal liver and has a better prognosis. Highly experienced Japanese surgeons now question whether surgery is indicated in HCC since tumors of less than 5 cm recurred in 54% of patients within 15 months in cirrhotics and in 39% of noncirrhotic livers within 2 years.

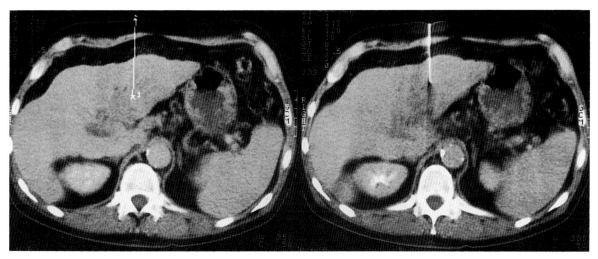

Fig. 14.**1   a** and **b Procedure for CT-guided biopsy of liver tumor in cirrhosis.** Note the irregular liver outline and the mass in the left lobe in alcoholic cirrhosis

Liver Cell Adenoma

This is a benign tumor of hepatocytes that develops in normal liver tissue and is usually 5 cm to 15 cm in diameter. With the tumor, normal cells are distributed in cords or plates. This is a very vascular tumor. It contains no portal tracts or Kupffer cells. The tumor occurs mostly in women on oral contraceptives. The treatment for this tumor is surgical removal.

Hemangioma of the Liver

This is a common tumor usually of a small size (less than 4 cm diameter) composed of vascular channels lined by flat endothelial cells in a fibrous stroma. It is usually asymptomatic, and therapy is not indicated.

Focal Nodular Hyperplasia

This is an isolated malformation with a characteristic gross appearance of a well-circumscribed nonencapsulated mass with a stellate central scar and slender septa radiating to the periphery. The central scar is composed of collagen and contains medium-sized arteries with media hyperplasia. Hepatocytes around septa contain copper associated with protein. A central artery supplies the tumor, which contains marked arterial vascularization on selective arteriography.

Metastatic Liver Tumors

Metastases are the most common liver tumors in Europe and the United States and are twenty times more common than primary liver neoplasms. The latter are more common in Africa, Japan, and Eastern countries. The liver is the most common site of metastatic tumor deposits. Commonly, these tumors arise from sites of drainage of the portal vein but also from other sites such as the breast and lung. Survival in metastatic liver disease depends on the extent of liver involvement and the presence or absence of systemic metastatic tumors. In one series, liver metastases from colon carcinoma, which was confined to one lobe and involved an area of less than 25% of the liver, caused death in 6 months when untreated. If 25% to 75% of the liver was involved, survival was 5.5 months, and if more than 75% of the liver was involved, death occurred in 3.4 months (26). Metastases from gastrointestinal cancer, pancreas, breast, or ovaries are present in the liver in 60% of patients dying from these neoplasms, and 40% of patients dying from renal or lung metastases have liver metastases.

Patients with untreated metastatic liver disease from colonic tumors have a mean survival time of 5 months. Patients with metastases from gastric tumors survive for 2 months, and patients with metastases from pancreatic carcinoma survive for 3 months.

Liver surgery offers the only hope of cure in metastatic liver disease, but only 20% of patients are suitable for surgical removal of metastases. Because of the poor prognosis, an aggressive approach to therapy is justified in metastatic liver disease. Carcinoid metastases from the gastrointestinal tract or bronchus have a better prognosis than adenocarcinoma. Carcinoids are solid tumors arising from chromaffin tissue.

Colonic carcinoid commonly causes multiple liver metastases.

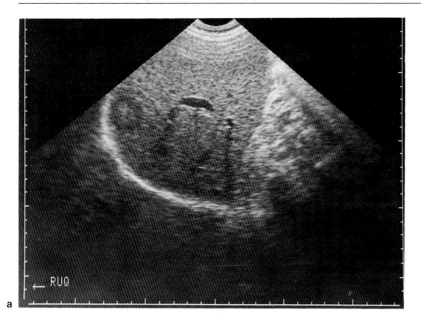

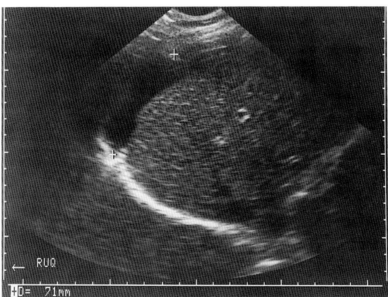

Fig. 14.**2   a Early tumor, right lobe of liver** (arrow)
b The lesion was obliterated with 5 mL of absolute alcohol, and repeat ultrasound shows a small fluid collection above the site of the lesion at 5 weeks. The lesion could not be demonstrated at that time. In the interval, the patient underwent an elective cholecystectomy

The tumor masses have no capsule and are composed of polygonal cells with abundant cytoplasm arranged in nests and sheets separated by a fibrous and vascular stroma.

Technique of Percutaneous Therapy

Establishing a Histological Diagnosis

Percutaneous fine-needle aspiration biopsy or Trucut biopsy for histological diagnosis is essential prior to therapy.

Echo-guided biopsy is a valuable and safe examination for the histological diagnosis of small liver nodules. It has a sensitivity greater than 90%. A study of 145 cases showed a sensitivity of 91% and a specificity of 100%. Cytoaspiration is less accurate than tissue core histological examination using a Surecut or preferably a Urocut needle, which is a modified Trucut needle. Echo-guided biopsy is most important before interventional therapy of small tumor masses (7, 8, 13, 15).

Combined cytological smears and tissue core biopsies are preferable to aspiration biopsy alone for accurate diagnosis (8).

Preparation of the Patient

Routine blood chemistry is used to exclude a bleeding or coagulation disorder. Percutaneous therapy is only carried out on patients with platelet counts of more than $40\,000/\mu L$ and a prothrombin time of more than 35%. Ultrasound is used to exclude ascites, which is a contraindication to percutaneous therapy. Informed consent is obtained from the patient. The procedure is performed in the fasting patient.

Technique of Alcohol Injection

The percutaneous injection of alcohol into a tumor mass is carried out under aseptic conditions and ultrasonic guidance using a 21-gauge, 20-cm needle with an ultrasonic tip. The needle tip is placed at the tumor center after local anesthesia of the abdominal wall anteriorly or in the right intercostal area. We use a linear array real-time scanner with a 3.5 MHz transducer for tumor localization and needle positioning. The *total volume* of alcohol necessary to obliterate the tumor is a little more than the tumor volume calculated from the tumor radius using the volume of a sphere according to the following equation:

$$V = \tfrac{4}{3}\,(r + 0.5)^3$$

V is the volume of the tumor in milliliters, and r is the tumor radius. The addition of 0.5 is to allow for obliteration of liver tissue at the periphery of the lesion to ensure cure of the tumor. The volume of alcohol is given in divided doses two or three times weekly over several weeks depending on patient tolerance, tumor location, number of lesions, the response of the tumor to sclerosis, and whether the aim of therapy is cure or palliation. The alcohol injection is made slowly into the lesion in amounts of 5–10 mL at one session. Care is taken not to spill alcohol into the peritoneum where it causes severe abdominal pains. After completing the injection, the needle is kept within the tumor for 30–60 seconds to minimize spill of alcohol from the lesion (13, 14).

Assessing the Response to Intratumoral Alcohol Injection

Tumor response is evaluated by contrast CT, MRI, digital arteriography, tumor biopsy, and levels of alpha-fetoprotein if the latter is elevated before therapy.

Carefully positioned alcohol injections cause tumor obliteration by necrosis in over 80% of tumors examined histologically (13).

Digital arteriography at 1–3 months after cessation of alcohol injections shows tumor obliteration in 85% of all tumors treated. Contrast CT shows failure of contrast uptake by the tumor in most cases treated aggressively. Ultrasound following therapy shows conversion of the tumor from hyperechoic to isodense lesions, or from hypoechoic to hyperechoic lesions. However, such changes at ultrasound do not indicate tumor obliteration. Tumors showing low signal intensity on T1-weighted MRI imaging before treatment showed an increased signal intensity on necrosis after therapy. All tumors show a high signal intensity on T2 weighting compared with the normal liver before therapy, and after necrosis, a low signal intensity compared to the normal liver.

In one recent study (Shina et al. 1990), survival rates at 1, 2, 3, and 4 years after tumor sclerosis were 85, 70, 55, and 50%, respectively. Survival is also influenced by underlying liver disease and is significantly higher in Child Class A than in Child Class B or C. Patients with a single tumor did not survive longer than patients with more than one tumor nodule. Tumor size had some influence on survival. Patients with tumors of 3.0 cm diameter or less survive longer than those with larger tumors.

Studies by Okuda (1986) seem to indicate that all solitary nodules in patients with chronic liver disease should be considered premalignant and should be removed or obliterated by percutaneous alcohol injection.

Complications of Percutaneous Alcohol Injection

Reported complications of this treatment include pain, fever, mild alcohol intoxication, and tumor necrosis causing intraperitoneal hemorrhage. Patient survival is reported to be as good or better than surgical resection, however, patients with Child Class C are usually excluded from surgical resections. Patients with good liver function have the best prognosis with this form of therapy. In cirrhotics, liver disease, rather than hepatoma, is the factor determining the prognosis (9, 10, 13, 14).

Recurrent treatments by alcohol sclerosis can control if not stop tumor growth, and the patient dies of complications of cirrhosis rather than hepatoma.

Since liver function is only minimally disturbed by local injection of a tumor, the therapy may be used in the presence of severe liver dysfunction when other forms of therapy are contraindicated.

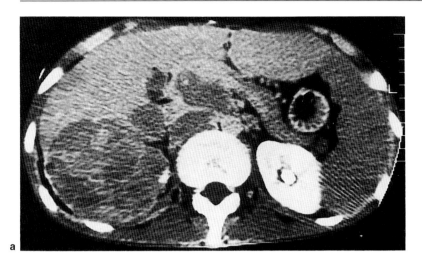

a

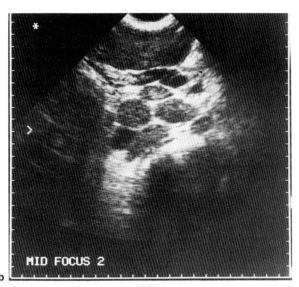

b

Fig. 14.**3 a CT scan of a 16-year-old boy showing mass in the right lobe of liver**
b Ultrasound showed portal nodal masses
c and **d** Celiac arteriogram showing vascular hepatoma with other nodules apart from the main tumor
e The lesion was embolized at weekly intervals for 3 weeks using injections of absolute alcohol, and a CT scan shows a sterile "abscess" containing gas at the end of the 3rd week
f CT at 3 months shows obliterated tumor
g Final hepatic arteriogram shows obliteration of the tumor vessels
The patient survived 1 year and 4 months after the original diagnosis

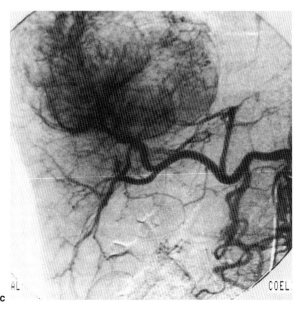

c

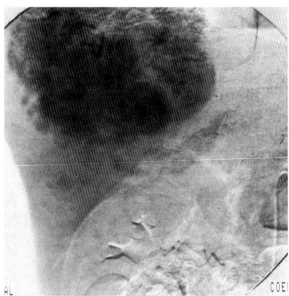

d

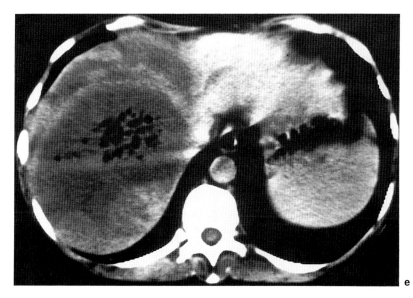

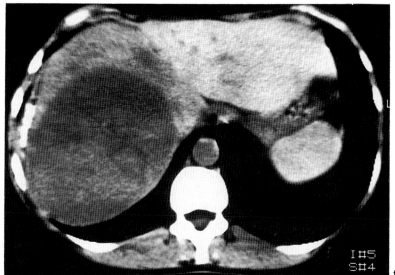

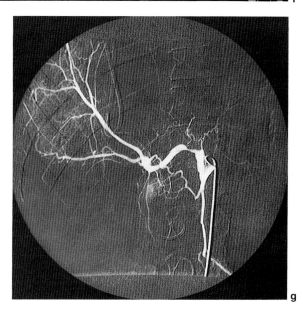

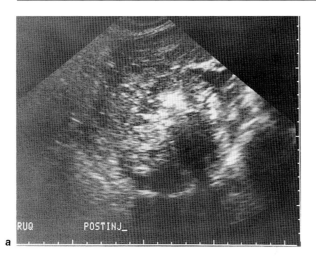

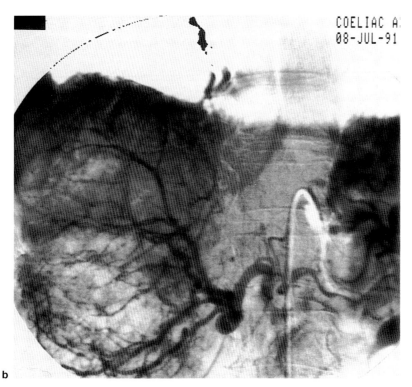

Fig. 14.**4   a Ultrasound of the liver showing large solitary colonic secondary deposit.** Surgery was refused
b Hepatic arteriogram showing moderate vascularity

c The lesion was embolized with absolute alcohol on two occasions at monthly intervals, and a CT scan at 7 days after the first embolization shows sterile gas containing necrotic tumor
d CT scan at 3 months shows sterile nontumor mass

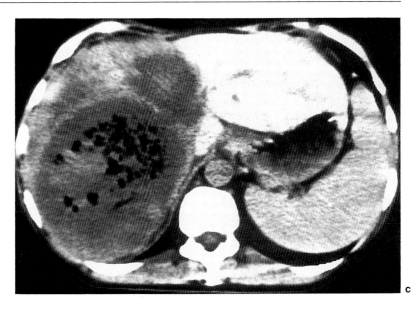

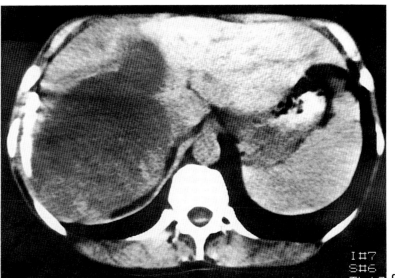

Fig. 14.**4c -d**

Percutaneous Alcohol Injection of Liver Metastases

Isolated hepatic metastases from colonic cancer are uncommon, but because of the large number of new cases of colonic carcinoma each year, isolated metastases are frequently encountered. A solitary liver deposit or at most up to four deposits in one lobe of the liver with no systemic spread and no lymph node involvement is ideal for hepatic resection or its alternatives, percutaneous tumor sclerosis, embolization, or chemoembolization. Early presymptomatic detection of liver metastases is achieved by serial postoperative follow-up of patients with large-bowel tumors by means of CEA assay. Position and number of tumor deposits are determined by MRI or CT portography, both of which are more sensitive than conventional CT or ultrasound. In patients who refuse liver surgery or are considered inoperable because of tumor position or size, other methods are valuable in reducing tumor size, obliterating tumors, and improving quality of life.

The technique of treating metastases is the same as that for primary liver carcinoma. *Ascites, bleeding, and coagulation disorders are contraindications.* Response to therapy is monitored by ultrasound, CT scan-

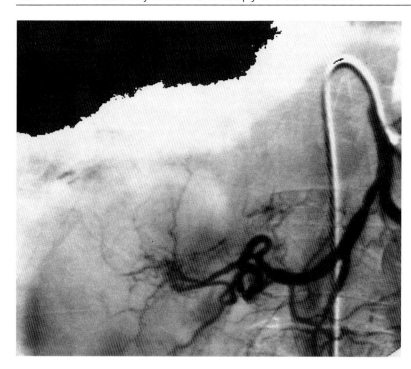

Fig. 14.**4**
e Final arteriogram showing obliteration of tumor vessels. The patient,
a 73-year-old woman, survived for
2 years and 7 months

ning, and measurements of levels of tissue carcinoembryonic antigen (CEA) from biopsy material.
Biopsy tissue levels of CEA are valuable as an indica-
tor of tumor ablation when cytology is inadequate (8).
Livraghi (1991) reported an excellent response to therapy in endocrine metastases with a maximum recur-
rence-free follow-up of 33 months. Fine needle biopsy for diagnosis in carcinoid liver metastases is contraindicated because it may cause fatal carcinoid crisis (2). We have used intratumor injections of alcohol
to treat metastases up to 10 cm in diameter with excellent results in solitary deposits, or in up to four masses
in one lobe to a total diameter of 10 cm. Tumor ablation by this method reduces liver size and improves
the quality of life. Prolongation of life may be
achieved when the technique is combined with tumor
embolization (see below). The volume of alcohol injected is determined by tumor diameter and calculated
volume. Major hepatic surgery, which still carries a
significant morbidity and mortality from intraoperative hemorrhage, bile leaks, and postoperative infection even with the use of ultrasonic dissection, is
avoided. Liver failure, a major cause of morbidity and
mortality in metastatic liver disease due to extensive
resections of normal liver when surgical therapy is the
primary treatment, is also avoided. This method of
treatment of suitable liver tumors is cheap and widely
available, but randomized trials are needed to establish it as an alternative to surgery (5).

Embolization of Liver Tumors

The indications for hepatic arterial embolization of
liver neoplasms are unresectable tumors, failure of
chemotherapy or radiation therapy, and when no other
effective treatment is available.

Preparation of the Patient

A *histological diagnosis* is established by fine needle
biopsy under ultrasound control. *Bleeding time, prothrombin time, partial thromboplastin time, platelet
count, serum uric acid,* and a *liver profile,* which
should include bilirubin, alkaline phosphatase, aspar-
tate transferase, and lactate dehydrogenase, are obtained before embolization and daily for 3 days after
embolization and on alternate days for 7 days. *Gallbladder ultrasound* is performed prior to therapy and
at 24 and 48 hours after therapy.

   Intravenous antibiotics are commenced prior to
embolization and are continued for 7 days.

   Allopurinol, probenecid, and diuretics are administered for 7 days commencing on the day of therapy.

Technique of Embolization

The patient is studied in the fasting state maintaining
hydration by intravenous fluids. Hepatic arterial studies are carried out to assess the blood supply to the
liver and document the patency of the portal vein. *Portal vein thrombosis is a contraindication* to embolization. *Child C cirrhosis is also a contraindication.* All

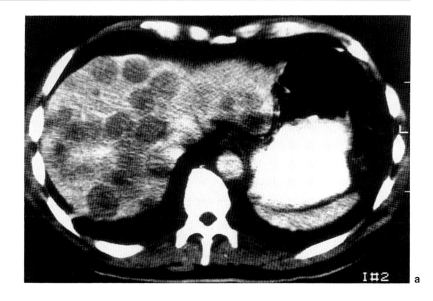

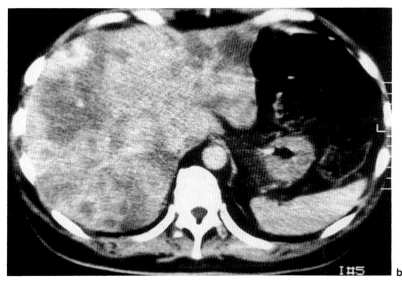

Fig. 14.**5   a CT scan showing hepatic metastases from melanoma of the skin of the fore-arm**

b CT scan 1 month post hepatic artery embolization with alcohol. The tumors are obliterated. The liver has increased in size due to hypertrophy of normal hepatocytes

procedures are performed under local anesthesia with analgesia for pain relief after embolization. Following catheterization of the hepatic artery via the femoral artery, subselective catheterization is performed using a coaxial catheter technique. The catheter tip is placed as close as possible to the tumor site. The tip should lie beyond the gastroduodenal artery and, if possible, beyond the origin of the cystic artery from the proper hepatic artery. Embolization of the proper hepatic artery is not a useful procedure in the treatment of liver neoplasm because of the development of collateral arteries to the liver. A similar phenomenon occurs after surgical hepatic artery ligation.

The ideal embolic agent should cause complete tumor necrosis following intra-arterial injection. It should not pass into the venous drainage of the tumor and hence, into the general circulation. It should have

a direct toxic effect on tumor tissue and should not harm normal surrounding liver cells. Various embolic agents have been used for liver tumor embolization including particles of Gelfoam, Ivalon sponge, chemoembolization with gelatin sponge soaked in solutions of mitocycin C, doxorubicin, or cisplatin, Lipiodal targeted chemotherapy combined with embolization, Gelfoam powder with alcohol and terbol.

In recent years we have used undiluted absolute alcohol (100%) for embolization of liver neoplasms occasionally combined with direct percutaneous intratumor alcohol injections.

Following superselective catheterization of the tumor blood supply, amounts of alcohol varying from 5 mL to 30 mL have been injected intra-arterially to necrose liver neoplasms.

The fluid is injected into the feeding arteries as close as possible to the neoplasm while avoiding the gastroduodenal and cystic arteries. Intra-arterial alcohol causes gastric ulceration if injected into the common hepatic artery. Gallbladder necrosis may also occur if the cystic artery receives alcohol from the intrahepatic injection. A coaxial catheter prevents reflux of alcohol into the common hepatic artery after hand injection. Alcohol injection of all vessels feeding the tumor is essential. Peripheral arterial embolization with alcohol causes tumor necrosis since all liver tumors are supplied by the arterial circulation. The proper hepatic artery remains patent and serves as a route for reembolization if tumor growth at the periphery of the neoplasm recurs. Alcohol sclerosis of the tumor reduces tumor size by tumor vessel necrosis and causes cessation of tumor growth unless some peripheral tumor vessels that receive blood supply from an ectopic site such as a renal, suprarenal, or inferior phrenic vessel are spared. Some interventionalists embolize the gastroduodenal artery before the hepatic artery to prevent embolization of the duodenum or head of pancreas.

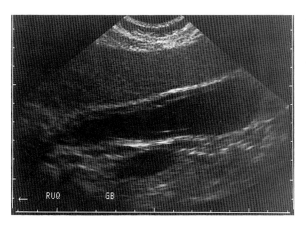

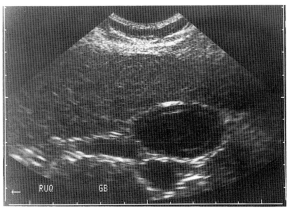

Fig. 14.**6   a** and **b Ultrasound of the gallbladder 3 days post hepatic artery embolization** showing thickening of the gallbladder wall by edema or elevation of the mucosa. The patient did not require surgery

Effects of Successful Tumor Embolization

Successful tumor embolization causes immediate severe pain over the liver area. This may be accompanied by immediate severe nausea and vomiting. These side effects indicate successful tumor obliteration. Biochemistry shows marked evelation of liver function tests at 24 hours. These return to normal over 10 days. Tumor necrosis causes elevation of uric acid levels, and urate nephropathy and renal failure are prevented by bicarbonates, allopurinol, and diuretics. Postembolization pain may last for 3 days and is treated by intravenous pethidine as required. Nausea and vomiting are controlled by antiemetics such as prochlorperazine. The severity of this *postembolization syndrome* is closely related to the success of tumor therapy. A CT scan at 48 hours should show liver tumor necrosis with gas in the neoplasm. Antibiotic prevents this sterile tumor from developing into an abscess.

In our experience with alcohol embolization, systemic effects were not observed and the toxic effect of 100% alcohol on the liver tumor was confined to the local area of liver embolized. When the postembolization syndrome had resolved, usually within 3–5 days, no other complications were observed. We have not observed acute gallbladder necrosis using alcohol as an embolic agent. Injection of alcohol into the gastroduodenal artery caused gastric ulceration and endoscopically observed hemorrhagic gastritis in one patient when the superselective catheter was dislodged into the common hepatic artery during alcohol injection. Another patient developed acute renal failure after embolization of parasitic arterial vessels from the renal artery. The patient recovered following 5 days peritoneal dialysis. Transient chest pain and dyspnea developed in another patient following embolization of the right inferior phrenic artery, which was supplying a tumor in the right lobe of the liver after occlusion of the hepatic artery at a previous embolization. All patients treated by us with alcohol embolization experienced regression of the tumor, a marked decrease in liver size, an increase in physical well-being and quality of life, and prolonged survival after failure of systemic chemotherapy.

Which Tumors Should Be Embolized?

Any primary or secondary liver tumor may be embolized if the portal vein is patent. Even colonic tumor metastases, which are often avascular as judged by contrast CT, may be reduced in size by alcohol embolization. The tumor microcirculation is obliterated, and patient survival is prolonged. Embolization of hepatoma in Child Class C cirrhosis is not indicated. Tumor recurrence is related to the presence of undestroyed viable tumor cells at the tumor periphery with neovascularization. This is treated by further embolization. We have noted the development of calcification within the center of embolized tumors. Transcatheter embolization may be combined with intra-arterial injection of chemotherapeutic agents such as mitocycin C, doxorubicin, or cisplatin. This has been termed *chemoembolization. Oily chemoembolization* may be used. Lipiodol is injected into the tumor by arterial catheter followed by chemotherapeutic drugs, and the tumor vessel is then embolized. Tumor recurrence after surgical resection may also be treated by embolization.

Lipiodol Targeted Chemotherapy

Lipiodol combined with a chemotherapeutic agent by emulsification is injected into the hepatic artery to the liver carcinoma. The Lipiodol emulsion is held by the tumor tissue, which is exposed to a higher dose of drug therapy than following intra-arterial injection, or systemic chemotherapy (7, 12, 18).

Combined with surgical resection of hepatoma, this form of treatment has a reported 70% five-year survival (12, 22, 28).

Reported complications include fever, transient nausea and abdominal pain, elevation of aminotransferase levels, leucopenia, alopecia, gastric ulcerations, pancreatitis, jaundice, and pulmonary edema. Liver failure may follow this therapy in advanced cirrhosis.

Iodine-131 Lipiodol Therapy

Part of the iodine component of Lipiodol is replaced by ^{131}I radionuclide, and the radioactive Lipiodol is injected into the tumor via the hepatic artery to selectively irradiate the hepatoma ^{131}I has a biological half-life of 8 days during which the tumor may be rendered necrotic. The patient's abdomen is shielded to prevent radioactivity risk from the retained radionucleide (4).

Toxicity to the thyroid, bone marrow, and lungs have not been described.

Conclusions

Earlier diagnosis of small liver tumors by monitoring patients at risk offers earlier treatment with a better prognosis than in symptomatic tumors. Several methods of treatment are now available. All have the potential to improve survival and provide significant palliation with a good quality of life when surgery is precluded by underlying liver disease or inoperability in single metastasis. Combined forms of therapy are now available, although it is not possible at present to select the most successful form of treatment for small hepatocellular carcinomas based on tumor biology, tumor blood flow, liver function, and tumor size. Surgery is now increasingly used in metastatic liver disease confined to one lobe and embolization combined with intratumoral irradiation and chemotherapy have proved successful in prolonging survival and increasing the quality of life in survivors without the morbidity of major surgery.

References

1. Arakawa M, Kage M, Sugihara S, Nakashima T, Seunaga M, Okuda K. Emergence of malignant lesion within an adenomatous hyperplastic nodule in a cirrhotic liver. Observations in five cases. Gastroenterology 1986; 91:198–208.
2. Bissonnette RT, Gibney RG, Berry BR, Buckley BR. Fatal carcinoid crisis after percutaneous fine needle biopsy of hepatic metastasis case report and literature review. Radiology 1990; 174:751–752.
3. Bondestram S, Jansson SE, Taavitsainen M, Standcrtskjold-Nordestam CG. Ultrasound guided fine needle biopsy of mass lesions affecting the hepatobiliary tract. Acta Radiol 1981; 22:549–551.
4. Bretagne J, Rauol J, Bourguet P, et al. Hepatic artery injection of I 131 labeled Lipiodol. Radiology 1988; 168:547–550.
5. Cottone M, Marceno MP, Maringhini A, et al. Ultrasound in the diagnosis of carcinoma in association with cirrhosis. Radiology 1983; 147:517–519.
6. Dusheiko GM, Hobbs KEF, Dick R, Burroughs AK. Treatment of small hepatocellular carcinomas. Lancet 1992; 340:285–288.
7. Furuta T, Kanematsu T, Matsumata T, et al. Lipiodilization prolongs survival rates in postoperative patients with recurrent hepatocellular carcinoma. Hepatogastroenterology 1990; 37:494–497.
8. Ebara M, Ohto M, Shinagawa T, et al. Natural history of minute hepatocellular carcinoma smaller than three centimetres complicating cirrhosis. A study of 22 patients. Gastroenterology 1986; 90:289–298.
9. Ebara M, Ohto M, Sugiura N, et al. Percutaneous ethanol injection or the treatment of small hepatocellular carcinoma: study of 95 patients. Gastroenterology 1990; 5:616–626.
10. Gandolfi L, Solmi L, Muratori R, Bertoni F. Echo guided fine needle liver biopsy in the diagnosis of hepatocellular carcinoma with particular reference to small lesions. Ital J Gasteroenterol 1987; 19:43–60.
11. Kudo M, Tomita S, Tochio H, et al. Small hepatocellular carcinoma: Diagnosis with US, angiography with intraarterial CO2 microbubbles. Radiology 1992; 182:155–160.
12. Kurodo IC, Saskurai M, Monden M, et al. Limitation of transcatheter arterial chemoembolisation using iodised oil for small hepatocellular carcinoma. A study in resected cases. Cancer 1991; 67:81–86.
13. Lee MJ, Muller PR, Dawson SL, et al. Measurement of Tissue Carcinoembryonic antigen levels from fine needle biopsy specimens: Technique and clinical usefulness. Radiology 1992; 184:717–720.
14. Livraghi T, Festi D, Monti F, et al. US-guided percutaneous alcohol injection of small hepatic and abdominal tumors Radiology 1986; 161:309–312.
15. Livraghi T, Vettori C. Percutaneous ethanol injection therapy of hepatoma. Cardiovasc Intervent Radiol 1990; 13:146–152.
16. Livraghi T, Vettori C, Lazzaroni S. Liver metastases: Results of percutaneous ethanol injection in 14 patients. Radiology 1991; 179:709–712.
17. Livraghi T, Bolandi L, Lazzaroni S, et al. Percutaneous ethanol injection in the treatment of hepatocellular carcinoma in cirrhosis. A study of 207 patients. Cancer 1992; 69:925–929.
18. Novell JR, Dusheiko G, Markham NI, et al. Selective regional chemotherapy of unresectable hepatic tumours using lipiodol. Hepatic Biliary Pancreatic 1991; 4:223–236.

19. Okuda K. What is the precancerous lesion for hepatocellular carcinoma in man. J Gastroenterol Hepatol 1986; 1:79–85.
20. Okuda K. Hepatocellular carcinoma: recent progress. Hepatology 1992; 15:948–963.
21. Otho M, Tsuchya Y, Kimura K. Ultrasonically guided puncture of the liver, pancreas, portal and biliary tree. In: Bolondi L, Gandolfi L, Labo G, eds. Diagnostic Ultrasound in Gastroenterology. Padova: Piccin 1984:449–521.
22. Park C, Choi SI, Kim H, et al. Distribution of lipiodol in hepatocellular carcinoma. Liver 1990; 10:72–78.
23. Sheu JC, Huang GT, Chen DS, et al. Small hepatocellular carcinoma intratumour ethanol treatment using new needle and guidance systems. Radiology 1987; 163:43–48.
24. Shiina S, Tagawa K, Unuma T, et al. Percutaneous ethanol injection therapy of hepatocellular carcinoma: analysis of 77 patients. AJR 1990; 155:1221–1226.
25. Solmi L, Muratori R, Brambati M, Gandolfi L. Comparison between the 21 gauge Urocut needle and the 21 gauge Surecut needle in echo guided percutaneous biopsy of neoplastic liver lesions. Surg Endosc 1989; 3:38–42.
26. Stugerbaker PH. Surgical decision making for large bowel cancer metastatic to the liver. Radiology 1990; 174:621–626.
27. Tanbaka S, Kitamura T, Ohshima A, et al. Diagnostic accuracy of ultrasonography for hepatocellular carcinoma. Cancer 1986; 58:344–347.
28. Watanabe A, Yamamoto H, Ito T, Nagashima H. Diagnosis, treatment and prognosis of small hepatocellular carcinoma. Hepatogastroenterology 1986; 33:52–55.
29. Weiss L. Principles of metastasis. Orlando: Academic Press, 1985:4–159.

15 Minimally Invasive Therapy of Malignant Biliary Obstruction

The therapy of malignant biliary obstruction remains difficult and, except in rare circumstances, does not achieve a 100% cure. The disease is often advanced before symptoms are evident, and vital structures are invaded, which render operation for successful tumor removal impossible.

The resectability rate of bile duct carcinoma rarely exceeds 30%, and the distinction between curative and palliative surgery is often not possible even when the patient is treated at centers for advanced biliary surgery (9, 10). Tumor removal is the only hope of cure. Palliative surgical procedures, such as segment III bypass surgery in hilar obstruction or use of the U-tube technique, should no longer be used as nonsurgical methods cause less morbidity and mortality than palliative surgical procedures. Similarly, cholecystojejunostomy for periampullary neoplasms should no longer be used as palliative therapy (33, 40). *The primary aim of palliative treatment is restoration of bile flow from the liver to the intestine.* The value of preoperative biliary drainage is still in dispute. Some authors consider it valuable in reducing operative morbidity and mortality while others report significant complications from the drainage procedure itself (40, 46).

Restoration of bile flow to the intestine in malignant biliary obstruction is now performed endoscopically or percutaneously with less morbidity and mortality than surgery in pancreatic head carcinoma and bile duct neoplasms. Ampullary carcinoma is an exception in that successful tumor removal by duodenopancreatectomy may be curative. There is, however, a 10% mortality with this form of surgery. Local ampullary excision and radical surgery have a reported similar survival rate (45, 49), which has encouraged endoscopists to perform endoscopic ampullectomy. However, local excision carries a higher mortality compared to radical surgery (18.8% vs. 27.7%) (37, 40). This higher mortality for tumor excision may be related to poorer patient condition prior to treatment in the local excision group. Local endoscopic ampullectomy has a much lower morbidity and mortality.

Pathology of Malignant Biliary Obstruction

Primary Bile Duct Carcinoma

A primary bile duct carcinoma is usually a well-differentiated adenocarcinoma. Subepithelial spread along the bile duct occurs in about 10% of cases; this is difficult to recognize at surgery. The tumor may be papillary, nodular, or diffuse. The papillary type is more common at the ampulla of Vater. The nodular form forms a mass projecting into the bile duct lumen. It is more common in the upper and mid–bile duct. It may form as a sclerotic mass at the liver hilum or as an intraduct mass in the mid–bile duct. The diffuse form may involve a long length of the bile duct with luminal narrowing and skip lesions, and it may be confused with sclerosing cholangitis. Squamous cell carcinoma and cystadenocarcinoma of the bile duct are rare, and bile duct sarcoma usually only occurs in children. Bile duct carcinoma may occur in choledochal cyst, Caroli disease, congenital hepatic fibrosis, polycystic disease of the liver, and cystic fibrosis. Biliary papillomatosis is now recognized as having a low malignancy potential.

Biliary carcinoma may be a component of familial adenomatous polyposis coli (1, 4, 14, 19, 29, 32, 39).

Periampullary and Pancreatic Carcinoma

Periampullary tumors may arise from the bile duct mucosa, the papilla of Vater, the head of the pancreas, or the duodenum. Carcinoma of the pancreas is the most common of these tumors and has a significantly worse prognosis than other periampullary tumors and it is less well differentiated than bile duct, papillary, or duodenal carcinoma. The origin of these carcinomas cannot be determined on the basis of histological criteria only. Pancreatic carcinomas arise from the duct system and rarely from the acini. Fibrous tissue proliferation is common with this tumor. It is an aggressive neoplasm and infiltrates the portal vein, mesenteric vessels, and duodenum with early metastases to the regional lymph nodes. Rarer periampullary tumors include carcinoid, cystadenocarcinoma, lymphoma, islet-cell tumors, adenocanthoma, sarcoma, and melanoma (29, 33, 37, 40, 45, 49, 52, 53).

Gallbladder Carcinoma

Carcinoma of the gallbladder has the worst prognosis of all the intra-abdominal neoplasms. It is more common in women and in the presence of gallstones, particularly large gallstones (3-cm diameter) (23, 38, 48) and in porcelain gallbladder. Ninety percent of gallbladder carcinomas are adenocarcinomas, and 5% are squamous cell tumors. Well-differentiated adenocarcinomas of the gallbladder are highly aggressive. Gallbladder melanoma, leiomyosarcoma, and mixed tumor are rare. Papillary adenocarcinomas have a better prognosis and are more localized than other adenocarcinomas. Squamous cell gallbladder carcinomas metastasize late and have a better prognosis than adenocarcinoma. At the time of diagnosis, the histological type is less important in judging prognosis than the extent of the tumor. Four stages are recognized by histology:

Stage 1:   carcinoma in situ – intramucosal tumor
Stage 2:   microinvasive tumor – muscle invasion
Stage 3:   locally invasive tumor – all layers of gallbladder wall without cystic node spread
Stage 4:   invasive – invasion of the liver and other structures by lymph node metastases

Tumors of the neck of the gallbladder invade the common hepatic duct by direct extension. Spread occurs early via the veins to the liver and may selectively obstruct the ducts of segment IV and V in the liver. Percutaneous transhepatic cholecystostomy and endoluminal biopsy of the gallbladder wall may be used for staging these tumors.

Cystic Duct Carcinoma

Carcinoma of the cystic duct is very rare and accounts for 7.5% of all extrahepatic bile duct carcinomas. It is considered a separate entity from gallbladder carcinoma as its prognosis is much better. Cystic duct tumors may compress the common bile duct and mimic the Mirizzi syndrome (51, 56).

Percutaneous Therapy of Malignant Biliary Obstruction

The diagnosis of obstruction is made in most instances by ultrasound or CT scanning. Hilar obstruction is caused by bile duct carcinoma, gallbladder carcinoma, cystic duct carcinoma, hilar metastatic carcinoma, or hilar lymphoma (11, 18). FN PTHC or ERCP as diagnostic procedures have lost much of their importance when careful imaging of the biliary tract is performed in suggested obstruction. High-resolution ultrasound is used to diagnose the cause of obstruction in most cases of obstructive jaundice (26).

The interventional procedure chosen in biliary obstruction depends on the available expertise in the hospital or clinic. Whether endoscopic or percutaneous therapy is chosen, the procedure is palliative only, and it is essential to establish a histological diagnosis of the cause of obstruction before therapy is initiated. This may be achieved by fine needle aspiration or core biopsy of the site of bile duct obstruction or by bile cytology. The latter is the easiest method, but has a low yield of about 30% positive diagnosis with no false positives. Intraluminal brush or forceps biopsy is best for bile duct stenoses, while percutaneous biopsy is ideal if an extrabiliary mass is present. Both percutaneous and endoscopic stent insertion in malignant obstruction may be very successful in relieving biliary obstruction. Even in expert hands, these procedures may also be very difficult to perform because of the ampullary anatomy and the empty lower common bile duct in hilar disease at ERCP, difficult duct catheterization and passage through tumor obstruction during PTHC and catheterization or endoscopic catheterization. During endoscopic or transhepatic stenting of obstruction, a one-stage procedure should be carried out unless there is evidence of cholangitis. In the latter instance, temporary external drainage is performed until the infection resolves. Endoscopic drainage is performed by nasobiliary catheter. Transhepatic drainage is performed using a 9-Fr pigtail catheter containing multiple side holes. Care is taken to position the catheter so that all of the section of the catheter containing side holes lies within the bile duct and no side holes traverse the liver parenchyma. Intraparenchymal side holes cause bleeding from the catheter. *Only in rare exceptions are long-term drainage catheters used in our practice.* External drainage catheters are inserted anteriorly from the epigastrium via the left hepatic duct and fixed by suture to the skin of the anterior abdominal wall. With the anterior approach there is less danger of catheter dislodgment in the patient confined to bed (43). External catheters are irrigated daily without prior aspiration and by infusion of 20 mL to 40 mL normal saline.

Patients discharged on external drainage are instructed in catheter care and irrigation. Signs of catheter occlusion such as leakage around the catheter at the skin or evidence of cholangitis are explained to the patient who is instructed to seek immediate catheter replacement. We do not perform external drainage as a preoperative procedure except in acute ascending cholangitis as indicated above. Others consider it a valuable procedure.

Direct cholangiography without drainage in biliary obstruction is one of the most common causes of cholangitis in current practice whether this is performed by endoscopy or transhepatic cholangiography.

Types of Malignant Hilar Obstruction
(Fig. 15. **1**)

There are three common types of hilar obstruction:

1. Type I: Common hepatic duct obstruction
2. Type II: Combined right and left hilar duct and common hepatic duct obstruction
3. Type III: Combined segmental duct and common hepatic obstruction

Percutaneous transhepatic therapy is the preferred route for the treatment of malignant hilar obstructions. This is especially the case in tumors of Type II and Type III. Type I tumor obstructions may be treated by endoscopic or percutaneous stent insertion. *Careful imaging by ultrasound and CT should precede any drainage procedures to discover segmental duct occlusions that may not be demonstrated by direct cholangiography (18).*

Type II and Type III obstructions are treated preferably by percutaneous transhepatic stent insertion. Multiple segmental duct occlusions occur more commonly in the right lobe of the liver since the segmental ducts on the right are closer to the hilum than in the left lobe. The left hepatic duct has a longer segment without branches. If two or more ducts are involved by tumor obstruction in the right lobe above the hilum, we prefer to initiate drainage of the left lobe from an anterior approach and leave the right lobe undrained. Left lobe drainage is often sufficient to reduce bilirubin levels and relieve pruritus (11, 21, 26, 44).

In Type II obstruction there is a choice of bilateral right and left lobe drainage using a dual approach from the right axilla and the epigastrium. This double liver puncture doubles the possible complication rate of percutaneous stent insertion. A useful alternative is to insert two stents from the right axillary approach. The first stent drains the right duct system into the lower common bile duct and duodenum. A second stent is now inserted from the right to the left hepatic duct. This stent drains bile from the left lobe into the right duct system (43). Failed endoscopic stent insertion is an urgent indication for percutaneous stent insertion. *While failed percutaneous drainage does not adversely affect the success of endoscopic stent inser-*

tion, collapsed intrahepatic bile ducts and the presence of an endoscopically inserted stent can adversely affect the outcome of percutaneous stent insertion.

Contraindications to Treatment of Hilar Obstructions

Both *extensive metastatic deposits* throughout the liver and tumor involving multiple segmental ducts are contraindications to stent insertion by endoscopic and percutaneous transhepatic techniques because the liver responds poorly to the drainage procedure and the risk of complications is higher.

Ascites is also a contraindication since it may lead to peritonitis, cause difficulties in bile duct catheterization by the percutaneous route, and its presence usually indicates malignant peritoneal disease. The inability of the patient to lie supine without *dyspnea* is a contraindication to all transhepatic biliary procedures.

Percutaneous Stent Insertion in Biliary Obstruction

Preparation of the Patient

The patient is prepared as for any operative procedure. Coagulation studies should show a normal profile, or abnormalities should be corrected before the procedure is performed. Patients receiving anticoagulant therapy require reversal of the defect before bile duct puncture. Preprocedure antibiotics are necessary in patients with cardiac defects, including heart valve replacements, in order to avoid bacterial endocarditis.

The patient fasts for 8 hours before the procedure. Normal hydration is maintained by intravenous fluids. In all cases, antibiotics are given intravenously 1 hour before the procedure is performed. We do not use preprocedure analgesics or hypnotics for fine needle percutaneous transhepatic cholangiography (FN PTHC). Intravenous pethidine is given when duct catheterization and transhepatic track dilatation is commenced; it produces analgesia and sedation in doses of 50 mg to 100 mg.

Many methods of anesthesia and analgesia have been advocated for percutaneous biliary procedures including intercostal nerve block, which is a very simple and effective technique but does not eliminate the pain of transhepatic procedures. Epidural anesthesia is also an effective method of pain relief; for this, a well-trained anesthetist is required, which increases the cost of the procedure and adds the complications of this form of anesthesia. Some interventionalists advocate general anesthesia for some bile duct manipulations such as bile duct stricture dilatation. This increases the risks of the procedure but has the benefit

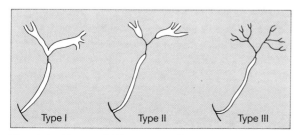

Fig. 15.**1**   **Types of hilar cholangiocarcinoma**

of complete pain relief for such dilatations, and pain is no longer a deterrent to repeated dilatations when or if these are necessary. The elimination of pain from the procedure has important results. The pain-free patient is more cooperative, the referring physician is more comfortable, and there is less morbidity from the procedure. The skin of the abdominal wall and right axilla is prepared by painting with antiseptic solution. This makes changing from a right axillary to an epigastric approach to the bile duct easier while sterility is maintained.

Percutaneous Bile Duct Puncture: Technique and Equipment

The patient is placed supine on the radiographic table, which incorporates high-resolution fluoroscopy (under table tube). All lead protection is removed to give direct access to the right axilla. The fluoroscopy and filming controls are covered by a sterile plastic cover (3M, USA or Siemens-Elema, Solna, Sweden). A single plane screening unit that is generally available in all radiology departments is the only X-ray equipment necessary for bile duct puncture and catheterization. We have not found it necessary to take lateral views of the liver for bile duct localization. The patient lies with the arms at his or her sides. Minimal fluoroscopy time screening is used, with the X-ray beam coned to the smallest area necessary for visualization of the needle, guide wire, and catheters during manipulations with the bile ducts. Using the axillary route of bile duct catheterization, the operators hands are never directly within the X-ray beam.

Ultrasound with 3.5 MHz and 5.0 MHz probes should be available in the fluoroscopy room for bile duct localization when necessary. Adequate space should be available for a sterile trolley, a drugs trolley, an assistant, a nurse, and an X-ray technologist.

The sterile trolley should contain:

Sterile gown and gloves
Local anesthetic without adrenaline
Needles for local anesthesia
Scalpel
Mosquito forceps
Containers of antiseptic and saline
Nonionic contrast medium such as Niopam 300, Ultravist 300, or Omnipaque 300
Syringes: 10 mL, 20 mL, 30 mL
Sterile surgical sheets
Sterile cover for X-ray controls
Sterile gauze and cotton wool
Chiba needle with ultrasonic tip
Guide wires
Dilators
Stents and pushers (Fig. 15.**2**)

Protection of Staff During the Procedure

The undercouch fluoroscopy unit results in the least amount of radiation to the patient, the operator, and the assistants. Standard full-length lead aprons are worn by all personnel present in the fluoroscopy room during the procedure, and through traffic of staff is forbidden during the procedure. Lead aprons should have all-around body protection because assistants present in the room spend a considerable amount of time with their backs to the fluoroscopy unit. Neck protection is also used. Because fluoroscopy times may be prolonged during catheter, wire, and stent positioning in the biliary tract, we strongly advocate special hand protection with thin lead-impregnated rubber gloves, which reduce radiation to the operators hands. Total fluoroscopy time for stent insertion varies from 20 minutes in some patients to a 60–90 minutes or longer in other patients. We have not used biplane fluoroscopy for this procedure although its availability would shorten the procedure; in some patients it also increases the radiation dose considerably.

Methods of Stenting of Biliary Tract Tumors

There are two basic methods of percutaneous stenting of biliary obstructions whether the right or left hepatic duct approach is used.

1. The *single-stage procedure* where FN PTHC, duct catheterization, stricture wiring, and stent insertion are completed as a single one-visit procedure. We prefer this method.
2. The *two-stage procedure*, favored by many authors until recently, where FN PTHC and duct catheterization are performed with external drainage for 48 hours followed by a second visit to the procedure room when the external drainage is replaced by stent insertion.

We only use a two-stage procedure if it proves impossible to negotiate a hilar obstruction with a guide wire at the initial cholangiography or there is evidence of gross biliary infection on FN PTHC, such as abscess demonstration communicating with the intrahepatic bile ducts.

A single-stage procedure should be undertaken if possible since it is preferred by the patient and the referring clinician, and it avoids introduction of infection from the external drainage catheter. It also favorably competes with endoscopic methods of stent insertion.

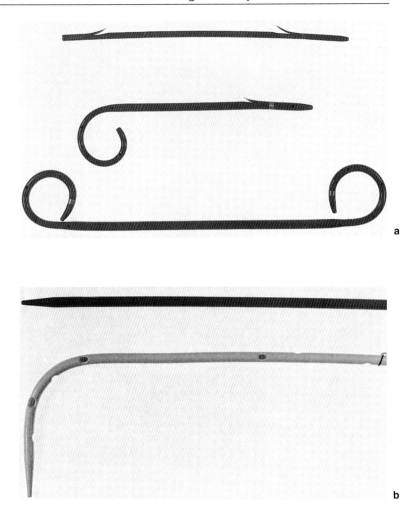

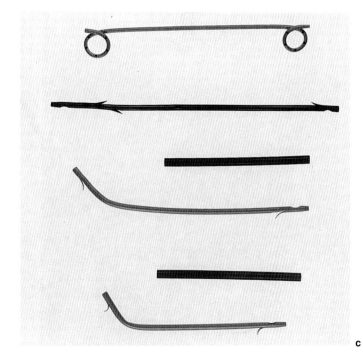

Fig. 15.**2   Stents for therapy of biliary obstruction**
a 7-Fr straight, 7-Fr single pigtail, and
10-Fr double pigtail for percutanous or
endoscopic stenting. Note metal
markers for stent visualization during insertion
b Distal end of Coon large stent with introducer
c 7-Fr long double pigtail, 10-Fr
straight, and 10-Fr straight fish-fin distal
curves

Guide Wires for Stenting of Biliary Obstruction

The interventional radiologist should have a superior knowledge of all available guide wires for negotiation of malignant biliary obstructions (Table 15.1).

The Terumo Radiofocus guide wire is valuable for negotiating strictures when other wires fail. This wire, however, may easily push the transhepatic catheter out of the bile duct if great care is not taken during its use.

Stents for Biliary Obstruction

There is now good evidence that long, large diameter stents remain patent longer than short, small diameter stents (8, 15, 26). Straight stents are reputed to stay patent longer than pigtail stents. We have not found this to be true in bile duct tumors. Metal mesh stents from several manufacturers are available (Table 15.2). These are very expensive and to date have not remained patent for longer periods than stents of other nonmetal materials. They require stricture dilatation before they are inserted across an obstruction. They also require insertion of a sheath through the liver into the bile duct for delivery of the stent on a balloon catheter. Therefore, insertion is not as simple as insertion of conventional stents.

In vitro studies have shown differences in patency rates for different stent materials. We have found that a 10-Fr double pigtail teflon stent inserted in an atraumatic manner and positioned correctly with the aid of metal markers incorporated within the stent at each end remains patent throughout the life of the most patients with malignant obstruction. In 107 patients treated by double pigtail 10-Fr teflon stents, 42

Table 15.1   Guide wires for biliary interventions

Lunderquist Ring Torque*
Amplatz Torque**
Amplatz Tapered Torque**
Amplatz Stiff*
Amplatz Superstiff*
Amplatz Extrastiff**
Lunderquist Rigid Wire*
Terumo M Glidewire***
Terumo M Stiff Glidewire***
Tadh 11****
Coons Superstiff**
Cope Mandril**
Flexifinder Blue*****
Flexifinder Black*****

* Cook, Denmark
** Medi-tech, Watertown, Mass., USA
*** Terumo, Japan
**** Peripheral Systems, Mountain View, Calif., USA
***** Flexmedics, USA

Table 15.2   Metal stents for internal biliary drainage

Gianturco Z stent (zigzag steel wire): self expanding (1)*
Wall: (steel woven tubular wire mesh): self expanding (2)
Palmaz: (steel latice tube): balloon expanding (3)*
Strecker: tantalum tubular wire mesh: balloon expanding (4)*
Accuflex elastalloy: (titanium) wire mesh self expanding (5)

* Inserted via a sheath
1. Cook, Denmark
2. Medivent, Lausanne, Switzerland
3. Johnson & Johnson, N.J., USA
4. Medi-tech, Watertown, Mass., USA
5. Medi-tech, Watertown, Mass., USA

patients had hilar obstructions. The stent was inserted from the right axilla (30 cases) or epigastrium via the left hepatic duct (12 cases). Five patients had a right hepatic duct to left hepatic duct double pigtail drainage in addition to the 10-Fr stent. Pruritus was relieved in all cases. Jaundice resolved clinically in 38 of 42 patients. All patients died eventually; 41 without recurrence of pruritus and 37 without recurrence of jaundice. In one patient, the stent remained patent for 19 months and was replaced by a second stent.

There were two procedure-related deaths in 107 patients treated. One was due to an unrecognized intrahepatic hematoma. The second was related to known myocardial infarction at 24 hours post stent insertion. There were no deaths in the hilar obstruction group related to stent insertion or stent occlusion.

Approximately 25% of hilar obstructions are endoscopic stent insertion failures related to the difficulty of endoscopic catheterization of the collapsed empty common bile duct.

Technique of Stent Insertion

1. Right Axillary Approach (Fig. 15. 3)

The most successful method of stent insertion with the least morbidity, in our experience, involves the use of the Chiba needle for "clean" FN PTHC followed by insertion of a fine .018 wire through the Chiba needle into the bile ducts. A relatively central duct is chosen, and intraparenchymal injections of contrast medium are avoided if possible during opacification of the bile ducts. We also opacify the ducts completely down to the site of obstruction.

When the fine wire is inserted into the bile duct, the Chiba needle is removed and a coaxial catheter (Accustick, Medi-tech, USA) is inserted over the wire into the bile duct. The fine guide wire is removed and replaced by a .038 guide wire after removal of the central catheter of the coaxial system. The .038 guide

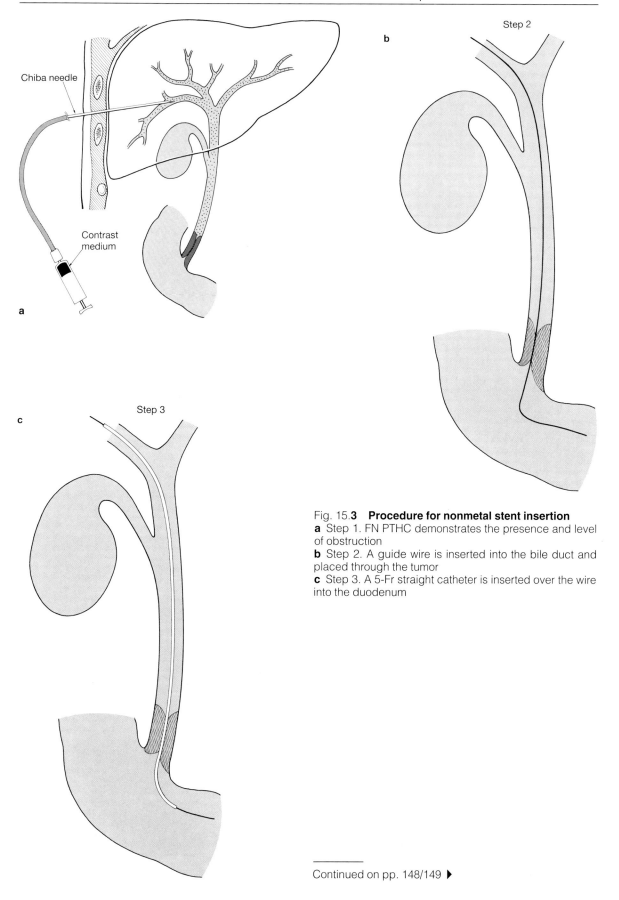

Chiba needle

Contrast
medium

a

Step 2

b

Step 3

c

Fig. 15.**3 Procedure for nonmetal stent insertion**
a Step 1. FN PTHC demonstrates the presence and level
of obstruction
b Step 2. A guide wire is inserted into the bile duct and
placed through the tumor
c Step 3. A 5-Fr straight catheter is inserted over the wire
into the duodenum

Continued on pp. 148/149 ▶

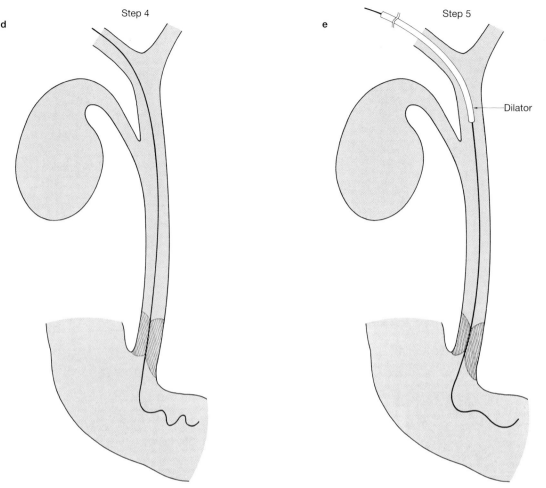

Fig. 15.**3**
d Step 4. A Lunderquist rigid wire is inserted into the catheter

e Step 5. The catheter is removed and a dilator inserted into the bile duct

wire is used to negotiate the hilar stricture. When this is achieved, it is passed well down into the duodenum. The coaxial outer sheath is replaced by a 5-Fr catheter, which is passed through the stricture into the duodenum. The .038 guide wire is now removed and replaced by a Lunderquist stiff guide wire, which is passed through the stricture and into the duodenum. A 7-Fr teflon dilator is now inserted over the rigid wire into the bile duct to dilated a track through the liver. While the Lunderquist wire is within the biliary tract, an assistant fixes the wire externally to prevent it passing further into the duodenum, which it may perforate if the wire is not controlled externally. The dilator is removed and the stent and a pusher inserted over the Lunderquist wire into the bile duct, across the stricture, and into the duodenum. The wire and pusher are now used to position the stent correctly within the bile duct above the stricture and in the duodenum or upper jejunum below. The Lunderquist wire is withdrawn followed by the pusher. *No external drainage is used after stent insertion.* Contrast is observed draining

into the intestine after successful stent insertion (Figs. 15.**4** and 15.**5**).

Postoperative Care

The patient is monitored carefully for signs of hemorrhage; antibiotics are continued for 5 days. If symptom free, the patient is discharged to primary care within 48 hours.

2. Left Hepatic Duct Catheterization

Following failure to cross a hilar stricture from the right lobe of the liver, the left hepatic duct is catheterized from the epigastrium using the same technique as described above. When the left hepatic duct is negotiated with the guide wire, there is seldom difficulty in crossing a hilar obstruction. The wire is passed to the duodenum and the procedure continued as described above. Advantages of the left hepatic duct route are that the pleura and diaphragm are avoided, chest complications do not occur, hemorrhage and

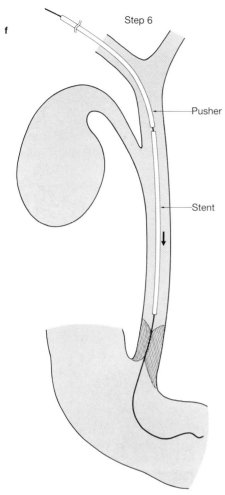

Step 6

Pusher

Stent

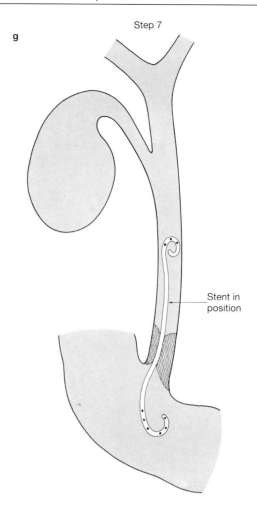

Step 7

Stent in position

Fig. 15.**3**
f Step 6. The stent is inserted across the tumor with the aid of a pusher

g Step 7. Correct positioning of the stent is achieved with the Lunderquist wire and the pusher. The wire is removed and then the pusher
Leakage does not occur around the liver if the obstruction is relieved by correct positioning of the stent across the obstruction.

other complications are less common, and biliary obstruction may be relieved for a longer period (21, 26, 44). The main disadvantage of left duct route stent insertion is the increased radiation dose to the hands of the radiologist.

3. Bilateral Duct Drainage from the Right Axilla

Following successful right-sided stent insertion as above, the pusher is used as a route of reentry for a guide wire into the right hepatic duct. An 18-gauge needle is introduced over the wire into the right duct system. The wire is removed and the needle is inserted across the liver into the left lobe and slowly withdrawn until bile enters the needle on suction with a syringe.

A guide wire is now inserted down the needle into

the left duct system. A double pigtail stent is now inserted over the wire into the left duct, and the wire is withdrawn leaving one loop of the pigtail in the left duct system and the second loop within the right hepatic duct. Bile from the left lobe now drains into the right duct system and from the right duct to the duodenum via the right-sided stent.

4. Bilateral Hepatic Drainage from the Right Axilla and Epigastrium

This requires percutaneous catheterization of the right and left hepatic ducts with the increased risk of two liver punctures and catheterizations for stenting. In order to prevent serious sepsis, bilateral drainage is essential in Type II hilar obstructions. Sepsis is more likely to occur if the percutaneous procedure has followed failed endoscopic drainage.

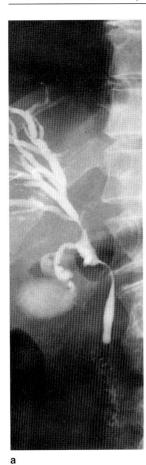
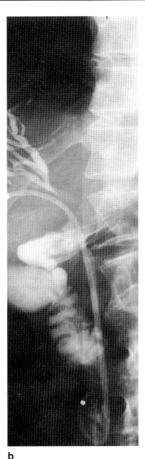

a   b

Fig. 15.**4   a FN PTHC showing hilar ductal carcinoma in a 67-year-old man**
b Percutaneous insertion of a 10-Fr teflon stent across the obstruction as a one-step procedure. The patient remained symptom free for 13 months

5. Percutaneous Insertion
of "Metal" Stents (Fig. 15.**6**)

All metal stents are inserted through a sheath. This sheath must always be inserted through the liver and into the biliary tract over a dilator. The average period before occlusion of a 10-Fr teflon stent in 137 patients studied over 3 years was 23 weeks and varied from 12 weeks to 1.5 years. Most patients died before stent occlusion could occur. This makes us reluctant to insert "metal" stents as a routine procedure because of their high occlusion rate due to tumor growth through the wire mesh of the stent. There is also a problem with removing these stents even for experienced biliary surgeons, while the teflon stent may be easily removed by endoscopic snaring when its lower end lies in the duodenum or jejunum. Metal stent occlusion requires insertion of a second stent alongside or through the occluded stent or reboring of the occluded stent. Metal stents are also very expensive, and those available to date are inserted sometimes with difficulty (6) and require further refinements in manufacture and design. The available stents include:

1. **Gianturco Stent** (Cook, Ind., USA; Angiomed, Germany)

This stent is constructed of stainless steel wire or laser cut steel plate in the form of a cylinder 8–10 mm in diameter and 3 cm long. The stent is housed in a 12-Fr cartridge and inserted across a stricture via a 12-Fr introducting sheath. When positioned, it continues to expand until the present stent diameter is reached. Multiple stents are inserted in long strictures; the first is placed at the lower limit of the obstruction. A pusher is used to transfer the stent from the cartridge to the sheath and across the stricture. Early results with this stent showed more promise in benign stricture treatment than in the treatment of biliary tumors (Irving, et al. 1989). In 16 malignant strictures, jaundice recurred in eight cases within 3 weeks to 8 months. All patients treated in this series required a two-stage procedure. The bile duct was catheterized and a Ring Lunderquist catheter inserted and drainage established "for several days" (26). Coons (1989) used this type of stent in 16 cases of malignant biliary obstruction and reported "biliary reconstructions" in cholangiocarcinoma with complex intrahepatic duct involvement. He reported a 10% occlusion rate at 6 months but indicated that the occlusion rate may be higher than stated. He also reported better results with benign strictures.

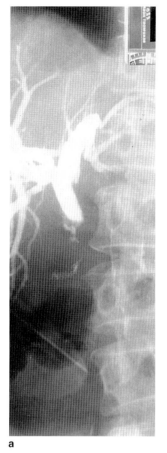 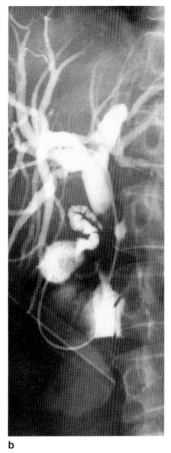 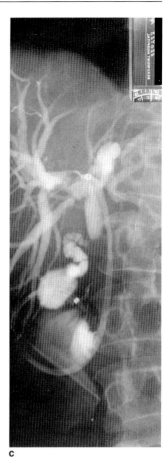

a   b   c

Fig. 15.**5   a FN PTHC showing hilar obstruction in known carcinoma of the gallbladder in a 62-year-old woman**
b A 10-Fr teflon stent was inserted from the right axilla. The patient survived for 9 weeks without recurrence of jaundice

Rossi et al. (1990) used this stent to treat benign bile duct strictures in 17 patients with good results in 14 of the 17 patients on follow-up for 21 months and concluded that these stents should only be used in selected cases of benign disease after several failures with balloon dilatation.

2. **Wallstent** (Schneider, Lausanne, Switzerland, Minneapolis, Minn., USA)

The biliary Wallstent is made of stainless steel wire woven into a tubular mesh. When fully open the stent has a diameter of 10 mm and is 8 cm in length. The stent is loaded in compressed form on a delivery catheter (9 Fr). It is held on the catheter, compressed and elongated by a plastic membrane. The stent is introduced through a 7-Fr sheath. The stent is positioned 2 –3 cm distally before membrane release since it retracts during its release. Balloon dilatation of the stricture in the bile duct before and after stent release is necessary for stent insertion and adequate immediate expansion. When the covering membrane is broken, the stent lies free of the introducing catheter. The stent shortens as it expands. Stent dilatation by balloon after insertion accelerates stent expansion and bile flow after relief of the obstruction. Gillams et al.

(1990) reported recurrent jaundice in 16 of 40 patients within 4 months of Wallstent insertion in malignant disease of the biliary tract. Fatal hemorrhage occurred in one patient within 72 hours of stent insertion, and septicemia occurred in four patients. Adam et al. (1990) treated 41 patients with malignant biliary obstruction with this stent and advised that it should be inserted via a 9-Fr sheath to avoid difficulties due to friction on membrane release for stent delivery. In four of their patients, jaundice was not relieved by stent insertion, and in only ten patients did bilirubin levels return to normal. In all other cases jaundice was significantly improved. Lameris et al. (1991) used this stent for palliation of malignant bilary obstruction in 69 patients. There were no complications of stent insertion. Twenty-eight patients with hilar obstruction received stents as did 41 patients with bile duct obstruction. Survival time varied from 1 to 15 months with hilar obstruction and from 1 to 8 months with common bile duct obstruction. Complications included septicemia in eight cases, bleeding from the pancreas after balloon dilatation of tumor in one patient who required transfusions, acute cholecystitis occurred in two patients with hilar obstruction,

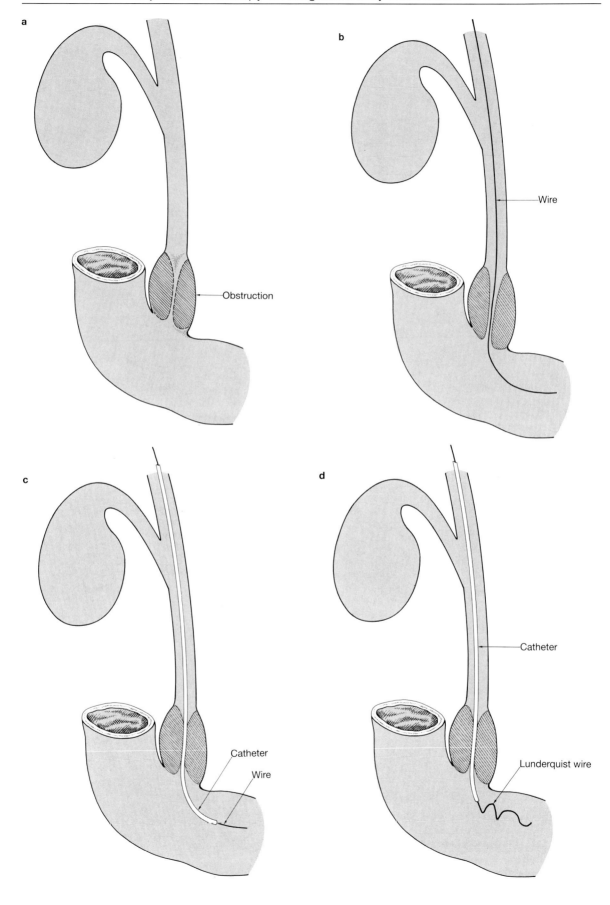

a

Obstruction

b

Wire

c

Catheter

Wire

d

Catheter

Lunderquist wire

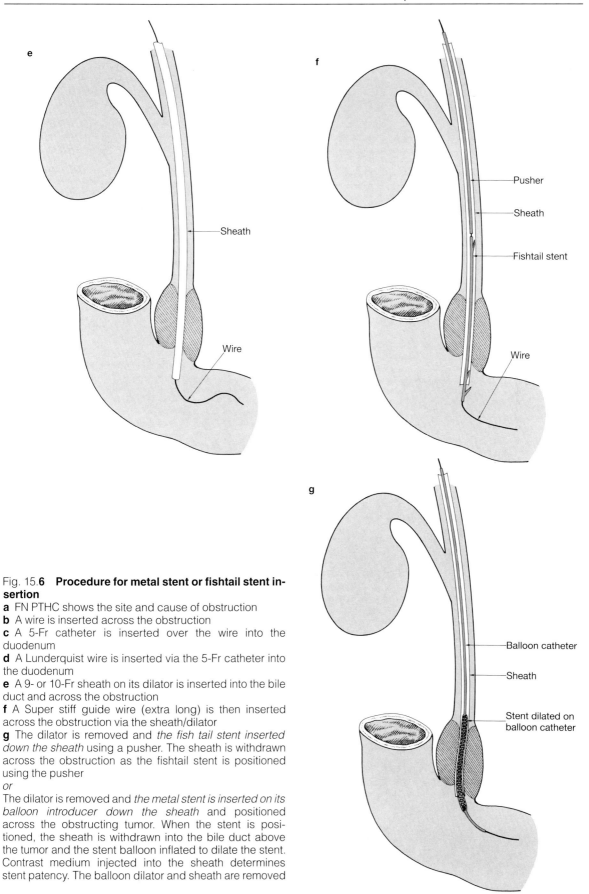

Fig. 15.6   Procedure for metal stent or fishtail stent insertion
a FN PTHC shows the site and cause of obstruction
b A wire is inserted across the obstruction
c A 5-Fr catheter is inserted over the wire into the duodenum
d A Lunderquist wire is inserted via the 5-Fr catheter into the duodenum
e A 9- or 10-Fr sheath on its dilator is inserted into the bile duct and across the obstruction
f A Super stiff guide wire (extra long) is then inserted across the obstruction via the sheath/dilator
g The dilator is removed and *the fish tail stent inserted down the sheath* using a pusher. The sheath is withdrawn across the obstruction as the fishtail stent is positioned using the pusher
or
The dilator is removed and *the metal stent is inserted on its balloon introducer down the sheath* and positioned across the obstructing tumor. When the stent is positioned, the sheath is withdrawn into the bile duct above the tumor and the stent balloon inflated to dilate the stent. Contrast medium injected into the sheath determines stent patency. The balloon dilator and sheath are removed

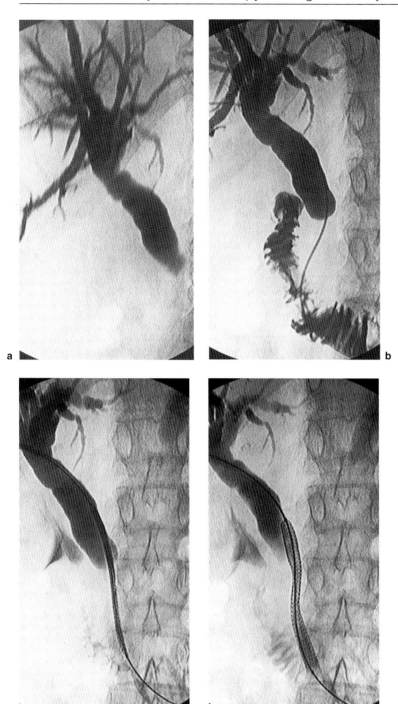

Fig. 15.**7 a FN PTHC showing carcinoma of the head of the pancreas in
an 84-year-old woman**
b, **c**, and **d** showing the steps for insertion of a metal stent, 8 cm, across the
tumor. This Strecker stent was dilated to
8 mm in diameter and remained patent
without cholangitis or other complications during the patient's life. She
survived 5 months

duodenal ulceration by the stent occurred in two
cases, and bile duct perforation by the stent at the site
of a tumor caused death in one patient 3 weeks after
stent insertion. Jaundice recurred in 10 cases. These
authors indicated the danger of inserting short stents
at the lower end of the bile duct.

Lammer (1990) treated 29 malignant biliary obstructions using the Wallstent. Jaundice recurred in 13% of
cases. Complications included hemorrhage from a
pseudoaneurysm of the hepatic artery, bile peritonitis,
and bile pleural effusion.

3. **Palmaz Stent** (Johnson and Johnson, Warren,
N.J., USA)

The Palmaz Stent is a balloon-expandable device
made in the form of a slotted, seamless stainless steel
tube, 3.1 mm in diameter and 30 mm in length, crimp

mounted on an angioplasty balloon catheter; it requires a 10-Fr sheath for insertion.

After positioning across the bile duct stricture, the stent is deployed by balloon inflation. Limited experience with the Palmaz stent in the bile duct has been reported (36).

4. Strecker Stent (Medi-tech, Watertown, Mass., USA) (Fig. 15.7)

The Strecker stent is a balloon-expandable device made from tantalum wire mesh mounted on a balloon catheter without any covering. The stent is held in place by two silicon rings that fix the stent to the catheter at the stent ends. It is available in lengths of 4, 6, or 8 cm and has a distended diameter of 8 mm. It is inserted through a 9-Fr sheath. The stent does not retract on balloon dilatation. Bethge et al. (1992) reported the use of this stent in 34 patients with malignant biliary obstruction. In 17 cases the transhepatic route was used successfully for stent deployment. Two stents showed incomplete expansion after balloon dilatation. They did not discuss the duration of stent patency.

5. Accuflex Stent (Medi-tech, Watertown, Mass., USA)

The Accuflex stent ist a self-expanding device made from elastalloy of titanium and woven from a single wire into a cylindrical mesh 3 cm or 6 cm in length mounted within its own sheat, which is 10 Fr in diameter. It has an expanded diameter of 10 mm without any shortening on expansion. The stent is inserted across the obstruction and released by simply withdrawing its covering sheath. It is a very easy stent to insert after balloon dilatation of a bile duct obstruction.

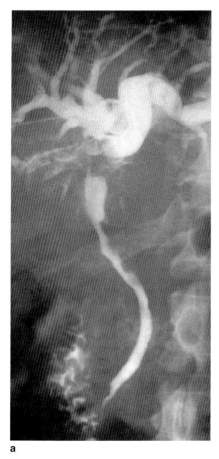 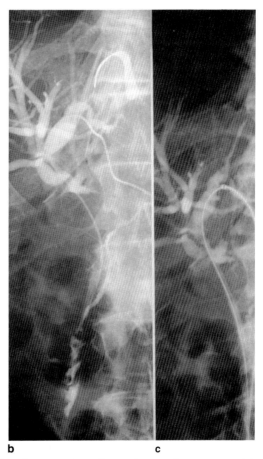

a   b   c

Fig. 15.**8   a FN PTHC showing almost complete hilar obstruction due to metastatic carcinoma.** Attempts at guide wire insertion from the right failed
b and **c** FN PTHC from the left by an anterior injection enabled the common bile duct to be catheterized and a 10-Fr Teflon stent was inserted. The patient survived 20 weeks without recurrence of jaundice

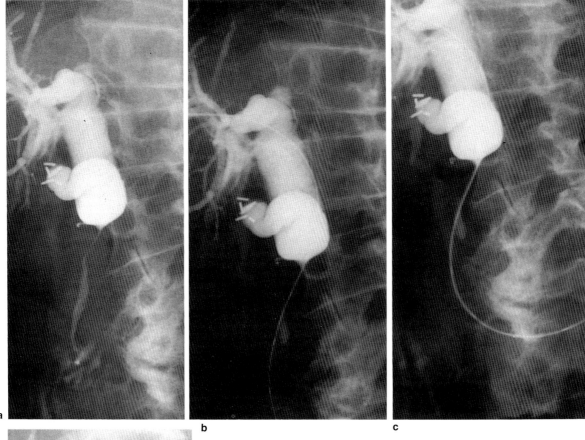

a

b   c

Fig. 15.**9   a FN PTHC showing carcinoma of the head of the pancreas**
b, **c**, and **d** showing the procedure for insertion of a 10-Fr Teflon stent

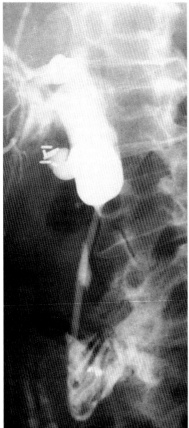

d

Stenting of Common Bile Duct Carcinoma

Primary cholangiocarcinoma is rarer in the common bile duct than at the liver hilum. The rat-tail stricture produced by this tumor usually produces no difficulty in crossing the lesion with a guide wire at FN PTHC. We always insert the wire well into the duodenum before commencing stent insertion. A 5-Fr straight catheter is inserted over the guide wire and the position of the catheter confirmed by fluoroscopy before the wire is replaced by a stiff wire used for stent insertion. Following dilatation of a liver track, the stent is inserted over the wire through the tumor and into the duodenum using a pusher. The stiff guide wire and the pusher are now used to position the stent correctly within the bile duct. Drainage of contrast medium to the duodenum is observed, and the guide wire and the pusher are removed. No external drainage is used.

Stenting of Periampullary Neoplasms (Fig. 15.9)

Most tumors in this region are pancreatic carcinomas. Some are ampullary carcinomas, and a few are primary bile duct neoplasms. Ulcerating periampullary neoplasms may be difficult to treat endoscopically due to difficulty in ampullary catheterization. Following FN PTHC, insertion of a wire into the common bile duct, and replacement of the fine wire by a standard semistiff wire, attempts are made to pass the wire into the duodenum through the tumor. This is achieved by varying the position of the lower end of the 5-Fr catheter to allow probing of the tumor in different areas until the lumen is found and the guide wire passed into the duodenum. In some tumors a semistiff glide wire (Terumo) is best for this purpose. After passing the tumor, a decision is made whether to use a "metal" stent or a standard stent. A standard stent is placed as described above.

Percutaneous Cholecystostomy for Stent Insertion in Periampullary Tumors (Fig. 15.10)

Percutaneous cholecystostomy is a valid method of biliary tract demonstration when FN PTHC fails. The bile ducts are always demonstrated when there is periampullary obstruction and when the biliary tract is normal. It is not useful in hilar obstruction.

Following the demonstration of periampullary obstruction by fine needle percutaneous cholecystostomy, the gallbladder is catheterized using a 5-Fr Thistle catheter. Three loops of this catheter are coiled in the gallbladder, and a second puncture of the fundus of the gallbladder is made using a Chiba needle. A fine guide wire is now inserted and coiled in the gallbladder. The Chiba needle is now replaced by a catheter (Accustick), and an .035 guide wire is inserted and coiled in the gallbladder. Dilators are used to dilate a track into the gallbladder (5 Fr, 6 Fr, 7 Fr, 8 Fr, 9 Fr). A steerable catheter is now used to direct the guide wire into the cystic duct and common bile duct and through the tumor into the duodenum. For this manipulation a Glide wire or semistiff Glide wire is best. When the common bile duct is entered the steerable catheter is removed and replaced by a 5-Fr straight catheter. The Glide wire is replaced by a stiff guide wire, which is used for stent insertion with a pusher as described above. This is a safe procedure in the absence of a diseased gallbladder wall.

When the stent is positioned, its proximal end must lie within the common bile duct and not in the cystic duct. Leaving the stent tip in the cystic duct will cause acute obstruction with cholecystitis or mucocele. The procedure is only useful when there is high insertion of the cystic duct, but it can be used when the junction of the common hepatic and cystic ducts lies lower down near the duodenum provided it lies above the upper limit of the tumor.

In this situation, a short stent with a single pigtail is ideal. When free flow of contrast medium is demonstrated via the stent across the obstruction into the duodenum the 5-Fr Thistle catheter is removed over a guide wire and the pusher is removed after complete emptying of the gallbladder. This does not cause leakage from the gallbladder in the absence of biliary obstruction.

Percutaneous Insertion of Metal Stents

Metal stents are inserted through a sheath without exception. Self-expanding stents exert a force on the tumor obstruction until their expanded diameter is reached. Balloon-expandible stents reach their expandible diameter after dilatation by balloon catheter. Dilatation of malignant strictures by balloon catheter or conventional dilator, such as the Van Andel catheter (Cook), which is available in sizes 3–12 Fr is recommended by some authors to assist stent insertion particularly with the balloon-expandible stents. Whether dilating a stricture before stent insertion is necessary or not depends on how hard the tumor mass is as judged during the initial insertion of a guide wire through it. Following FN PTHC and passage of a wire through a stricture, it is necessary to dilate a track to the bile duct to receive the necessary sheath size for stent insertion. For the Wallstent, a 9-Fr sheath is recommended. Gianturco–Rosch Z stent requires a 10-Fr sheath for its insertion. The Palmaz stent requires a 10-Fr sheath for its insertion. The Strecker stent requires a 9-Fr sheath for deployment across a stricture.

As with nonmetallic stents, it is best to insert these prostheses at the same time as the initial diagnosis of tumor obstruction is made by FN PTHC. Dawson et al. (1991) recommend that, whenever possible, metal stents should be deployed above the papilla to preserve sphincter function and preclude duodenal reflux. They also recommend external drainage of the biliary tract after stent deployment for 2–7 days.

Occlusion of Metal Stents

Recurrence of biliary obstruction after placing a metal stent may be due to (1) tumor overgrowth at the stent ends with the use of short stents. This is avoided by using long stents and centering the stent in the tumor stricture. (2) Tumor ingrowth and mucosal hyperplasia are unavoidable with metal stents. Covering the metal stent with silicone or polymer showed no difference in patency at 24 weeks with the Palmaz stent in animals. Common bile duct tumors showed the lowest

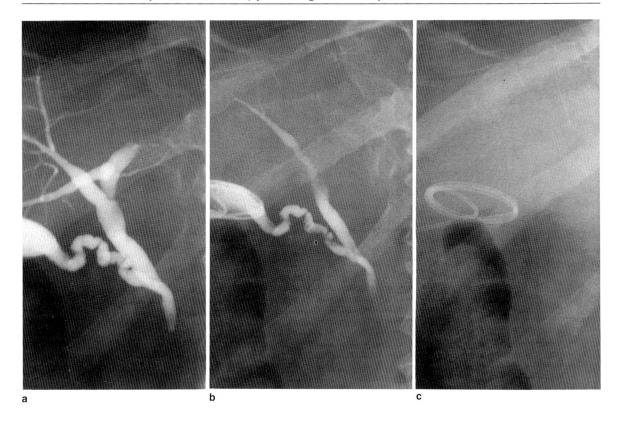

a   b   c

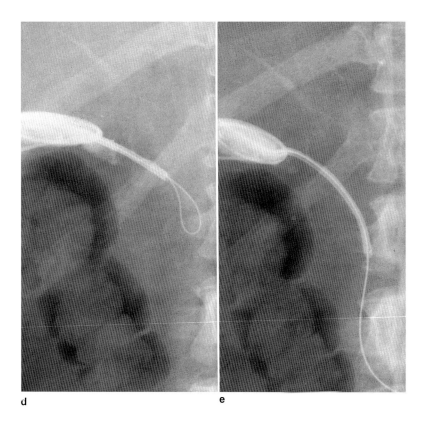

d   e

Fig. 15.**10**

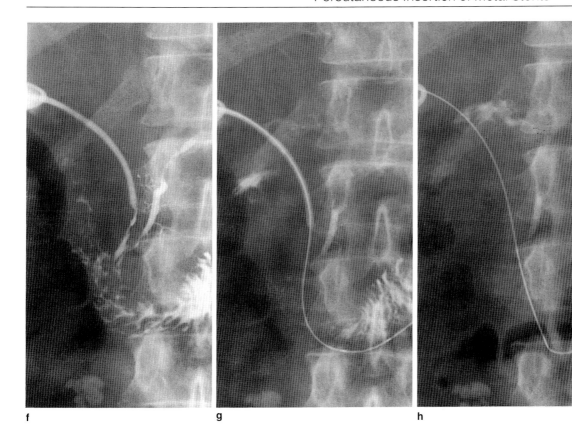

f   g   h

rate of occlusion compared to hilar tumors when the
Wallstent was inserted by experienced interventionalists (20). Stent occlusion with jaundice recurrence and
cholangitis requires urgent therapy including intensive care, antibiotic therapy, and reestablishment of
bile flow by wire and balloon stent dilatation, basket
clearance, insertion of a second teflon stent, or endoscopic stenting. (3) Stent migration occurs within the
first few days of stent positioning or during positioning. After that time, the stent becomes embedded in
the duct wall and does not migrate and cannot be removed, even by surgery (Figs. 15.**11** – 15.**16**).

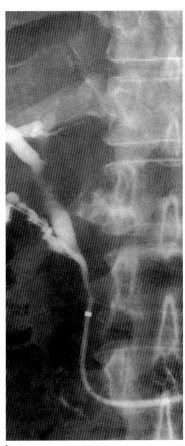

Fig. 15.**10**
**a FN PTHC showing nondilated intrahepatic ducts and lower common
bile duct obstruction due to lymphoma in a 59-year-old man**
b Fine needle percutaneous cholecystostomy was performed and the common bile duct catheterized via the cystic duct because of the absence of dilated ducts in the liver
c The gallbladder was drained externally for 24 hours after insertion and coiling of a 5-Fr catheter within it
d and **e** At 24 hours the fundus of the gallbladder was punctured and a track
dilated to the lumen. A steerable catheter was used to insert a Terumo guide
wire through the cystic duct
f Contrast injection demonstrates the common bile duct narrowing
g The bile duct was catheterized over the Terumo wire using a 5-Fr catheter
h The Terumo wire was exchanged for a rigid wire
i A 10-Fr single pigtail stent was inserted over the wire across the stricture and
positioned outside the cystic duct. The gallbladder catheter was removed. The
patient died from disseminated lymphoma at 10 weeks without recurrence of
jaundice

i

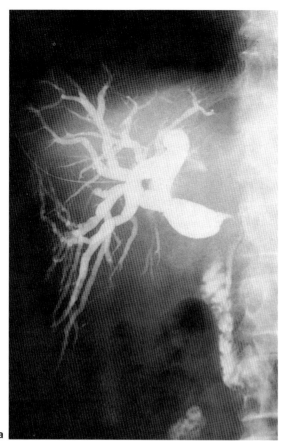 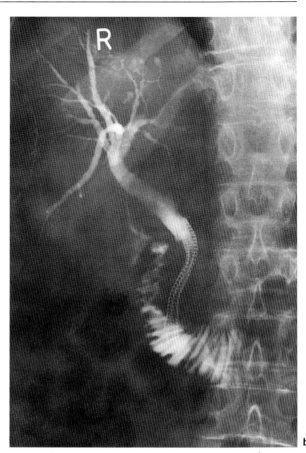

a

b

Fig. 15.**11**   **a FN PTHC showing carcinoma of the head of the pancreas**
b A metal stent, 10 mm in diameter and 10 cm long, was inserted percutaneously across the tumor. The stent remained patent at 5 months

Complications of Percutaneous Stenting of Biliary Obstruction

The major complications of percutaneous transhepatic stent insertion are liver laceration, hemorrhage, systemic sepsis, cholangitis, and bile leakage into the peritoneum. Other complications include duodenal perforation, acute cholecystitis, hemothorax, pneumothorax, empyema, biliary pleural fistula, malignant pleural effusion, and tumor spread along access routes. The pulmonary complications are avoided if the anterior, left hepatic duct route is used. Duodenal perforation is caused by the guide wire during stent insertion, and it is avoided by external fixation of the Lunderquist wire during stent insertion to prevent it perforating the duodenal wall. Liver laceration and vessel injury causes hemorrhage, a major cause of morbidity and mortality. Care in initial FN PTHC and use of a single liver puncture for cholangiography and stent insertion may decrease the incidence of hemor-

rhage. Bile leaks into the peritoneum are rare after successful stent drainage in biliary obstruction.

Systemic sepsis is a serious complication related to pus in the bile, and it requires intensive antibiotic therapy and major intensive care therapy. Cholangitis follows inadequate drainage or stent occlusion and requires removal of a blocked stent and drainage of obstructed liver segments. The cause of acute cholecystitis after stenting is unknown (42). It may be related to cystic duct obstruction by the stent wall.

Most reports indicate that a two-stage procedure was used in most cases for "metal stent" insertion following external drainage for "several days." We believe that stent insertion for drainage should be a "single-visit" procedure unless infected bile is encountered on initial catheterization of the biliary ducts. This avoids the possibility of introducing external infection to the bile.

A single-visit procedure also competes favorably with endoscopic stent insertion. Even though the metal stents are compressed into a relatively small

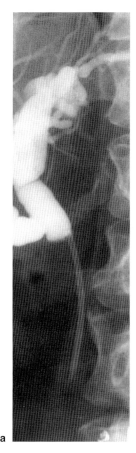
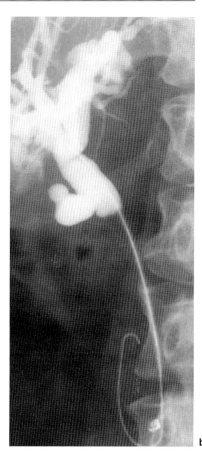

Fig. 15.**12   a FN PTHC showed upper common bile duct occlusion**
b A wire could not be passed through the obstruction. A 7-Fr dilator was pushed through the obstruction followed by a guide wire
c A 10-Fr stent was inserted across the obstruction into the duodenum
d Fine needle biopsy was performed at 24 hours
e Adenocarcinoma cells were aspirated

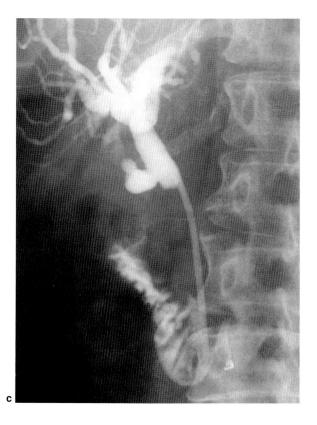
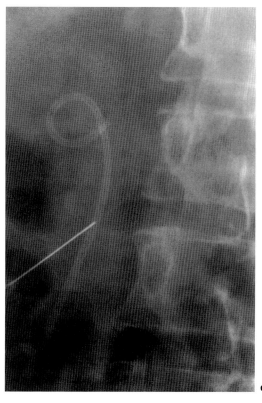

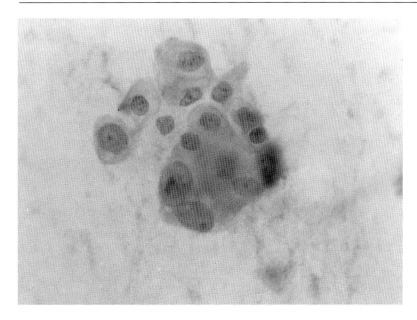

Fig. 15.**12e**

diameter during passage through the liver, similar complications have been reported after their insertion as with nonmetallic stents (3, 22, 26, 34, 36, 43).

Factors that Determine the Duration of Stent Drainage

Regardless of the type of stent inserted percutaneously or endoscopically into the biliary tract, (metal or nonmetal), or the stent configuration (straight, pigtail, double pigtail fishtail, mushroom, double mushroom), or the length of the stent shaft, there are certain factors that determine the duration of the flow of bile through the prosthesis and therefore the relief of biliary obstruction. Technical advances have broadened the spectrum of successful bile duct drainage. Endoscopic drainage has not replaced percutaneous drainage, and surgery still has an important place in the restoration of bile flow in malignant biliary obstruction and with one exception, primary bile duct carcinoma, offers the only hope of cure in malignant biliary obstruction. *The condition of the patient on presentation with malignant biliary obstruction regardless of the method of restoration of bile flow ultimately determines the duration of survival.* Percutaneous external drainage is associated with a significant incidence of infection and other complications in some patients but not in others. Surgical therapies have their own problems even though surgical therapy is more likely to be performed in those patients in better clinical condition.

Successful percutaneous stent insertion begins with successful FN PTHC without complications, minimal attempts at needling of the intrahepatic ducts, no perihepatic contrast accumulations, and care-

ful positioning of the needle for both cholangiography and duct catheterization.

Ideally, a duct is punctured for cholangiography, and the same duct is used for catheterization of the biliary tract and stent insertion. This duct should lie in close proximity to the first division of the right or left hepatic duct, and the needle should not traverse the pleural space when the axillary approach is used. From the punctured bile duct it should be easy to pass a guide wire into the common bile duct without problems of duct angulation, which may cause difficulties in wire insertion through a periampullary obstruction. Passing a wire through a hilar, bile duct, or periampullary neoplasm causes trauma to the duct mucosa, and in difficult cases, there is venous bleeding that causes clot formation within the duct above the obstruction. Making a passage through a periampullary neoplasm also causes some bleeding into the intestine, which may be more severe if a dilator is used. Using the single duct approach requires the use of a fine needle coaxial system as described by Cope (1982) that makes it possible to exchange the fine needle and an .018 guide were for an .038 guide wire when access is gained to the biliary tract.

Fig. 15.**13   a** FN PTHC demonstrated common bile ▶ **duct obstruction using an anterior approach**
b A guide wire was inserted from the right axilla
c A 9-Fr dilator was inserted through the obstruction
d A metal stent, 8 mm in diameter and 8 cm long, was positioned across the obstruction. There is some stent narrowing at the level of the tumor

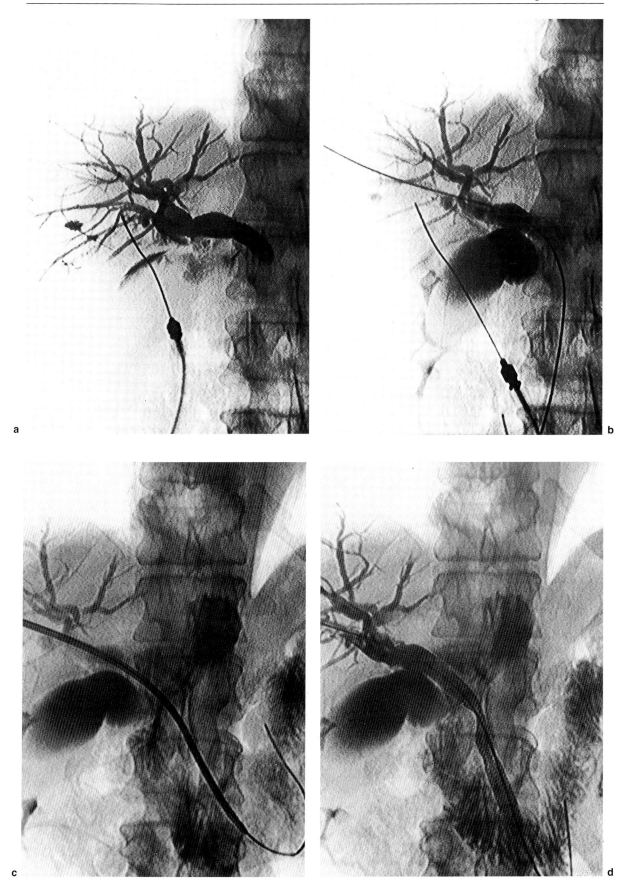

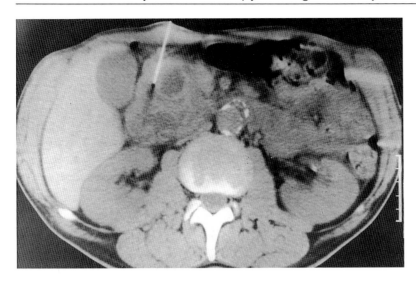

Fig. 15.**14   CT-guided core biopsy of complex mass in the head of the pancreas**

Negotiation of malignant hilar, common duct, or periampullary obstruction requires a selection of guide wires for continuous success in stent insertion. The Lunderquist Ring guide wire is one of the most successful in our experience. Tortuous obstructions may require the Terumo M wire or the Tadh II wire for successful passage through tight or tortuous obstructions.

It is better to switch to a left hepatic duct approach if difficulty is encountered in stricture passage after three or four attempts from the right duct system.

When an obstruction is passed by the guide wire, a 5-Fr catheter is inserted over the wire into the duodenum.

The .038 wire is exchanged for a stiff wire over which dilators are inserted until the required diameter is reached for nonmetal stent insertion or the diameter of sheath insertion for metal stent insertion is reached. Careful positioning of the stent with its middle third crossing the obstruction is essential to maintain stent position. The latter is maintained by combined manipulations with the stent pusher and the stiff guide wire when using nonmetal stents. With the latter we have never found it necessary to dilate the stricture before stent insertion. The question of pre–stent insertion dilatation of malignant obstruction when using metal stents is not settled. With tight strictures, it is best to dilate the tumor obstruction before stent insertion to encourage early bile flow and avoid the need for external drainage after stent deployment.

The Palmaz stent and Strecker stent must be dilated by balloon catheter after insertion to achieve stent expansion. The self-expanding Wallstent may also be dilated to achieve its final diameter, particularly in the presence of a tight stricture. Metal stents must be positioned carefully if early stent failure is to be avoided. The middle third of the stent should lie across the obstruction. Dawson et al. (1991) recommend external drainage universally after metal stent insertion and clamping the external drain for 24 hours prior to its removal. Failures with metal stents occur early from incorrect positioning, using a stent that is too short, stent obstruction by normal mucosa when short stents are inserted near the lower end of the common bile duct, or using straight stents in a curved bile duct. Later tumor overgrowth at the stent ends or through the stent wall causes obstruction. The former may be overcome by using longer stents or by tandem stenting. The ingrowth of tumor tissue or mucosal hyperplasia is an unavoidable cause of stent occlusion, which may be partly caused by balloon dilatation damaging the mucosa and leading to mucosal hypertrophy with luminal narrowing. Lameris (1991) showed that with the Wallstent, patency was longer in common bile duct tumors than in hilar tumors. With correctly placed stents, hilar obstruction occurs at the upper end of the stent by tumor overgrowth. In hilar and common bile duct tumors above the papilla, the metal stent is positioned above the papilla to preserve papillary function and lessen cholangitis associated with duodenal reflux. When two stents are inserted from the right and left hepatic ducts, the delivery sheaths and catheters are inserted across the stenoses and released one after another. If the hilar stenosis is long and extends into the common hepatic duct or common bile duct, a stent is first placed in the duct below the obstruction, and the two stents are released from the right and left duct systems with their lower ends within the first stent. With bile duct carcinoma, metal stent perforation of the duct has followed endoluminal irradiation. This has not occurred in our experience with Teflon stenting prior to endoluminal irradiation with iridium-192. Because this therapy may cure a localized bile duct carcinoma, it is best not to insert a metal stent in such patients.

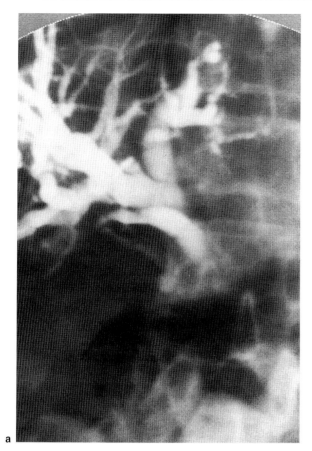

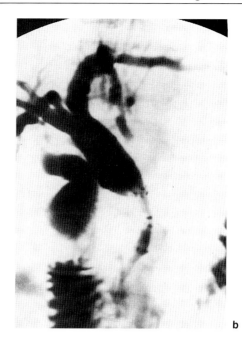

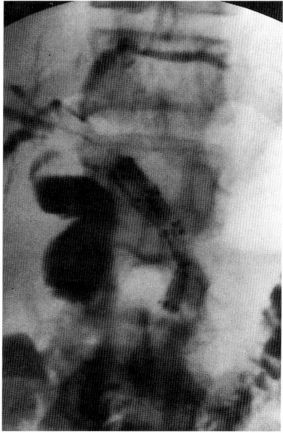

Fig. 15.**15   a FN PTHC in lower common bile duct carcinoma.**
b Cholangiogram after insertion of a long Z stent
c The biliary system has drained at three minutes. The patient survived for 5 months and was free of jaundice

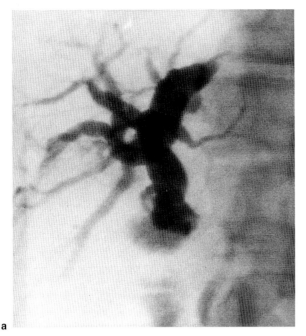

a

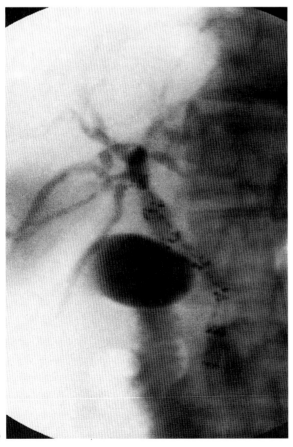

b

Fig. 15.**16 a FN PTHC in neoplastic obstruction of the upper common bile duct from gastric carcinoma.** **b** Cholangiogram after Z stent insertion showing free drainage and normal caliber bile ducts. The lower end of the stent lies above the papilla

References

1. Aabakken L, Karesen R, Serck-Hanssen A, Osnes M. Trans-papillary biopsies and brush cytology from the common bile duct. Endoscopy 1986; 18:49 –51.
2. Adam A, Benjamin IS. The staging of cholangiocarcinoma. Clin Radiol 1992; 46:299–303.
3. Adam A, Chetty N, Roddie M, et al. Self-expandable stainless steel endoprostheses for treatment of malignant bile duct obstruction. AJR 1991; 156:321–325.
4. Alexander F, Rossi RL, O'Brian M, et al. Biliary carcinoma. Am J Surg 1984; 147:503–509.
5. Anthony PP. Tumours and tumour-like lesions of the liver and biliary tract. In: Mac Sween RNM, et al, eds. Pathology of the liver. 2nd ed. Edinburgh: Churchill Livingstone, 1987:574–645.
6. Alvarado R, Palmaz JC, Garcia OJ, et al. Evaluation of polymer coated balloon expandable stents in bile ducts. Radiology 1989; 170:975–978.
7. Barth KH. Percutaneous biliary drainage for high obstructions. Radiol Clin N Am 1990; 28:1223–1235.
8. Bethge N, Wagner HJ, Knyrim K, et al. Technical failure of biliary metal stent deployment in a series of 116 applications. Endoscopy 1992; 24:395–400.
9. Bismuth H, Castaing D, Traynor O. Resection or palliation: priority of surgery in the treatment of hilar cancer. World J Surg 1988; 12:39–47.
10. Blumgart LH. Cancer of the bile duct. In: Blumgart LH, ed. Surgery of the liver and biliary tract. Edinburgh: Churchill Livingstone, 1988:829–853.
11. Bonnel D, Ferrucci JT Jr, Mueller PR, et al. Surgical and radiological decompression in malignant biliary obstruction. A retrospective study using multivariate risk factor analysis. Radiology 1984; 152:347–351.
12. Bret PM. Les techniques d'abord direct, dites invasives: opacification Directe, Prelevements, traitements par voie percutanee. In: Doyon D, Amiel M, eds. Voies Biliares. Paris: Masson, 1984:67–99.
13. Burcharth F, Efsen F, Christeansen LA, et al. Nonsurgical internal biliary drainage by endoprosthesis. Surg. Gynecol Obstet 1981; 153:867–860.
14. Cameron JL, Broe P, Zuidema GD. Proximal bile duct tumours. Ann Surg 1982; 196:412–419.
15. Carrosco CH, Zornoza J, Bechtel WJ. Malignant biliary obstruction complications of percutaneous biliary drainage. Radiology 1984; 152:343 –346.
16. Cohan RH, Illescas FF, Saeed M, et al. Infectious complications of percutaneous biliary drainage. Invest Radiol 1986; 21:705–709.
17. Coons H, Carey PH. Large bore long biliary endoprostheses for improved drainage. Radiology 1983; 148:89–92.
18. Coons HG. Self expanding stainless steel biliary stents. Radiology 1989; 170:979–983.
19. Dalton-Clarke HJ, MC Pherson GAD, Pearse E, et al. Fine needle aspiration cytology and exfoliative biliary cytology in the diagnosis of hilar cholangiocarcinoma. Europ J Surg Oncol 1986; 12:143–145.
20. Dawson SL, Lee MJ, Mueller PR. Metallic stents in malignant biliary obstruction. Sem Intervent Radiol 1991; 8:242–251.
21. Dawson SL, Neff CC, Mueller PR, et al. Fatal haemorrhage after inadvertent transpleural biliary drainage. AJR 1983; 141:33–35.
22. Dooley J, Dick R, Irving D, et al. Relief of bile duct obstruction by the percutaneous transhepatic insertion of an endoprosthesis. Clin Radiol 1981; 32:163–172.
23. Foster J. Carcinoma of the gallbladder. In: Way LW, Pellegrini CA, eds. Surgery of the gallbladder and bile ducts. Philadelphia: Saunders, 1987:471–485.
24. Gibney RG, Cooperberg PL, Scudamore CH, Nagy AG. Segmental biliary obstruction: false-negative diagnosis with direct cholangiography without US guidance. Radiology 1987; 164:27–30.
25. Gibson RN. Transhepatic biliary endoprostheses. J Intervent Radiol 1989; 4:7–12.
26. Gilliams A, Dick R. Dooley JS, et al. Self-expandable stainless steel braided endoprosthesis for biliary strictures. Radiology 1990; 174:137–140.

27. Gmelin E, Weiss HD. Tumours in the region of the papilla of Vater. Eur J Radiology 1981; 1:301–306.
28. Gray R. Percutaneous biliary drainage with emphasis on hilar lesions. Can J Gastroenterol 1990; 4:579–587.
29. Gulsrud PO, Feinberg M, Koretz RL. Rapid development of cirrhosis secondary to squamous cell carcinoma of the bile duct. Digest Disease Science 1979; 24:166–169.
30. Hall-Craggs MA, Lees WR. Fine needle aspiration biopsy: pancreatic and biliary tumours. AJR 1986; 147:399–403.
31. Hamlin JA, Friedman M, Stein MG, Bray JF. Percutaneous biliary drainage: complications of 118 consecutive catheterisations. Radiology 1986; 158:199–202.
32. Hodgson HJ, Maton PN. Carcinoid and neuroendocrine tumours of the liver. Baillieres Clin Gastroenterol 1987; 1:35–61.
33. Houthoff HJ. Surgical pathology of hepatobiliary and pancreatic tumors. In: Lygidakis NJ, Tytgat GNJ, eds. Hepatobiliary and pancreatic malignancies. Stuttgart: Thieme, 1989:21–45.
34. Irving D, Adam A, Dick R. Gianturco expandable metal biliary stents: Results of a European clinical trial. Radiology 1989; 172:321–326.
35. Jones BA, Langer B, Taylor BR, Girotti M. Periampullary tumours: which ones should be resected? Am J Surg 1985; 149:46–52.
36. Karani J, Fletcher M. Brinkley D, et al. Internal biliary drainage and local radiotherapy with Iridium 192 wire in treatment of hilar cholangiocarcinoma. Clin Radiol 1985; 36:603–606.
37. Klaskin G. Adenocarcinoma of the hepatic duct at its bifurcation within the porta hepatis. Am J Med 1965; 38:241–256.
38. Knox RA, Kingston RD. Carcinoma of the ampulla of Vater. Br J Surg 1986; 73:72–73.
39. Koo J, Wong F, Cheng FCY, Ong GB. Carcinoma of the gallbladder. Br J Surg 1981; 68:161–165.
40. Lai ECS, Tompkins RK, Roslyn JJ, Mann LL. Proximal bile duct cancer. Ann Surg 1987; 205:111–118.
41. Lameris JS. Ultrasound guided percutaneous transhepatic cholangiography and drainage in malignant biliary disease. In: Lygidakis NJ, Tytgat GNJ, eds. Hepatobiliary and Pancreatic Malignancies. Stuttgart: Thieme, 1989:115–124.
42. Lameris J, Stoker J, Nigs H, et al. Percutaneous use of self expandable stents in patients with malignant biliary obstruction. Radiology 1991; 179:703–707.
43. Lammer J. Biliary endoprosthesis: Plastic versus metal stents. Radiol Clin N Am 1990; 29:1211–1222.
44. Lee MJ, Mueller PR, Saini S, et al. Occlusion of biliary endoprostheses: Presentation and management. Radiology 1989; 170:975–978.
45. Leese T, Neoptolemus JP, West KP, et al. Tumours and pseudotumours of the region of the ampulla of Vater: an endoscopic clinical and pathological study. Gut 1986; 27:1186–1192.
46. Levin B. Diagnosis and medical treatment of malignant disorders of the biliary tract. Sem Liver Dis 1987; 7:328–333.
47. Lillemoe KD, Pitt HA, Kaufmann SI, Cameron JL. Acute cholecystitis as a complication of percutaneous transhepatic drainage. Surg Gynec Obstet 1989; 168:348–352.
48. Lygidakis NJ, Brummelkamp WH, Tytgat GH, et al. Periampullary and pancreatic head carcinoma: facts and factors influencing mortality, survival and quality of postoperative life. Am J Gastroenterol 1986; 81:968–974.
49. Manabe T, Sugie T. Primary carcinoma of the cystic duct. Arch Surg 1978; 113:1202–1204.
50. Mc Lean GK, Burke DR. Role of endoprosthesis in the management of malignant biliary obstruction. Radiology 1989; 170:961–963.
51. Mc Pherson GAD, Benjamin IS, Hodgson HJF, et al. Preoperative percutaneous transhepatic biliary drainage; the results of a controlled trial. Br J Surgery 1984; 71:371–375.
52. Mizumoto R, Kawarada Y, Suzuki H. Surgical treatment of hilar carcinoma of the bile duct. Surg Gynecol Obstet 1986; 162:153–158.
53. Robertson JFR, Imrie CW, Hole DJ, et al. Management of periampullary carcinoma. Br J Surg 1987; 74:816–817.
54. Rossi, P, Bezzi M, Salvatori FM, et al. Recurrent benign biliary strictures: management with self expanding metallic stents Radiology 1990; 175:661–665.
55. Smith PLO, Mueller PR. New perspectives in biliary endoprostheses; metal stents. Biliary Radiol Rev 1992; 1:143–155.
56. Trede M. Treatment of pancreatic carcinoma: the surgeon's dilemma. Br J Surg 1987; 74:79–80.
57. Uflacker R, Mourao GS, Piske RL, Lima S. Percutaneous transhepatic biliary drainage: Alternatives in left hepatic duct obstruction. Gastrointest Radiol 1989; 14:137–142.
58. Wagner JS, Adson MA, Van Heerden JA, Ilstrup DM. The natural history of hepatic metastases from carcinoma of the colorectal carcinoma. Ann Surg 1984; 199:502–507.
59. Walker JM, Kanzer BF. Cacinoma of the cystic duct mimicking the Mirizzi Syndrome. Am J Gastroenterol 1982; 77:936–938.
60. Weber J. Percutaneous Transhepatic Biliary Drainage. In: Lygidakis NJ, Tytgat GNJ, eds. Hepatobiliary and pancreatic malignancy. Stuttgart: Thieme, 1989:125–135.
61. Weinbren K. Tumours of the bile duct; pathological aspects. In: Blumgart LH, ed. Surgery of the liver and biliary tract. Edinburgh: Churchill Livingstone, 1988:793–806 and 1093–1114.
62. Wood CB. In: Van der Velde CJH, Sugarbaker Ph, eds. Liver metastasis. Basic aspects, detection and management. New York: Martinus Nijhoff, 1984:47–54.
63. Yee ANC, Ho CS. Complications of percutaneous biliary drainage benign vs malignant diseases. AJR 1987; 148:1207–1209.

16   Endoscopic Therapy of Malignant Biliary Obstruction

The only hope of cure in primary malignant biliary obstruction is radical resection. This is possible in only a small percentage of patients and then only in highly specialized surgical centers. Primary bile duct carcinoma is only rarely treatable by surgical excision, and attempts at preoperative staging are less than useful. Many patients with this disease are very old and often unfit for major surgery. Resections for carcinoma of the head of pancreas and bile duct carcinoma have a high morbidity and mortality. Biliary decompression by surgical bypass also has a high mortality rate in the elderly. Nonsurgical methods of palliation provide relief of jaundice with fewer complications and less mortality. Endoscopic stent insertion, percutaneous stenting, or the combined approach at stenting using large bore stents have improved clinical results in recent years. The ultimate duration of survival depends on the clinical state of the patient at stenting (2, 4, 6).

Technique of Endoscopic Stent Insertion

Preparation of the Patient

Imaging methods are used to define the site and cause of the obstruction. The coagulation screen should be normal. The patient should be in a normal state of hydration with an adequate urinary output. Prophylactic antibiotics are given to lessen the effects of biliary sepsis.

Diagnostic ERCP

Diagnostic ERCP is performed with a 2.8-mm channel duodenoscope. The exact site of obstruction and the cause are determined using forceps or brush biopsy if necessary.

Endoluminal Tumor Biopsy

When a suggested tumor is demonstrated, biopsy via the endoscope is performed with sawtooth forceps or by endoluminal brushing of the wall of the bile duct at the tumor site. The biopsy forceps is positioned at the tumor site by daughter scope and viewed directly for biopsy, or biopsy is performed aided by fluoroscopy.

The forceps is seen grasping the wall at the site, and the biopsy "bite" produces a tug on the opacified bile duct wall.

It is decided at this stage whether stenting is possible.

Patients with multiple strictures in the hilar ducts or intrahepatic metastases derive little benefit from stent insertion.

Pus in the bile is an indication for nasobiliary catheter insertion and delayed stenting when infection has resolved.

When malignant duct stenosis is demonstrated, the length of the stricture and its relation to the right and left hepatic ducts is noted. A stent of appropriate length and shape is then selected. The stent should be of sufficient size to allow free flow of bile through the obstruction. At present, straight stents are favored by the experts, and stents of 10 Fr or 12 Fr in diameter remain patent when correctly positioned across a tumor for longer periods than the smaller 7-Fr stents. The larger stents are more difficult to insert using the larger diameter endoscope. The 7-Fr stent may be inserted using the standard 2.8-mm channel side-viewing endoscope. When the main hepatic ducts show strictures, two small 7-Fr stents may be inserted to drain both lobes of the liver. The 7-Fr stent may be inserted without sphincterotomy and its added hazards. Larger stents require larger endoscope channels (4.2 mm), and a sphincterotomy is often necessary for stent insertion (4, 6, 7, 8, 9).

Endoscopic Sphincterotomy for Stent Insertion

Sphincterotomy aids the flow of bile and pancreatic juice when the stent is in position. It is easier to pass the papilla with a stent after sphincterotomy. Periampullary strictures and tumors may produce difficulties in cannulation of the bile duct, and the empty bile duct of a hilar obstruction may be difficult to cannulate. Standard sphincterotomy may be impossible in a periampullary tumor because of difficulties in duct cannulation. In this circumstance sphincterotomy using the needle knife is necessary. Short 2-mm cuts are made with the needle extended 2–3 mm outside its sheath and the needle raising the roof of the papilla at 11 o'clock.

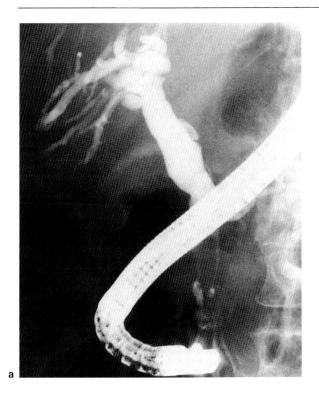
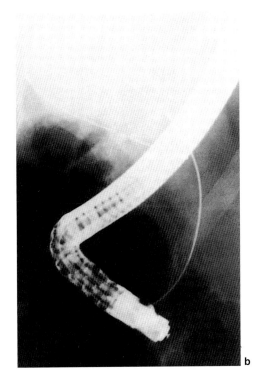
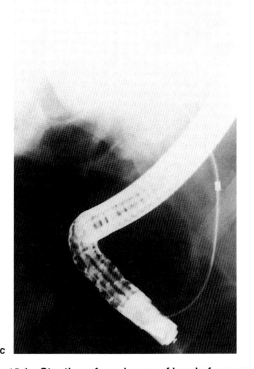
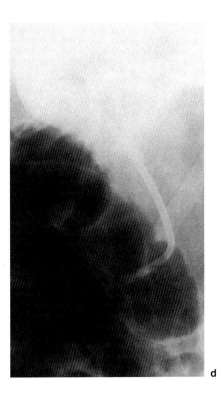

Fig. 16.**1   Stenting of carcinoma of head of pancreas**
a ERCP shows long strictures in the bile duct and pancreatic duct
b A guide wire is inserted into the bile duct
c A catheter is inserted over the wire
d A 12-Fr straight stent is in position across the biliary stricture

This is a difficult and hazardous form of sphincterotomy with the risk of perforation. If duct cannulation fails, the combined technique using a transhepatically inserted guide wire may be used for stenting. After sphincterotomy, the obstructing tumor is biopsied. A negative result does not, however, exclude tumor.

Stricture Stenting

Stenting of Periampullary Tumors

After cannulating the bile duct, injecting contrast medium, and establishing a diagnosis of malignant lower biliary obstruction, a decision is made regarding the size and type of stent.

A 7-Fr stent may be inserted by 2.8-mm duodenoscope. A 10-Fr or larger stent requires a 3.8-mm or 4.2-mm channel duodenoscope. We do not routinely dilate malignant strictures before stent insertion. Others consider dilatation essential to prevent stent impaction in the tumor.

The smaller channel endoscope is easier to position correctly and control than the large channel endoscopes. It is therefore easier for the inexperienced endoscopist to insert a 7-Fr prosthesis than one of 10-Fr or 12-Fr. Ampullary carcinomas, which are curable by resection, may be palliated by a small 7-Fr stent while awaiting surgery. Relief of jaundice due to pancreatic or lower bile duct carcinoma requires introduction of a large (10-Fr or 12-Fr) stent. After bile duct catheterization, a guide wire is inserted through the catheter into the bile duct and its tip passed into an intrahepatic duct without force. Excessive force produces false passages or an intrahepatic hematoma, or causes perforation of the liver capsule. The catheter is now removed from the bile duct using the "wire in–catheter out" maneuver. The endoscope tip is kept close to the papilla. The endoprosthesis is next inserted over the wire (7-Fr prosthesis) or over a previously inserted guiding catheter (10-Fr or 12-Fr prosthesis) and down the endoscope using a catheter pusher. The prosthesis is pushed through the tumor stricture with the pusher taking care to prevent a loop forming in the duodenum outside the endoscope. If a loop begins to form, the wire is withdrawn into the endoscope a short distance to remove the loop.

The prosthesis must be positioned accurately across the tumor by fluoroscopy and contrast injection if needed.

The wire is now withdrawn, followed by the pusher, once the proximal stent tip is lodged in the duodenum (6, 7, 9, 10, 14, 15).

Stenting of Hilar Tumors

Hilar obstruction may be due to bile duct carcinoma or to invasion from portal lymph node carcinoma. If only the common hepatic duct is strictured, a single stent is inserted with its proximal end in a right or left hepatic duct. When both the right and left main hepatic ducts are strictured, ideally, both ducts should be stented. This is, however, not possible in 60% of patients. The alternatives are to stent the right duct from below and the left duct percutaneously from above, or to only stent one duct. This usually relieves jaundice and pruritus but may be associated with cholangitis from the undrained lobe of the liver. An endoprosthesis caliber of 7 Fr is adequate for hilar duct stenting in bilateral right and left hepatic duct strictures. The procedure for hilar stenting is similar to that used for periampullary stenting. The guide wire is lodged in a peripheral hepatic duct. The catheter is removed. The 7-Fr stent is inserted over the wire by pusher through the endoscope, through the papilla, and through the hilar stricture. The wire and pusher are removed as above after the lower end of the stent has been passed into the duodenum from the endoscope (8, 10, 13, 15, 16).

The *combined transhepatic endoscopic technique* of transhepatic long guide wire insertion into the duodenum via a transhepatic needle/catheter may also be used to insert a stent endoscopically. The wire is withdrawn through the endoscope, and using the advantage of a taut wire by traction at both ends, the stent is inserted over the wire using the pusher to position it across the tumor stricture.

Postprocedure Care of the Patient

Antibiotics are given for 72 hours or longer if there is any suggestion of cholangitis. Pruritus should resolve within 48 hours if the stent is draining bile. Jaundice due to biliary obstruction resolves within 7–10 days (4, 4, 10, 15).

Complications of Stenting of Biliary Obstruction

Early complications occur in 20–30% of cases within 48 hours.

Cholangitis is the most common early complication. It is more common after stenting of hilar obstructions than of periampullary tumors. It is more common with the use of 7-Fr stents than 10-Fr stents.

Early stent occlusion by blood clot or incorrect positioning within the duct lumen causing stent occlusion or stent dislodgement may occur. Symptoms may mimic cholangitis. Stent positioning may be easily checked by abdominal radiography. HIDA scanning or repeat ERCP are used to confirm stent occlusion.

Late complications of stenting of biliary obstruction include stent occlusion in 20 30% of cases after a me-

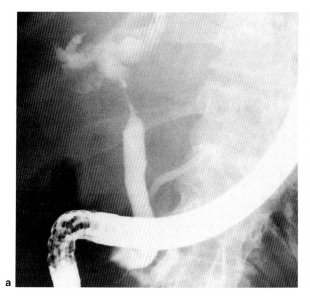

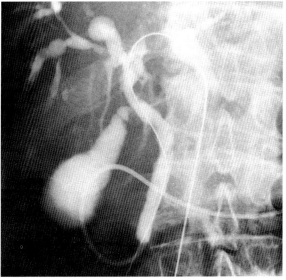

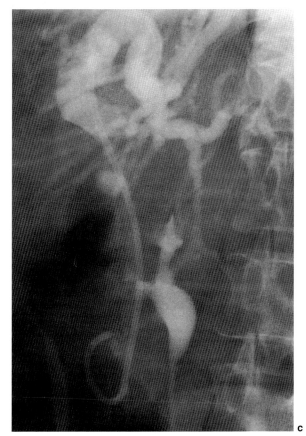

Fig. 16.**2   a Hilar cholangiocarcinoma**
b Nasobiliary catheter in right hepatic duct for radiation therapy. Percutaneous wire insertion into the duodenum via the left hepatic duct for stenting
c Stent inserted into the left duct

dian stent patency of 32 weeks for 10 Fr and 10–12 weeks for a 7-Fr or 8-Fr stent.

Stent occlusion causes cholangitis and jaundice. The stent is immediately removed by grasping the duodenal end by wire basket and replacing it with a new stent.

Rarer complications include duodenal obstruction by tumor, upward or downward migration of the stent, bile duct perforation, duodenal ulceration, or perforation by the stent. Acute cholecystitis may occur at any time due to tumor obstruction of the cystic duct.

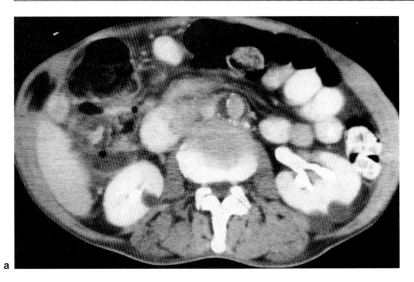

a

Fig. 16.3   **a CT scan showing ampullary carcinoma invading the duodenum**
b ERCP showing biliary obstruction at the papilla
c Nasobiliary catheter inserted into the common hepatic duct. The wire in the common bile duct is a guard wire. The wire at the lower end is the radioactive needle wire in correct position. The pusher guide wire is visible being removed from the nasobiliary catheter

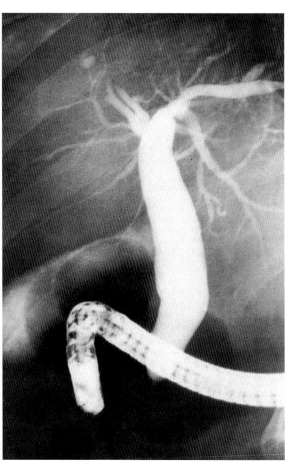

b

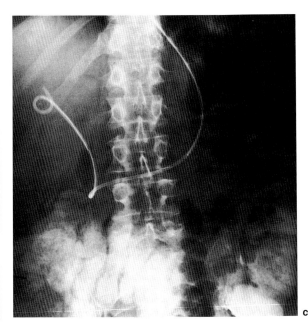

c

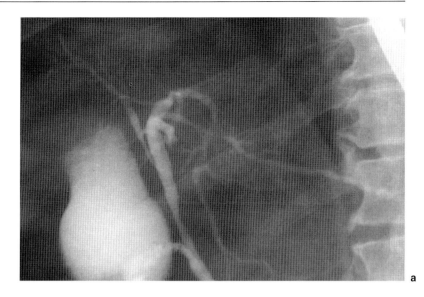

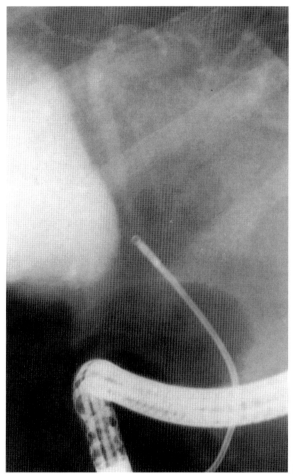

Fig. 16.**4   a ERCP showing narrowing in the common
hepatic duct**
b Forceps biopsy inserted for biopsy of the margin of the
lesion,—an early cholangiocarcinoma

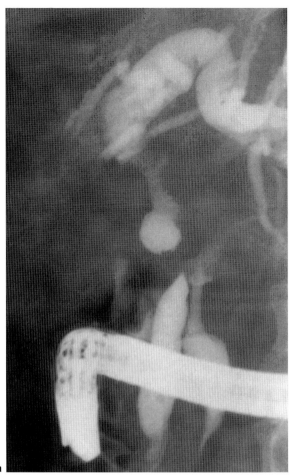
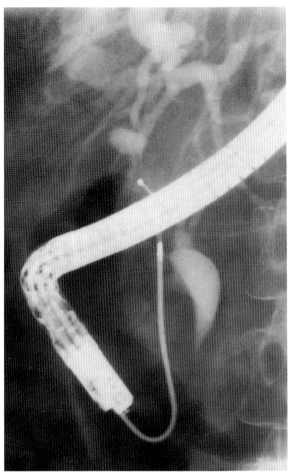

Fig. 16.**5**   **a Long stricture, common hepatic duct**   **b** Brush biopsy of the lesion

Failure of Stent Insertion

Failed stent insertion may be due to inability to enter the duodenum due to stenosis by neoplasm, failed sphincterotomy, or failure to pass a wire through the tumor obstruction.

Results of Stent Insertion

Pancreatic tumors (6, 8, 9)

Large stents (10 Fr or larger) in pancreatic carcinomas remain patent for 21–26 weeks when inserted by experts (1, 2, 6). Stent insertion was successful in 80% to 95% of cases and had a 30-day mortality of 5–10%. Early cholangitis occurred in 12% of cases and late stent occlusion occurred in 17–29% of cases. Mean survival time was 21–26 weeks.

Hilar tumors (1, 4, 6, 7, 8, 9, 15)

In malignant hilar obstruction, stent insertion was successful in 70% to 80% of cases. The higher insertion success was for common hepatic duct obstructions. Drainage was successful in 50% to 90% of cases (higher for the common hepatic duct).

The 30-day mortality was 7–20%. Early complications occurred in 15% of cases, and survival time ranged from 12 to 20 weeks.

Conclusions

Endoscopic stent insertion is a valuable procedure in malignant biliary obstruction when performed competently. Then, stent size determines the outcome of the procedure. This is limited by endoscope channel size unless metal stents are inserted. Preliminary stud-

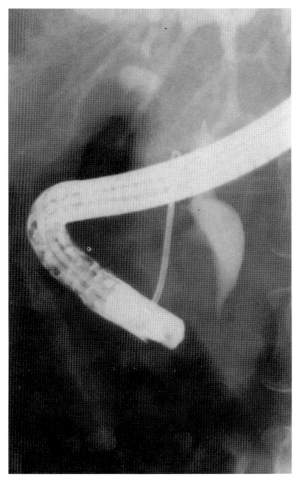

Fig. 16.**5c**   Forceps biopsy of the lesion

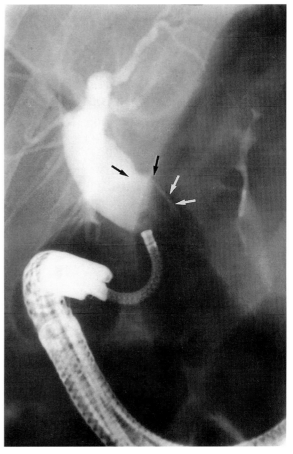

Fig. 16.**6   Polypoid lesion, upper common bile duct** (arrows)
The mother/daughter scope is in position for direct inspection of the lesion—an endoluminal carcinoma—and for biopsy under direct vision

ies with endoscopically inserted metal stents are still limited and show some initial technical problems with stent deployment. It is also important to remember that these stents cannot be removed once inserted. Balloon-expandable and self-expanding metal stents may be the way forward in the endoscopic therapy of malignant biliary obstruction.

Endoluminal Iridium-192 Irradiation of Biliary Tumors

Endoluminal irradiation with iridium-192 needles delivers a high radiation dose to a small volume of tissue in a short period of time with less morbidity than external radiotherapy. A transhepatic or endoscopically inserted catheter is positioned across the tumor site. We use a nasobiliary catheter and insert the catheter into the duct with its tip above the tumor obstruction.

The radioactive source is inserted after inserting a short length of guide wire. The guide wire prevents the iridium being expelled into the bile duct accidently during iridium needle positioning by guide wire. The length of radioactive source used depends on the length of the malignant stricture. The duration of treatment depends on the activity of the source. After therapy is completed, a stent is inserted across the obstruction. We have used this treatment with success in bile duct carcinoma, pancreatic head carcinoma, and hilar cholangioma. There were no complications directly related to the therapy in 22 patients treated. Post-treatment prosthesis insertion increases the duration of stent patency. The therapy relieved pain in pancreatic head tumors and converted bile duct carcinoma into a non-neoplastic biliary stricture.

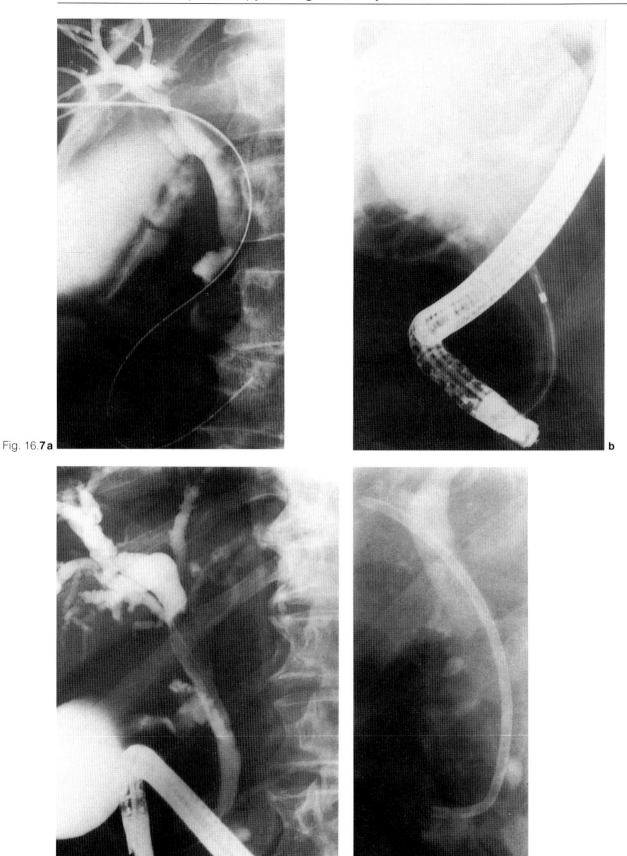

Fig. 16.**7a**

b

Fig. 16.**8a**

b

References

1. Carr-Locke DL. Endoscopic exchange in biliary prosthesis procedures. Lancet 1988; 2:903.
2. Classen M, Geenan MJ, Kawai K. Nonsurgical biliary drainage. Berlin: Springer, 1984.
3. Cotton PB. Progress report, ERCP. Gut 1977; 18:316 –343.
4. Cotton PB, Williams CB. Practical gastrointestinal endoscopy. 3rd ed. Oxford: Blackwell, 1990:85 – 117.
5. Hannigan BF, Keeling PWN, Stavin B, Thompson RPH. Hyperamylasemia after ERCP with ionic and nonionic contrast media. Gastrointest Endosc 1985; 31:109 – 110.
6. Huibregtse K. Endoscopic biliary and pancreatic drainage. Stuttgart: Thieme, 1988.
7. Jacobson IM, ed. ERCP: diagnostic and therapeutic applications. Amsterdam: Elsevier, 1989.
8. Laurence BH. Endoscopic stenting in malignant biliary obstruction. In: Bennett JR, Hunt RH, eds. Therapeutic endoscopy and radiology of the gut. London: Chapman and Hall 1990: 286 – 308.
9. Liguory C, Sahel J. Endoscopie digestive Practique. Padova: Piccin, 1988:230 – 241.
10. Lux G. Retrograde cholangiopankreatikographie (ERCP). In: Fruhmorgen P, ed. Diagnostische und therapeutische Endoskopie in der Gastroenterologie. Berlin: Springer, 1991: 128 – 147.
11. Mirsa RP, Divivedi M. Pancreaticobiliary ductal union. Gut 1989; 31:1144 – 1149.
12. Ohto M, Ono T, Tsuchiya Y, et al. Cholangiography and Pancreatography. Tokyo: Igaku Shoin, 1978.
13. Pott G, Schrameyer B. ERCP. Toronto: Decker, 1989:3 – 188.
14. Siegel JH. Endoscopic retrograde cholangiopancreatography. New York: Raven Press, 1992:25 – 122.
15. Sivak MV, ed. Gastrointestinal endoscopy. Philadelphia: Saunders, 1989.
16. Tulassay Z. Serum enzyme changes after ERCP. Endoscopy 1989; 21:197 – 198.
17. Warwick F, Anderson RJL, Braganza JM. Sclerosing cholangitis-like changes in pancreatic disease. Clin Radiol 1985; 36:51 – 56.

◄ Fig. 16.**7** **a Transhepatic wire insertion into the duodenum in failed duct cannulation by endoscopy**
b Subsequent stent insertion across a lower bile duct carcinoma

Fig. 16.**8** **a Polypoid neoplasm, common hepatic duct**
b 12-Fr stent inserted while awaiting endoluminal radiation therapy

Interventional Procedures in Diseases of the Hepatic Vasculature and Portal System

180

17 Interventional Procedures in Vascular Diseases of the Liver

Interventional vascular procedures are performed using Seldinger technique catheterization of the femoral artery (24) or by a transvenous route via the right jugular vein, an antecubital vein, or the femoral vein. Percutaneous transhepatic venous access to the portal vein and percutaneous transhepatic puncture of hepatic artery aneurysms are other important techniques of vascular intervention.

Selective Arteriography of the Liver

We use the transfemoral route for access to the liver arteries. Under local anesthesia, the femoral artery is punctured with a short beveled needle below the inguinal ligament following a 5-mm vertical (not transverse) skin incision over the artery. The short beveled needle prevents the guide wire from dissecting of the artery during insertion and the vertical skin incision from inadvertently sectioning of femoral artery if the artery lies in an anomalous superficial position. A 7-Fr catheter is adequate for most interventions. Catheters for embolization should have an end hole only. We introduce this via a vascular sheath. The sheath makes changing the catheter easier, and a long sheath may be used to assist selective catheterization when there is atheroma and vessel tortuosity, particularly in the elderly. The simplest catheter for abdominal visceral arteriography is a single curve catheter (2).

It is introduced into the celiac or superior mesenteric artery from above the vessel. To selectively catheterize the hepatic artery following celiac axis catheterization, a J (3-mm radius) stainless steel guide wire with a 3–4 cm soft tip is advanced into the hepatic artery, and with the rigid part of the guide wire well into the vessel, the catheter is advanced over the wire into a superselective position.

The success of this method of hepatic artery catheterization depends on how far the catheter tip lies in the celiac axis before the guide wire is inserted.

Another method of hepatic artery catheterization uses a hepatic curve catheter. This catheter is inserted to the aortic arch and rotated clockwise to reform the hepatic curve. At the level of the celiac artery the catheter shaft lies on the right side of the aorta, and the tip lies anteriorly. It is gently pulled down and into the celiac artery with a counterclockwise rotation of the

catheter shaft, and its tip slides easily into the common hepatic artery. A J or C guide wire lying just outside the catheter tip during this maneuver prevents intimal damage. For superselective catheterization we use a Tracker 18, 3 Fr, or a Mag 3-Fr catheter introduced through a single curve 7-Fr catheter (Table 17.1). An open curve catheter with a large radius passes further into the hepatic artery than any type of double curve catheter (4, 13). Attempts at single vessel selective or superselective catheterization require great care to avoid intimal dissection since this precludes intervention through the catheter. We are of the

Table 17.1 Catheter shapes for visceral selective arteriography

1. Large radius loop catheter. 7 Fr*

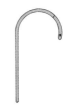

2. Simmons catheter **a** Hepatic **b** Splenic**

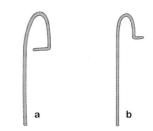

a   b

3. Tracker catheter***

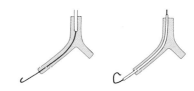

*   Balt, Montmorency, France
**   Cook, Denmark
***   Target Therapeutics, San Jose, Cal., USA

opinion that embolization procedures should be completed within 60 minutes of femoral artery catheterization.

An adequate knowledge of one or two methods of catheterization with the correct catheter shape and a knowledge of guide wires and careful preparation for a particular procedure are essential for success. The successful interventional radiologist does not try for hours with an ineffective technique.

Hemobilia

Hemobilia, or bleeding into the biliary tract, occurs when trauma or disease causes an abnormal communication to develop between an intrahepatic blood vessel and a bile duct (21). Most hemorrhage of clinical consequence is arterial in origin except in portal hypertension when portal vein trauma may cause significant bleeding. Glisson (1645) discussed the possibility of bleeding from the biliary tract in a case of penetrating liver trauma after a duel (10). Iatrogenic liver trauma is the major cause of hemobilia in current practice (7, 18, 21). Diagnostic and interventional procedures in the liver including liver biopsy, percutaneous transhepatic cholangiography with drainage, and endoscopic drainage of hilar obstructions are common causes. Iatrogenic bleeding is usually from the right lobe of the liver following conventional "blind" liver biopsy or percutaneous drainage via a right axillary approach.

Fine needle biopsy using 19–21-gauge needles rarely causes hemorrhage, but the risk is greater with 14–18-gauge needles (31). There is a direct correlation between the size of the needle and the complication rate (19). The risk is greater in the presence of dilated bile ducts.

Percutaneous drainage of the left lobe of the liver may also cause hemobilia from the left hepatic ducts. Attempts at endoscopic guide wire insertion for intrahepatic duct catheterization prior to stenting of hilar neoplasms may cause hemobilia by injury to the blood vessels in the right or left lobe by false passage formation. Endoscopic or transhepatic sphincterotomy may cause injury to a branch of the gastroduodenal artery, usually the posterior superior pancreaticoduodenal artery, with torrential ampullary hemorrhage (23). During interventional procedures in the biliary tract, there is almost always some bleeding into the bile ducts, which may be visible on cholangiography or at endoscopy. This is most common when attempts are made to pass a guide wire through a neoplastic obstruction.

Generally, a clot cast in the bile ducts indicates venous bleeding since slow bleeding causes clot formation, while fast bleeding from arterial injury remains fluid and mixes with bile (14). Pulsating blood from a transhepatic catheter or from the ampulla of Vater at endoscopic catheterization indicates arterial injury. This is an indication for arterial catheterization and embolization of the bleeding point in the liver or branch of the gastroduodenal artery. Bleeding at endoscopic sphincterotomy is more common when the bile duct is not dilated. Peripheral duct puncture for transhepatic catheterization has been recommended in order to avoid injury to a major artery. In iatrogenic hemobilia a pseudoaneurysm develops within the liver parenchyma, and increasing pressure within the false cavity causes its contents to burst into an adjacent bile duct with subsequent gastrointestinal hemorrhage. In most cases blood enters the gastrointestinal tract in a fluid state and, because of the fibrinolytic capacity of the bile clots, rapidly dissolves (22). However, clot obstruction of the bile duct may occur, cause jaundice, and require removal by endoscopy or surgery. Retained clot fragments in the bile may lead later to choledocholithiasis (14).

Penetrating injuries and blunt abdominal trauma are other important causes of hemobilia. Stabbing may cause pseudoaneurysm formation with hemobilia, while bullets and missiles cause serious liver trauma. Blunt trauma with central liver rupture is now treated conservatively with CT scan monitoring. Perihepatic packing is used in serious liver injuries for a 48-hour period after which the packs are removed to avoid sepsis. Patients who continue to bleed with packs in situ usually have a traumatic arterial injury that is treated by embolization (9). Surgical hepatic arterial ligation has now been abandoned (9). Arterial injury by dissection or suturing at liver or biliary surgery causes an arteriovenous fistula or pseudoaneurysm that erodes into a bile duct. Usually the right hepatic artery is injured because of its location, or there is an anomalous artery present.

Intraoperative injury to ducts in the liver during the removal of intrahepatic stones may cause arterial injury with profuse hemobilia. Arteriosclerotic aneurysms of the hepatic artery are rare (11, 26). Incidental hepatic artery aneurysms discovered at diagnostic arteriography should be embolized if they are greater than 1.0 cm in diameter because of the dangers of rupture. Mycotic aneurysms are now rare except in intravenous drug users. These aneurysms are multiple and resemble those aneurysms seen in arteritis. Rarely, hemorrhage occurs from the gallbladder in systemic hypertension, hemocholecyst, from the cystic artery after perforation of a gallstone from the gallbladder into the duodenum or colon, or from the gallbladder during percutaneous cholecystostomy. Biliary hemorrhage in liver tumors is rare (18). Tropical hemobilia due to worm infestations of the bile ducts (common in the Orient) is rare in the United States and Europe.

Interventional Procedures in Hemobilia

Selective and superselective arteriography of the liver vessels is the definitive procedure for establishing the site of the bleeding artery. Superselective injection may show a lesion not shown by celiac injection. Selective embolization is the treatment of choice (Fig. 17.**1**). It is safer and preferable to surgery in life-threatening hemobilia.

The surgical alternatives include the need to identify the bleeding site on the operating table, hepatic artery ligation, or acute major liver resections, such as right or left hepatectomy or lobectomy. These are formidible emergency procedures in all but the major centers of liver surgery and carry a high morbidity and mortality.

Materials for Embolization in Hemobilia

Stainless Steel Coils

Stainless steel coils (minicoils and microcoils) may now be safely delivered via a 5-Fr or Tracker 18 (Target Therapeutics, La Jolla, Cal., USA) or a Mag 3-Fr catheter (Balt, France) using a guide wire as an introducer.

The coils are received from the manufacturer contained within a sheath that fits into the catheter hub. After expulsion into the artery, the coils reform in a diameter varying from 2 mm to 15 mm according to the size used. Coil size is determined by the diameter of the vessel to be embolized. Dacron strands attached to the coils act as a focus for thrombus formation, and the coil produces permanent vessel occlusion by caus-

ing an arteritis and a periarteritis (1, 3). The use of these coils is the fastest method of permanent vessel occlusion. They are suitable for therapy in hemobilia if selective catheterization of the vessel causing the hemorrhage can be achieved. Vessel occlusion occurs within 1–2 minutes as witnessed by contrast medium injection following embolization. The embolization catheter must lie distal to the origin of the cystic artery to prevent gallbladder necrosis. During multiple coil insertions a coil may lodge at the catheter tip and fail to pass into the artery. If this happens, the catheter is removed and replaced via the introducting sheath. Saline infusions through the catheter between insertions of coils may prevent failure of coil release. Coils are reliable, easy to introduce, and cost less than detachable balloons. Microcoils may be used via a Tracker 18 or Mag 3-Fr catheter to embolize the gastroduodenal artery or pancreaticoduodenal arteries in bleeding after sphincterotomy, but it is essential that the catheter tip lies in a selective position within these vessels. The modern version of the Gianturco Wallace Anderson coils cause permanent vessel occlusion and are easier to insert into the catheter and vessel being occluded than Gelfoam.

Gelfoam

Gelfoam strips *not Gelfoam powder* may also be used in the treatment of hemobilia. Gelfoam is a gelatin sponge that is available in sterile sheets that may be cut into strips of various sizes for injection through the selective hepatic catheter. The small strips are rolled into cylinders and placed in the catheter hub. The embolus is injected gently into the artery with saline. Gelfoam forms an intravascular matrix for throm-

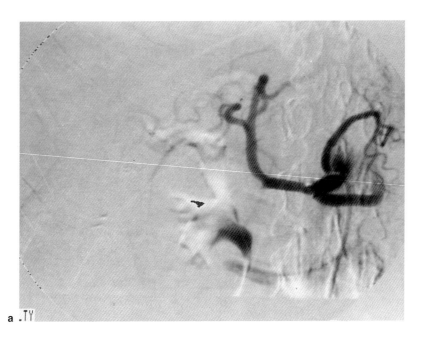

a .TY

Fig. 17.**1 Hemobilia following liver biopsy in primary biliary cirrhosis**
a Selective celiac arteriography shows normal arteries and absence of the right hepatic artery
b Superior mesenteric arteriography shows the right hepatic artery arising from this vessel and absence of opacification of the bleeding site. The patient had received 80 units of blood over 24 hours, and two previous arteriographic studies had failed to show the bleeding site
c The right hepatic artery was embolized with two minicoils. Hemobilia ceased and did not recur

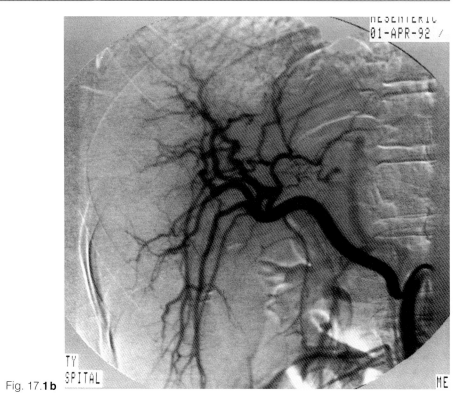

Fig. 17.**1b**

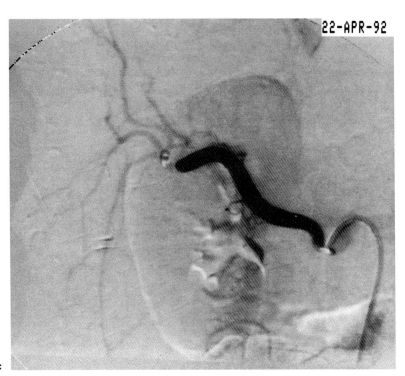

Fig. 17.**1c**

bus formation. The occlusion produced is not permanent. It lasts 3 to 5 weeks. Some authors recommend only inserting Gelfoam using a balloon catheter. The site of Gelfoam occlusion is less easy to demonstrate than that of the coil, which is radiopaque.

Other Occlusive Agents for Hemorrhage Control

Other occlusive agents include:

1. *Detachable miniballoons*
   Miniballoons have been used successfully in treating iatrogenic hemobilia from biliary drainage (2). Balloons as small as 1 mm in diameter are available. This method has been used extensively in neuroradiology.
   Balloon delivery catheter systems are expensive, and larger catheter systems are needed for balloon delivery (e.g., a 1-mm balloon is inserted on a 2-Fr catheter by a 9-Fr introducer catheter, and a 5- or 7-Fr catheter is used to dislodge the balloon). A 1-mm balloon is inflated with contrast medium to a maximum of 4 mm, or a 2-mm balloon is inflated to 8 mm maximum.
   Isotonic contrast medium is used for balloon inflation.
2. *Nondetachable balloon catheters*
   These catheters are used to safely introduce embolic material such as Gelfoam strips or liquid emboli and to prevent overspill into the general circulation or to directly occlude an artery.
3. *Polyvinyl alcohol (PVA Ivalon)*
   Ivalon is a plastic sponge material available as sheets, blocks, spheres, or powder. It expands on wetting. It is used in a similar fashion to Gelfoam.
4. *Bucrylate (isobutyl 2-cyanoacrylate)*
   Bucrylate is a suggested carcinogen and should only be used in life-threatening situations. It can be made opaque by adding tantalum powder or myodil. Contrast medium concentrations of 25–30% render it opaque to X-rays. It is injected by coaxial balloon catheter to prevent reflux of the embolic agent and to facilitate catheter changing if the embolizing catheter is blocked by bucrylate.
5. *Other embolic agents* are either obsolete (blood clot, tissue fragments) or not suitable as embolic agents for treating hemobilia (collagens, Ethibloc, silicon spheres, alcohol, hypertonic glucose, or other sclerosing agents).

Technique of Embolization

Informed consent is obtained from the patient or a close relative after explanation of the purpose of the investigation and treatment, the risks involved, the possible complications, and the benefits of a successful outcome. A *hematological screen* is obtained and any abnormalities corrected before proceeding. *Hy-dration of the patient* is maintained by intravenous fluids. Blood volume is corrected by transfusions. The patient in the acute situation is usually fasting. *Sedation and analgesia* are given as required.

Antibiotic cover is essential in all patients in whom embolization of the liver is performed. It is continued for 5–7 days depending on the presence of any liver ischemia. We perform DSA with a 7-Fr single curve catheter of the liver blood supply until the bleeding site is located.

The patency of the portal vein is established by arterial portography via splenic or superior mesenteric artery injection. Embolization of the hepatic artery distal to the gastroduodenal artery should only be performed if the portal vein is patent. *Hepatic segmental arteries may be embolized even if the portal vein is occluded.*

Selective studies of the hepatic, left gastric, superior mesenteric, and any anomalous arteries to the liver are performed rapidly with DSA.

The origin of the cystic artery is noted. Bleeding from the gastroduodenal artery is identified where appropriate after sphincterotomy.

When the site and cause of hemorrhage is demonstrated, embolization is performed with the catheter positioned as close as possible to the lesion. Microcoils injected through a Tracker 18 catheter inserted into the angiographic catheter allow positioning of the embolus at the bleeding site, thus avoiding the cystic artery (Fig. 17.**2**). Occlusion of the latter may produce gallbladder necrosis. After vessel occlusion all catheters are removed, and the patient is returned to the ward.

Complications of Embolization in Hemobilia

Gallbladder necrosis occurs if the cystic artery is occluded.

Hepatic pseudoaneurysms have a thin fragile wall and may *rupture* during embolization. This is diagnosed by extravasation of contrast medium at the site. When this occurs, emboli are introduced immediately to occlude the site of extravasation (16).

Hepatic necrosis is rare after coil occlusion of an aneurysm, pseudoaneurysm, or arteriovenous fistula when the portal vein is patent because of the rich interlobar anastomoses with the arterial supply of the liver, and the numerous collaterals to the liver via the inferior phrenic arteries, ascending arteries of the common bile duct, interhilar anastomoses, and other unnamed arteries.

Dissection of the hepatic artery during catheter positioning for embolization makes embolization impossible.

When this occurs, a fine needle may be inserted percutaneously directly into the liver lesion guided by color Doppler ultrasound and thrombin injections used to occlude the aneurysm (6, 11, 16).

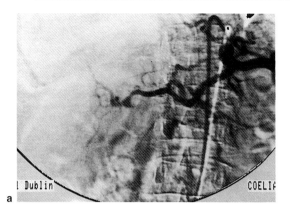

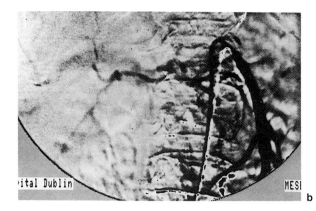

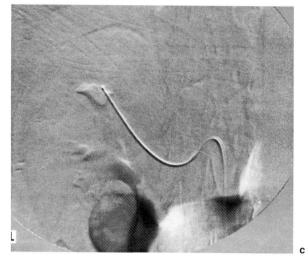

Fig. 17.**2   Hemobilia in an 87-year-old woman**
a Celiac arteriography was performed with difficulty because of arteriosclerosis
b Superior mesenteric arteriography also demonstrated aneurysm
c A Tracker catheter was inserted into the hepatic artery and a microcoil inserted. It failed to control hemorrhage. Cholecystectomy showed a gallstone eroding into the cystic artery. The patient made a successful recovery

Liver failure and/or renal failure are rare after successful careful embolization of the liver in hemobilia and are usually associated with tumor embolization.

When hemobilia is confirmed by endoscopy or cholangioscopy and a bleeding site is not demonstrated within the liver arteries after a careful search of all its arterial supply, we embolize the right or left lobe artery of the liver depending on the iatrogenic cause of the hemobilia.

References

1. Anderson JH, Wallace S, Gianturco C, Gerson LP. Mini Gianturco stainless steel coils for transcatheter vascular occlusion. Radiology 1979; 132:301–304.
2. Ayella RJ. An ideal catheter: the simple curve. Vasc Surg 1975; 3:147–150.
3. Barth KH, Strandberg JD, White RI Jr. Chronic vascular reactions to stainless steel coil occlusion devices. AJR 1978; 131:135–138.
4. Chung VP, Sos CS, Carrasco CH, Wallace S. Superselective catheterisation techniques in hepatic angiography. AJR 1983; 141:803–811.
5. Clements D, Nirula R, Evans A. Treatment of haemobilia by arterial embolisation. Hosp Update 1990; 16:928–929.
6. Cope C, Zeit R. Coagulation of aneurysms by direct percutaneous thrombin injection. AJR 1978; 147:383–387.
7. Czernik A, Thompson JN, Hemingway AP, et al. Hemobilia. A disease in evolution. Arch Surg 1988; 123:718–721.
8. Dan SHJ, Train JS, Cohen BA, Mitty HA. Common bile duct varices: cholangiographic demonstration of a hazardous portal systemic communication. Am J Gastroenterol 1983: 78:42–43.
9. Managing liver trauma conservatively [Editorial]. Lancet 1991; 338:1429–1430.
10. Glisson F. Anatomia hepatis, 1654.
11. Greiner N, Greselle JF, Douws C, et al. Hepatic artery aneurysms and pseudoaneurysms: diagnosis and percutaneous management with color flow Doppler ultrasound. Diag Intervent Radiol 1990; 2:115–118.

12. Holmlond D, Lundstrom B. Extrahepatic obstruction of the portal vein with bleeding from the gallbladder. Acta Radiol 1977; 18:680–684.
13. Levin DC. Catheters for selective arteriography: additional alternatives. Radiology 1983; 146:553–555.
14. Luzuy F, Reinberg O, Kauszlaric D, et al. Biliary calculi caused by haemobilia. Surgery 1987; 102:886–889.
15. Mitchell SE, Shumann R, Kaufman SL, et al. Biliary catheter drainage complicated by haemobilia. Radiology 1985; 157:645–648.
16. Mc Namara MP. Percutaneous procedures guided by color flow Doppler sonography. AJR 1989; 152:1123–1125.
17. Okazaki M, Ono H, Higashihara H, et al. Angiographic management of massive haemobilia due to iatrogenic trauma. Gastrointest Radiol 1991; 16:205–211.
18. Okazaki M, Higashihara H, Koganemaru F, et al. Intraperitoneal haemorrhage from hepatocellular carcinoma: emergency chemoembolisation or embolisation. Radiology 1991; 180:647–651.
19. Richardson A, Simmons K, Gutmann J, Little JM. Hepatic haemobilia nonoperative management in eight cases Aust NZ J Surg 1985; 55:447–451.
20. Salam, AA, Goldman M, Smith D, Hill HL. Gastric intestinal and gallbladder varices. South Med J 1979; 72:402–408.
21. Sandblom P. Haemorrhage into the biliary tract following trauma (traumatic haemobilia) Surgery 1948; 24:571–576.
22. Sandblom P. Iatrogenic haemobilia. Am J Surg 1986; 151:754–758.
23. Saeed M, Kadir S, Kaufmann SL, et al. Bleeding following endoscopic sphincterotomy; angiographic management by transcatheter embolisation. Gastrointest Endosc 1989; 35:300–303.
24. Seldinger SI. Catheter replacement of the needle in percutaneous arteriography. Acta Radiol 1953; 39:368–375.
25. Strickland SK, Khoury MB, Kiproff PM, et al. Cystic artery pseudoaneurysm: a rare cause of hemobilia. Cardiovasc Intervent Radiol 1991; 14:183–185.
26. Uflacker R. Transcatheter embolisation of arterial aneurysms. Br J Radiol 1986; 59:317–324.
27. Uflacker R, Mourai GS, Piske RL, et al. Haemobilia: transcatheter occlusive therapy and long term follow up. Cardiovasc Intervent Radiol 1989; 12:136–141.
28. Vlahos L, Kalovidouris A, Gouiliamos A, et al. Post-traumatic hemobilia. Eur J Radiol 1992; 13:199–201.
29. Walter JF, Passo BT, Cannon WB. Successful transcatheter embolic control of massive haematobilia secondary to liver biopsy. AJR 1976; 127:132–135.
30. Williams SM, Burnett DA, Mazer MJ. Radiographic demonstration of common bile duct varices. Gastrointest Radiol 1982; 7:69–70.
31. Yoshida J, Donoghue PE, Nyhus LM. Hemobilia: review of recent experience with a world wide problem. Am J Gastroenterol 1987; 82:448–453.

18 Portal Hypertension and Esophageal Varices

A. S. B. Chua and P. W. N. Keeling

The portal vein forms when the superior mesenteric vein joins the splenic vein. It receives tributaries from the stomach, intestine, spleen, and pancreas. Its main branches consist of the inferior mesenteric vein, the superior mesenteric vein, and the splenic vein, with lesser veins draining from the stomach.

The lower esophagus and the upper stomach is the site of anastomosis between the left gastric vein of the portal system and the azygous vein that drains into the vena cava of the systemic system. When portal hypertension develops, these vessels become engorged due to increased blood flow through them in an attempt to decompress the portal system. Portal hypertension is usually recognized only when a patient presents with one of its principal manifestations: ascites, variceal bleeding, or portosystemic encephalopathy.

Portal pressure is determined by the pressure in the portal vein or its branches and the pressure necessary to perfuse the liver. Portal hypertension results when there is increased portal blood flow, increased portal systemic resistance, or a combination of both. Under physiological conditions of vigorous exercise (decreases portal flow) and eating (increases portal flow), homeostatic mechanisms compensate for changes in portal blood flow to maintain portal pressure within a normal range by modulating portal vascular resistance. In the normal liver, only about 20% of the liver sinusoids are used at ordinary liver flows, but as more portal flow occurs, more sinusoids are used. Only when flow has achieved five to six times normal, and all sinusoids are used, is there an abrupt rise in portal pressure.

No amount of augmentation of the portal blood flow can account for portal hypertension if the liver is normal in the first place. One of the more common causes of portal hypertension is cirrhosis. In cirrhosis, the sinusoids are distorted with regenerative nodules and scar tissues causing the sinusoidal pressure to be elevated. It has also been postulated that the increased sympathetic activity associated with cirrhosis may also contribute to the elevated intrahepatic resistance to portal flow (47). A further factor in the maintenance of portal hypertension in cirrhosis is the presence of a hyperdynamic state (high cardiac output and low vascular resistance). The systemic circulation is characterized by peripheral vasodilation resulting in reduced peripheral vascular resistance and enhanced cardiac output while portal venous inflow increases as a result of increase splanchnic blood flow. The significant clinical complications of portal hypertension are presented in Table 18.1.

If esophagogastric varices did not form and bleed, portal hypertension would be of no clinical significance (34). Approximately one-third of patients with cirrhosis have esophageal varices, and about one-third of these patients bleed from them. Varices seldom bleed if portal pressure is less than 12 mmHg (7). However, there is no consistent evidence to show that rupture of the varices is a function of pressure increasing beyond this threshold. Factors that may assist in predicting that a varix may bleed include: the Child classification (Table 18.2) (group A less likely than group B or C), their size (the larger the varix the more likely it is to bleed), and several endoscopic signs (cherry red spots, red wale markings, and blue varices as opposed to white) (33, 43). An attractive theory to explain why varices rupture is based on the concept of variceal wall tension. This concept integrates local and hemodynamic factors when relating to variceal rupture. It uses LaPlace's equation:

$$T = P \times R/W$$

T = variceal wall tension, P = transmural pressure gradient, R = radius (size of varix), and W = wall thickness.

Thus, high pressure, a large varix, and thin walls are compounding factors leading to variceal rupture (1).

Bleeding from esophageal varices is a major cause of morbidity and mortality in chronic liver disease. Control of variceal bleeding involves first, methods of arresting an acute bleed and second, a more definitive management. The immediate management of acute variceal bleeding involves resuscitation measures such as blood transfusion, fresh-frozen plasma admin-

Table 18.1   Clinical complications of portal hypertension

Variceal bleeding
Ascites
Encephalopathy
Hypersplenism
Hepatorenal syndrome
Renal sodium and water retention
Altered enterohepatic circulation
Portal vein thrombosis

istration, and balloon tamponade. Blood transfusion is lifesaving, however, attempts to correct clotting factors and platelet count are of secondary importance in an emergency since their half-life is short and they are unlikely to affect variceal bleeding. Vitamin K i.m. should be routine. Stress-induced acute mucosal ulcers are frequent and ^{2}H-antagonist should be given.

The patient's condition must be stabilized; this is best achieved in the intensive care unit. Monitoring of pulmonary capillary wedge pressure is important to prevent overtransfusion and unnecessary overexpansion of blood volume and increasing portal pressures. Intravenous saline should not be used since it may induce edema and ascites. In addition, vasoactive drugs, emergency endoscopic sclerotherapy, and surgery have all been used successfully to arrest bleeding.

Acute Variceal Bleeding

The role of vasoactive drugs (vasopressin, glypressin, or somatostatin) in acute variceal bleeding remains controversial when endoscopic procedures are performed in many centers. Since endoscopy is the method of choice used in the diagnosis of upper gastrointestinal bleeding, endoscopic sclerotherapy is the first-choice treatment in stopping bleeding if variceal bleeding is found to be the cause of bleeding. However, there is a place for a drug that has few side effects and is effective in the interval before (to facilitate sclerotherapy) and after endoscopy (to prevent rebleeding). Intravenous glypressin, an analog of vasopressin, bolus injection of 2 mg every 4 hours (for 24–36 hours) was compared to placebo in a randomized study with 60 patients. In 28 of 31 glypressin patients, as opposed to only 17 of 29 placebo patients (P > 0.01), bleeding was arrested (35). The need for blood transfusion in the vasoactive therapy group was also reduced, and there was a significant difference in hospital mortality in favor of the treatment group. Nitrate vasodilators have been used to obviate the effects of glypressin on systemic circulation. Lin et al. (1990) demonstrated that all the abnormal systemic hemodynamic effects of glypressin induced by a 2-mg bolus dose were normalized by 0.6 mg of sublingual nitroglycerin (18).

The role of somatostatin or its analog, octreotide, remains unconfirmed. Two placebo-controlled studies reached opposite conclusions, however, two trials versus balloon tamponade showed that somatostatin is as effective as tamponade (2, 14).

Terblanche et al. (1989) recommended emergency endoscopic sclerotherapy, or if expertise is not available, drugs or balloon tamponade to control bleeding followed by sclerotherapy within 6–24 hours. The most commonly used balloon device is the Sengstaken–Blakemore tube. This device is inserted with both of the large balloons collapsed. It is pushed well

into the stomach, and the gastric balloon is inflated to prevent it being readily pulled into the esophagus. It may then be pulled back so that the gastric balloon is snug against the diaphragm (Fig. 18.**2**). This is the principle action that controls hemorrhage presumably by pressing the feeding veins (short gastric and coronary veins) against the diaphragm. The esophageal balloon may then be inflated for further compression. The tube is left in place for a maximum of only 24 hours because the pressure and pull cause tissue necrosis.

Emergency balloon tamponade has been shown to be superior to intravenous vasopressin/nitroglycerin in arresting active variceal bleeding in cirrhotics, but initial hemostasis does not guarantee survival in such patients (30% had recurrent bleeding within 72 hours, and there was a 30% early and late mortality) (41). Furthermore, if the balloon tamponade is inserted improperly, it has major side effects including asphyxiation, aspiration, esophageal erosions, ulceration, and rupture.

Injection Sclerotherapy

Endoscopic sclerotherapy, however, is more effective than balloon tamponade in controlling acute variceal bleeding (22). Sclerotherapy controls acute variceal bleeding in 80% to 90% of patients, however, rebleeding occurs in half of these patients within 2 years. Numerous studies show a better survival rate for those treated with sclerotherapy compared with those controls treated medically, but there are studies that show little difference between the two modalities. Such conflicting results arose from differing variables used in the studies including, different patient populations, different techniques of sclerotherapy, intravariceal versus paravariceal injection, and differences in the end point of sclerotherapy. The type of sclerosants used (5% ethanolamine oleate, 3% tetradecyl sulfate, and absolute alcohol) does not appear to be important, although alcohol has the advantages of low cost and availability (16). Sclerotherapy requires skill and is not without complications. Complications (strictures, ulceration, and perforation) associated with sclerotherapy vary in different centers and are clearly operator dependent (28, 36).

Sclerotherapy is followed by rebleeding in 50% of patients (usually prior to the variceal obliteration). In 40% of the patients with rebleeding, the etiology is esophageal ulceration. Sucralfate administration (1 g, four times daily) reduced the incidence of rebleeding, especially in patients with well-compensated hepatic reserve (45).

Sclerotherapy was originally performed with the rigid esophagoscopes, but now, flexible instruments are routinely used. A medium-sized endoscope, which can be angled within the esophagus, is ideal. Most operators use a "free-hand technique" with a standard endoscope and a flexible retractable sclerotherapy needle. The needle lies at the distal end of a long thin flexible plastic tube, whose proximal end is a luer connection. The whole device lies within an outer protective sheath through which the needle can be protruded and retracted.

The lower 5 cm of the esophagus is almost invariably the site of bleeding, and this area is also rich in large perforating vessels that supply the varices with blood from the periesophageal plexus (20). Sclerosants are injected into this area, starting close to the cardia and working upward for about 5 cm. Each injection consists of 1–2 mL of sclerosant, to a total of 15–30 mL. Precise placement of the needle within the varix (intravariceal) may improve results and lessen complications. Other endoscopists prefer injection into the lamina propria and submucosa along the varix, which will eventually produce a fibrous coat along the varix (paravariceal).

Comparing the two, intravariceal injection appears to be more effective in controlling active bleeding, faster at obliterating varices, and it requires fewer treatment sessions to achieve obliteration (30, 32). There appears to be little difference in the incidence of complications. Most patients probably end up with a combination of both intravariceal and paravariceal injection.

Sclerotherapy must be repeated every 2 weeks until the varices are obliterated (8). The ability to assess variceal pressure endoscopically could be a major aid in the evaluation of sclerotherapy and the prediction of rebleeding.

Endoscopic Variceal Ligation

Endoscopic variceal ligation using small elastic "O" rings appear to be effective in both emergency and elective treatment of esophageal varices. Stiegmann et al. (1992) in a randomized multicenter study, showed that patients with cirrhosis who have bleeding esophageal varices have fewer treatment-related complications and better survival rates when they are treated by esophageal ligation than when they are treated by sclerotherapy (37).

Variceal ligation is performed on patients who are actively bleeding or who have recently bled from the varices. The endoscope is passed with an overtube placed on the shaft of the endoscope. It is used to place the tube in the proper place within the esophagus. The overtube is semiflexible with a beveled distal tip and a rigid mouthpiece built in to the proximal end. It facilitates repeated passage of the endoscope without excessive trauma to the pharyngeal area. Once the overtube is in place, the endoscope is removed, the endoscopic variceal ligation device placed on its tip, and the whole thing repassed through the overtube into the distal esophagus.

The device is made up two plastic cylinders, a trip wire, and the small elastic O ring. The larger cylinder is fitted to the end of the endoscope, while the O ring is preloaded onto the smaller cylinder. The tripwire is passed through the biopsy channel and attached to the smaller cylinder. The smaller cylinder is then seated in the larger cylinder at the end of the scope. Pulling the trip wire in this setup will slide the smaller cylinder further into the larger one and strip off the O ring.

The endoscope tip is positioned over a variceal column, and suction is applied to draw the esophageal mucosa and varix up into the dead space created by the two cylinders at the endoscope tip. When the tissue is fully inside the cylinders, the trip wire is pulled and the O ring slips around the protruding varix. The endoscope is removed, reloaded with a fresh ring, and the procedure repeated.

The procedure is repeated as many times as needed until all varices are ligated at least once (this may vary from one to 12). The process is repeated after 1 week and every 2 weeks after that until all varices are visibly gone. The patients have repeat endoscopies every 3 to 6 months to ensure that no varices recur.

In the actively bleeding patient, variceal ligation has the advantage over injection sclerotherapy that the placement of the O ring need only be near a variceal column to be effective, while sclerotherapy should be done intravariceally if possible to avoid sclerosant causing necrosis in the esophageal wall. The overtube also protects the airway and prevents aspiration of the esophageal and gastric contents. Sinson et al. (1993) concluded that variceal banding is safe and effective and obliterates varices more quickly and with a lower rebleeding rate than injection sclerotherapy (5).

Emergency Surgery

Patients who do not respond either to sclerotherapy or to ligation should be considered for esophageal transection using the staple gun, or for portocaval shunting (39, 4). However, emergency surgical procedures carry a high mortality and morbidity risk and should be avoided whenever possible.

A portocaval shunt performed after the bleeding episode eliminates recurrent hemorrhage from varices (23). The mortality for grade C patients is 50%, and only 20% of survivors are alive 5 years later. Even in mild to moderate cirrhosis, this operation has a postoperative encephalopathy rate of 30% (44).

Emergency esophageal transection is performed using a staple gun. The stapling transection arrests hemorrhage in every patient and has a place in the emergency treatment of bleeding esophageal varices (19). However, a third of patients die from liver failure during this hospital admission.

Transjugular Intrahepatic Portosystemic Stent Shunts

More recently, transjugular intrahepatic portosystemic stent shunts (TIPSS) has been advocated as a safe and effective alternative for controlling acute bleeding (21, 27). This new development is exciting, and in 24 cases of the 343 cases reviewed, the indication was for acute bleeding varices. Twenty-three of the 24 acute bleeds were halted. However, controlled studies are needed to compare this technique with the more accepted modalities such as endoscopic ligation or sclerotherapy.

Liver Transplantation

Patients with cirrhosis and bleeding varices die from liver failure rather than blood loss per se. All the above-proposed treatment modalities do not cure the underlying cirrhosis. Survival rates of orthotopic liver transplantation have steadily improved, making it a viable option in the management of esophageal varices. Iwatsuki et al. (1988) reported an actuarial survival rate of 79% at 1 year and 71% at 5 years, regardless of the cause of cirrhosis (12). Patients with end-stage liver disease presenting with bleeding varices should be considered for liver transplantation as it is the only potentially curative treatment, especially if endoscopic sclerotherapy has failed. However, this is not routinely possible due to the limited number of liver donors and the high costs.

Prevention of Rebleeding from Varices

Long-term management of bleeding esophageal varices aims at reducing recurrent hemorrhage and improving survival. Patients who survived their episodes of variceal bleeding should be given some treatment to prevent rebleeding, either drug therapy, endoscopic sclerotherapy or ligation, surgery, or nonsurgical shunts.

Data from seven available randomized trials (748 patients total) that evaluated the effect of repeated endoscopic variceal sclerosis on the long-term survival of patients with variceal bleeding were assessed by meta-analysis. The patients had various causes of portal hypertension and varying severity of liver disease and were followed up for at least 1 year after the index bleed. Sclerotherapy patients received conventional treatment plus repeated sclerosis to achieve and maintain variceal obliteration, and controls received only conventional therapy. The results indicated that repeated sclerotherapy significantly improved survival when compared with conventional medical management of episodic bleeding (11). Endoscopic variceal rubber-band ligation is a newer technique and has been shown to have a relatively low incidence of complications and, in fact, is a safer alternative to standard sclerotherapy (6).

Sclerotherapy and beta-blockers are very similar, with mortality rates that are virtually the same and no significant difference in rebleeding rates (24, 31, 45). In addition, Jensen and Krarup (1990) demonstrated that the addition of propanolol during the period of sclerotherapy significantly reduces the incidence of variceal recurrence (15). Thus drug therapy could be considered as the first-choice treatment to prevent rebleeding because it is as good as sclerotherapy, avoids surgery, and has few side effects. Only four of the 52 patients treated with propranolol in King's College Hospital (45) had significant propranolol-related toxicity (impotence, dyspnea, encephalopathy, and complete heart block). However, 50% of patients rebled (24), and more effective drug therapy must be found. Furthermore, it will be interesting to see the results of a study comparing drug therapy with endoscopic variceal ligation.

In an uncontrolled prospective study by Paquet et al. (1989), Child grade A and B patients were selected for insertion of a distal splenorenal shunt after initial control of bleeding by sclerotherapy (25). Operative mortality in this selected group of patients was 8% and late mortality 12%. Five-year survival was 75% and encephalopathy, recurrent bleeding, or shunt thrombosis did not occur. Henderson et al.

Table 18.**2**   Child classification of cirrhosis in terms of hepatic functional reserve

Child grade	A	B	C
Degree of impairment	Minimal	Moderate	Severe
Serum bilirubin (mg/dL)	< 2.0	2.0–3.0	> 3.0
Serum albumin (g/dL)	> 3.5	3.0–3.5	< 3.0
Ascites	None	Easily controlled	Poorly controlled
Encephalopathy	None	Minimal	Advanced coma
Nutrition	Excellent	Good	Poor – wasting

(1990) studied 37 cirrhotic patients with recurrent variceal bleeding and biopsy-proven cirrhosis who randomly receeved sclerotherapy and 35 others who had distal splenorenal shunts (9). Crossover treatment was allowed if therapy failed. Survival was improved (P < 0.02) in the group receiving sclerotherapy despite the fact that 35% ultimately required shunts. Alcoholic cirrhotics who had sclerotherapy prior to surgery fared better than nonalcoholics treated with either sclerotherapy or shunting. They suggested that alcoholics with recurrent bleeding be treated with sclerotherapy first, then followed by shunting.

The innovative interventional radiologic technique of TIPSS has been quite revolutionary in the treatment of bleeding esophageal varices. McDermott et al. (1992) reviewed 343 patients (from 12 published abstracts), the majority of whom had the procedure performed because of recurrent bleeding from esophageal varices despite sclerotherapy (21). TIPSS was successful in decompressing portal hypertension in almost all cases. Thirty-six deaths were reported among the 343 patients; most were due to sepsis or multiorgan failure. Procedure-related complications were infrequent and included neck hematoma and bacteremia. TIPSS has already been used successfully in liver transplant candidates (37) and other groups are obtaining similar results (48). It may be the answer for both the acute and elective situation for the management of variceal bleeding in liver transplantation.

Prophylactic Therapy

Several controlled prospective studies have clearly shown that surgical decompressive shunting of varices that have not bled is contraindicated and of no value in patients with portal hypertension (3, 13, 29). The use of beta-blockers in the prevention of the first variceal bleed has been reported (10, 26, 42). The results using propanolol or nadolol appear favorable, especially in patients with well-compensated liver disease. Propanolol was effective in preventing variceal bleeding if the portal pressure was kept to less than 12 mmHg. Other promising pharmacological approaches to the management of portal hypertension are currently under evaluation. The role of calcium channel blockers, organic nitrates, serotonin blockers, or combination therapy of the above agents are presently being evaluated. Despite the publications of many controlled studies assessing the role of prophylactic sclerotherapy, there is still no definitive answer to this difficult question (17).

Conclusions

Different centers favor different management modalities, and the therapy practiced depends on the avail-

ability of resources and the endoscopist. We recommend initially stabilizing the patient and controlling the acute bleeding episode with vasopressin or glypressin and injection sclerotherapy with or without balloon tamponade. Sclerotherapy is then performed at two weekly intervals until the varices are obliterated. Thereafter, reassessment endoscopy is performed at 3 months, followed by endoscopic follow-up every 6 months. Patients should also be started on concurrent betablockers in a dose sufficient to maintain portal pressure at less than 12 mmHg. Patients in whom sclerotherapy has failed should be considered for liver transplantation. However, a transjugular intrahepatic portosystemic stent shunt could be inserted while the patient is waiting for a suitable donor organ.

References

1. Atterbury C, Groszmann RJ. Approach to the patient with cirrhosis and portal hypertension. In: Kelley WN, ed. Textbook of internal medicine. Philadelphia: JB Lippincott, 1989.
2. Averginos A, Klonis C, Rekoumis G, et al. A prospective randomized trial comparing somatostatin, balloon tamponade and the combination of both methods in the management of acute variceal haemorrhage. J Hepatol 1991; 13:78–83.
3. Conn HO, Lindenmuth WW. Prophylactic portocaval anastomosis in cirrhotic patients with oesophageal varices: interim results with suggestion for subsequent investigations. N Engl J Med 1968; 279:725–732.
4. Fleig WE, Stage F. Esophageal varices: Current therapy in 1989. Endoscopy 1989; 21:89–96.
5. Gimson AES, Ramage JK, Panos MZ, et al. Randomised trial of variceal banding ligation versus injection sclerotherapy for bleeding oesophageal varices. Lancet 1993; 242:391–394.
6. Goff JS, Reveille RM, et al. Endoscopic sclerotherapy versus endoscopic variceal ligation: Esophageal symptoms, complications and motility. Am J Gastroenterol 1988; 83(11):1240–1244.
7. Groszmann RJ, Bosch J, Grace ND, et al. Haemodynamic events in a prospective randomized trial of propanolol versus placebo in the prevention of a first variceal hemorrhage. Gastroenterology 1990; 99:1401–1407.
8. Higashi H, Kitaro S, Hashizuma M, et al. A prospective randomized trial of schedules for sclerosing esophageal varices. Hepatogastroenterology 1989; 36:337–340.
9. Henderson JM, Kutrer MH, et al. Endoscopic variceal sclerosis compared with distal splenorenal shunt to prevent recurrent variceal bleeding in cirrhosis. Ann Intern Med 1990; 112:262–269.
10. Ideo G, Bellati G, Fesco E, et al. Nadol can prevent the first gastrointestinal bleeding in cirrhosis: a prospective, randomized study. Hepatology 1988; 8:6–9.
11. Infante-Richard C, Esnaola S, et al. Role of endoscopic variceal sclerotherapy in the long term management of variceal bleeding: A meta-analysis. Gastroenterology 1989; 96:1087–1092.
12. Iwatsuki S, Starzl PE, Todo S, et al. Liver transplantation in the treatment of bleeding oesophageal varices. Surgery 1988; 104:697–706.
13. Jackson FC, Perrin E, Smith AG, et al. A clinical investigation of the portocaval shunt: survival analysis of the prophylactic operation. Am J Surg 1968; 115:22–25.
14. Jaramillo JL, DeLa Mata M, Mino G, et al. Somatostatin versus Sengstaken balloon tamponade for primary hemostasis of bleeding oesophageal varices. J Hepatol 1991; 12:100–105.
15. Jensen LS, Krarup N. Propanolol may prevent recurrence of oesophageal varices after obliteration by endoscopic sclerotherapy. Scand J Gastroenterol 1990; 25:352–356.

16. Kochler R, Goenka MK, Mehta S, et al. A comparison evaluation of sclerosants for oesophageal varices: a prospective randomized controlled study. Gastrointest Endosc 1990; 36:127–130.
17. Korula J. Prophylactic sclerotherapy. J Gastroenterol Hepatol 1988; 4:589–591.
18. Lin HC, Tsai YT, Lee FY, et al. Systemic and vasopressin plus nitroglycerin administration in patients with hepatitis B related cirrhosis. J Hepatol 1990; 10:370–374.
19. McCormack PA, Kaye GL, Greenslade L, et al. Oesophageal staple transection as a salvage procedure after failure of acute injection sclerotherapy. Hepatology 1992; 15:403.
20. McCormack TT, Rose J, Smith PM, et al. Perforating veins and blood flow in oesophageal varices. Lancet 1983; II:1442–1444.
21. McDermot V. Bleeding oesophageal varices and transjugular intrahepatic portosystemic shunting. Lancet 1992; 340:1231.
22. Moreto M, Zabaka M, et al. A randomized trial of tamponade or sclerotherapy as immediate treatment for bleeding oesophageal varices. Surg Gynecol Obstetr 1988; 167:331–334.
23. Orloff MJ, Bell RH Jr, Greenburg AG. Prospective randomized trial of emergency portocaval shunt and medical therapy in unselected cirrhotic patients with bleeding varices. Gastroenterology 1986; 90:1754.
24. Pagliaro L, Burroughs AK, Sorensen T, et al. Therapeutic controversies and randomized controlled trials (RCTs): prevention of bleeding and re-bleeding in cirrhosis. Gastroenterol Int 1989; 2:71–84.
25. Paquet KJ, Mercado MA, Koussouris P, et al. Improved results with selective distal splenorenal shunt in a highly selected population. Ann Surg 1989; 210:184–189.
26. Pascal JP, Cales P, multicentre study group. Propanolol in the prevention of first upper gastrointestinal tract hemorrhage in patients with cirrhosis of the liver and oesophageal varices. N Engl J Med 1987; 317:856–861.
27. Perarnau JM, Noelge G, Rossle M. Transjugular intrahepatic portosystemic stent-shunt: early results with an improved technique [abstract]. J Hepatol 1991; 13 (suppl 2):S59.
28. Pilay P, Starzl TE, Van Thiel DH. Complications of sclerotherapy for oesophageal varices in liver transplant candidates. Transplant Proc 1990; 22:2149–2151.
29. Resnick RH, Chalmers TC, Ishihana, et al. A controlled study of the prophylactic portocaval shunt: a final report. Ann Intern Med 1969; 70:675–688.
30. Rose JDR, Crane MD, Smith PM. Factors affecting successful endoscopic sclerotherapy for oesophageal varices. Gut 1983; 24:946–949.
31. Rossi V, Cales P, Burtin P, et al. Prevention of recurrent variceal bleeding in alcoholic cirrhotic patients: prospective controlled trial of propanolol and sclerotherapy. J Hepatol 1991; 12:283–289.
32. Sarin SK, Nand R, Sachder G, et al. Intravariceal versus paravariceal sclerotherapy. A prospective, controlled randomized trial. Gut 1987; 28:657–662.
33. Sarin SK, Sundaram KR, Ahuja RK. Predictors of variceal bleeding: an analysis of clinical, endoscopic and haemodynamic variables, with special references to intravariceal pressure. Gut 1989; 30:1757–1764.
34. Sherlock S. Oesophageal varices. Am J Surg 1990; 160:9–13.
35. Soderlund C, Magnusoon I, Tongren S, et al. Terlipressin (Triglycyl-lysine vasopressin) controls acute bleeding oesophageal varices: a double-blind randomized placebo-controlled study. Scand J Gastroenterol 1990; 25:622–630.
36. Soehendra N, Grimm H, Maydeo A, et al. Endoscopic sclerotherapy: personal experience. Hepatogastroenterology 1991; 38:220–223.
37. Sterneck M, Ring E, Gordon R, et al. Intrahepatic portocaval shunt: a bridge to liver transplantation in patients with refractory bleeding. Gastroenterology 1991; 100:A801.
38. Stiegmann GV, Goff JS, Patrice A, et al. Endoscopic sclerotherapy compared with endoscopic ligation for bleeding oesophageal varices. N Engl J Med 1992; 326:1527–1532.
39. Terblanche J, Burroughs AK, Hobbs KEF. Controversies in the management of bleeding oesophageal varices. N Engl J Med 1989; 320:1393–1398.
40. Terblanche J, Burroughs AK, Hobbs KEF. Controversies in the management of bleeding oesophageal varices. N Engl J Med 1989; 320:1469–1475.
41. Teres J, Planas R, et al. Vasopressin/nitroglycerin infusion vs. oesophageal tamponade in the treatment of acute variceal bleeding. Hepatology 1990; 11:964–968.
42. The Italian multicentre project for propanolol in prevention of bleeding in cirrhotic patients with large varices. A multicentre randomized clinical trial. Hepatolog 1988; 8:1–5.
43. The North Italian Endoscopic Club for the study and treatment of oesophageal varices. Prediction of the first variceal hemorrhage in patients with cirrhosis of the liver and oesophageal varices. N Engl J Med 1988; 319:983–989.
44. Villenueve JP, Pomier-Layrargues G, Duguay L, et al. Emergency portacaval shunt for variceal hemorrhage. Ann Surg 1987; 206:48.
45. Westaby D, Polson RJ, et al. A controlled trial of oral propanolol compared with injection sclerotherpy for the long-term management of variceal bleeding. Hepatology 1990; 11:353–359.
46. Westaby D, Polson RJ, Gimson AES, et al. Sucralfate for the prevention of early rebleeding following injection sclerotherapy for oesophageal varices. Hepatology 1989; 10:279–282.
47. Willet IR, Esler M, Jennings G, et al. Sympathetic tone modulates portal venous pressure in alcoholic cirrhosis. Lancet 1986; 1:939–942.
48. Zemel G, Ketzen BT, Becker GJ, et al. Percutaneous transjugular porto-systemic shunt. JAMA 1991; 266:390–393.

19 Transhepatic Portal Systemic Intrahepatic Stent Shunts (TIPSS)

Surgically created portal systemic shunts of many types have been used in the past to lower portal pressure and prevent hemorrhage from esophageal varices (8). The arrival of endoscopic sclerotherapy and its success in arresting variceal bleeding markedly reduced the need for such operations. Endoscopic variceal ligation introduced in recent years is reported to be more effective than injection sclerotherapy in obliterating varices (Fig. 19.1). Sclerotherapy or ligation of varices do not, however, reduce portal pressure or prevent new varices developing in the esophagus with recurrence of bleeding. Sclerotherapy of gastric varices can lead to serious complications. Failure to control bleeding by sclerotherapy and variceal ligation and recurrent variceal hemorrhages are indications for percutaneous stent shunt insertion as an alternative to a surgical shunt (2, 5, 8, 11). Neither portal vein thrombosis nor hepatic vein disease are absolute contraindications to the TIPSS procedure (9). The TIPSS procedure has also been used in the treatment of intractable ascites (4). The TIPSS procedure is a minor interventional procedure in comparison with mesocaval or distal splenorenal surgical shunt procedures.

Preparation for Percutaneous Stent Shunts

Coagulation abnormalities and low serum albumin levels should be corrected. The presence of ascites is not a contraindication to this procedure.

Technique of Shunt Insertion
(Figs. 19.1–19.3)

Before the procedure we use arterial portography to demonstrate the portal venous anatomy following superior mesenteric and splenic arteriography. A hepatic artery injection is used to exclude a vascular liver tumor or demonstrate reversed flow in the portal vein. The *bifurcation of the portal vein* in the liver is identified by ultrasound and the abdominal wall at the site marked with a metal marker to aid needling of the portal vein in the liver from the hepatic vein. Adequate i.v. analgesia and sedation are given and maintained during the procedure. Gentamycin, i.v., is given before the procedure and continued for 3 days (4).

The stent insertion procedure is summarized in Table 19.1.

1. Puncture of the Jugular Vein

The right internal jugular vein is punctured 4 cm below the angle of the mandible under local anesthesia using a sterile technique. The vein lies lateral and posterior to the carotid artery at this level. The vein is punctured anterior to the sternomastoid muscle while the carotid artery is displaced medially by the fingers of the left hand. The left internal jugular vein may also be used if the right vein is occluded for any reason, such as previous central line catheter insertions.

2. Introduction of a Vascular Sheath

After dilating the needle track into the internal jugular vein, the Seldinger technique is used to introduce over a guide wire a 10-Fr *vascular sheath on its dilator* into the inferior vena cava. All subsequent manipulations

Table 19.1   Hepatic–portal stent shunt procedure

1. **DSA portography** via splenic and superior arteries
2. **Mark the portal vein bifurcation** in the liver using ultrasound
3. **Catheterize the right jugular vein**
4. Insert a **10-Fr vascular sheath** into the IVC
5. Insert a **5-Fr angiographic catheter** into an hepatic vein
6. Insert a **16-gauge needle** into the hepatic vein
7. Puncture a **right main portal vein** in the liver
8. Insert a **guide wire into the portal/superior mesenteric vein**
9. Insert a catheter over the guide wire into the portal vein and **measure portal pressure**
10. Insert an angioplasty balloon catheter into the portal vein and **dilate the shunt track**
11. Insert a **metal stent or stents across the track dilate stent** to 8–10-mm diameter
12. **Measure portal vein pressure**

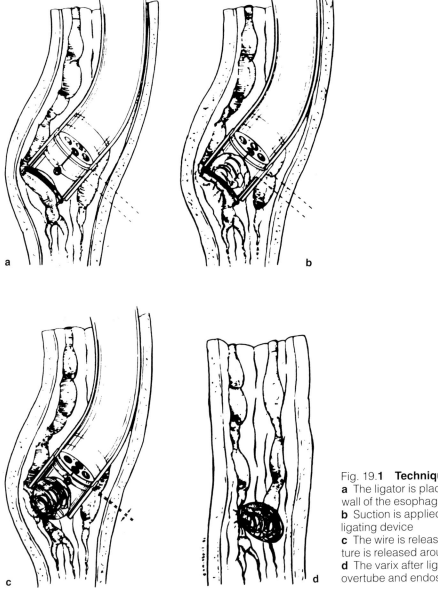

Fig. 19.**1   Technique of variceal ligation**
a The ligator is placed adjacent to the varix in the wall of the esophagus
b Suction is applied to draw the varix into the ligating device
c The wire is released, and the elastic band ligature is released around the varix
d The varix after ligation and withdrawal of the overtube and endoscope

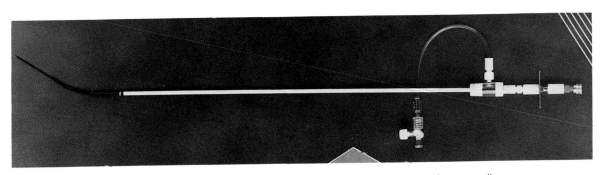

Fig. 19.**2   Equipment for TIPSS insertion** including 5-Fr catheter and transjugular catheter needle

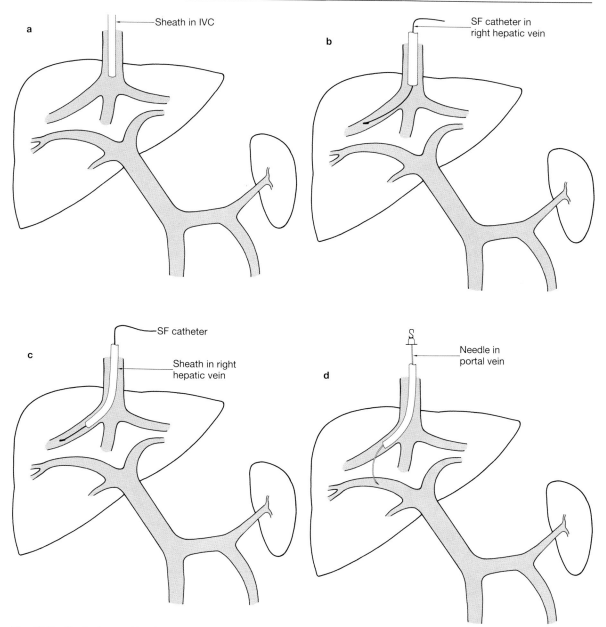

Fig. 19.**3** **Technique of TIPSS insertion**
a The internal jugular vein is catheterized and a 10-Fr vascular sheath is introduced over a guide wire into the inferior vena cava
b A 5-Fr angiographic catheter is now inserted via the sheath into a right or middle hepatic vein
c The sheath is now inserted into the hepatic vein over the catheter
d The needle is inserted through the sheath for 3–4 cm into the liver parenchyma with its tip directed anteriorly. Aspiration is performed as the needle is withdrawn until good blood flow occurs into the syringe, and contrast agent is injected to confirm that a suitable portal vein has been entered

(Continued on pp. 196/197)

are performed via this sheath. All catheter and guide wire manipulations are performed while monitoring carefully by fluoroscopy.

A 5-Fr angiographic catheter is now used to catheterize a suitable right or middle hepatic vein, and the vascular sheath is advanced into the hepatic vein.

3. Puncturing an Intrahepatic Portal Vein

A 16-gauge reverse-bevel curved transjugular liver biopsy needle (Cook, Denmark) is now introduced via the sheath into the hepatic vein and the needle tip exposed. The needle is inserted 3–5 cm into the right

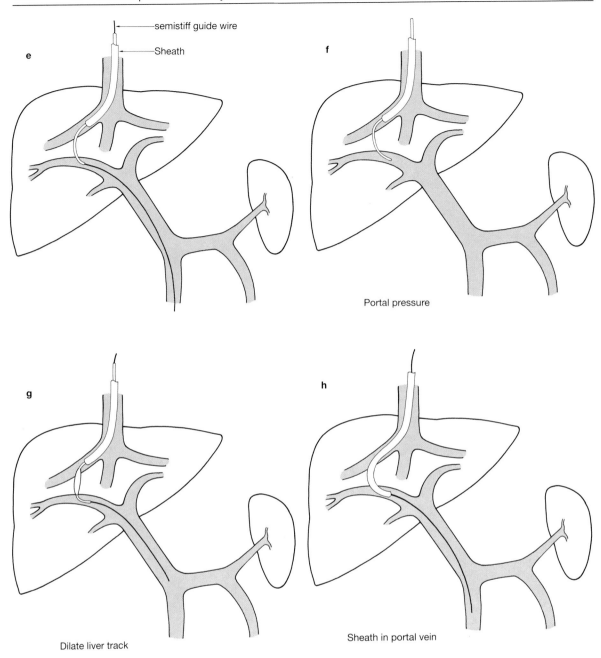

lobe in an anterior and medial direction from the hepatic vein 3–4 cm from its entrance into the inferior vena cava. This is done using fluoroscopy and a skin marker on the anterior abdominal wall at the level of portal vein bifurcation. Remembering that the portal vein bifurcation is outside the liver, efforts are made to needle the right main branch or the anterior segmental branch of the portal vein within the liver. The needle is aspirated while it is slowly withdrawn from the liver parenchyma until good blood flow occurs into the syringe. Contrast medium is now injected to assess the vein entered. The procedure is repeated if necessary until a suitable portal vein is entered. This is the most difficult part of this procedure. Once a suitable vein is catheterized in the liver, a semistiff long (160 cm) guide wire is inserted through the needle into the splenic or superior mesenteric vein. The needle is removed and a catheter passed over the

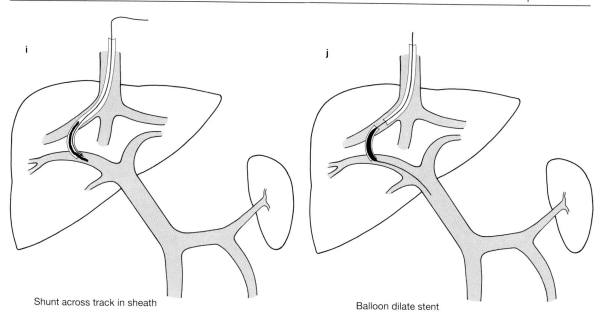

i

Shunt across track in sheath

j

Balloon dilate stent

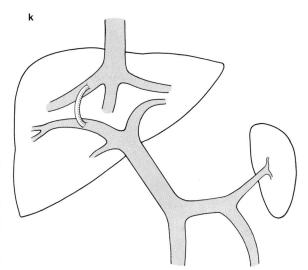

k

Fig. 19.**3**
e A semistiff guide wire is inserted into the splenic or superior mesenteric vein and portal vein
f IVC pressures are measured
g An 8-mm balloon catheter is inserted across the liver track until the balloon waist is no longer visible
h The sheath is advanced into the portal vein
i The stent shunt is inserted through the sheath taking care to position the end of the stent distally within the portal vein lumen and proximally within the hepatic vein or inferior vena cava
j The stent is dilated according to post–shunt pressure measurements
k The balloon catheter for stent dilatation and the sheath are withdrawn from the venous system, and the neck area is compressed for 5 minutes

guide wire into the portal vein, and the portal pressure is recorded.

4. Portal Pressure Measurements

Portal pressures are now measured in the main portal vein. Using a hand injection of contrast medium, a portal venogram is performed to study the number, sites, and direction of flow in portal branch collaterals. The

portal pressure measurement at this stage is essential in order to assess the degree of pressure reduction by the subsequent shunt.

5. Liver Track Preparation for Stent Insertion

An 8-mm angioplasty balloon is now inserted via the sheath on the semistiff guide wire into the portal vein and positioned across the parenchymal track. The balloon is inflated until the waist created by the track is no longer visible. Next, the sheath is advanced through the track into the portal vein.

6. Stent Shunt Insertion

The balloon angioplasty catheter is removed, and one or more (usually two) Palmaz stents are inserted across the track with the first stent tip lying within the portal vein and the second stent tip lying proximally in or adjacent to the inferior vena cava. Using a single long stent reduces the cost of the procedure. Dick et al (1992) used a 6 cm Wallstent (3). The stents are dilated by balloon catheter to 8–10 mm according to portal pressure measurements. The portal pressure after stent insertion should be reduced to 10–12 mmHg. Stent dilatation reduces its length. Allowance should be made for this during track stenting. Following successful stent deployment, a portogram is performed by injecting contrast medium into the main portal vein, and a record of the stent shunt obtained. Opacification of any gastroesophageal collaterals requires sclerosis of these veins. This is easily performed before sheath removal by selective injections of 100% alcohol. The catheter and vascular sheath are removed and the jugular puncture site in the neck compressed for 5–10 minutes. The patient is monitored for bleeding and, in the absence of complications, is discharged within 3 days.

Complications of Stent Shunts

The TIPSS procedure performed under local anesthesia carries a very low procedure-related complication rate when performed without percutaneous transhepatic portal vein catheterization.

During the search for a suitable portal vein branch within the liver, puncture of a bile duct or an artery may occur and lead to intrahepatic biloma or hematoma. *Intrahepatic biloma* should not occur if the biliary tract is unobstructed. Puncture of an artery with *intrahepatic hematoma* formation should not occur if stabbing motions are not used when the transparenchymal needle search for a suitable portal vein is performed. If an unsuitable hepatic vein is chosen for shunt insertion the needle may perforate the liver capsule. This is recognized immediately on contrast medium injection. The needle is withdrawn, another more central vein is chosen, and there are usually no ill effects, but in a small cirrhotic liver, *hemoperitoneum* may occur. We no longer use percutaneous transhepatic portal catheterization for portal vein localization because it may lead to death from hemorrhage (9, 11).

Delayed complications of TIPSS include *shunt stenosis* due to intimal growth through the wire mesh of the stent. This is treated by angioplasty or insertion of a second stent. Intimal hyperplasia may occur at the stent margins in the hepatic vein and cause stenosis or *occlusion of the shunt*. Careful positioning of the stent shunt so that its hepatic vein end lies adjacent to or within the hepatic inferior vena cava may prevent or delay proximal intimal hyperplasia. Because of the known risk of these two complications, it is essential to monitor stent shunts regularly with ultrasound, on which stent narrowing within the liver can be easily detected. Doppler studies also can be used to detect stent occlusion. Stent occlusion may be treated by re-stenting through the occluded lesion. Experience to date indicates that a stent shunt requires monitoring for life or until successful liver transplantation is performed. *Hepatic encephalopathy*, a recognized complication of surgical stents, also occurs after successful portal decompression by TIPSS and is related to failure of liver perfusion by diversion of portal blood away from the liver (7, 9).

Stent Shunt Follow-up

In the asymptomatic patient regular follow-up by Doppler ultrasound following TIPSS is essential. This should be performed monthly for 3 months, then every 3 months for 1 year. At the end of the first 6 months, phlebography is performed to assess shunt patency more accurately than with ultrasound, and any stenosis of the stent is treated by balloon angioplasty. This procedure is repeated at 12 months and at regular intervals or earlier if ultrasound findings differ from the previous examination. Excellent records of stent position, stent diameters along the shunt length, and blood velocity through the stent are essential. Recurrence of ascites previously absent may be an early indication of stenosis of the stent. Stent shunt insertion increases portal flow velocity as demonstrated by Doppler ultrasound. Intrahepatic portal flow is demonstrated, and the direction of flow in the intrahepatic portal veins is readily shown. Reversed flow in these veins contributes to hepatic encephalopathy reported after TIPSS. Portal vein thrombosis does not occur. Normal directional flow also occurs in the hepatic vein used for stent shunt insertion and in the hepatic vein's tributaries. A successful shunt insertion should decompress all gastroesophageal collaterals in order to prevent further variceal hemorrhage. Ultrasound is not valuable for assessing these collateral vessels after shunt procedures. This may only be achieved by catheter studies via the shunt or if necessary by percutaneous splenoportography, which does not produce the artifacts observed during catheter studies via the stent following high- or low-pressure contrast injections (7, 9). Catheter studies and ultrasound have a complimentary role in assessing the results and complications of percutaneous transjugular hepatic portal vein stent shunts (7, 12, 13).

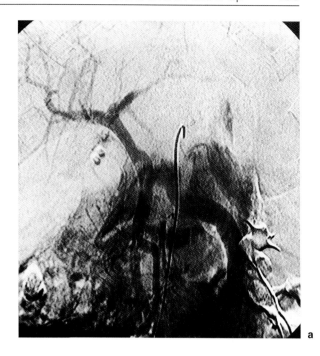

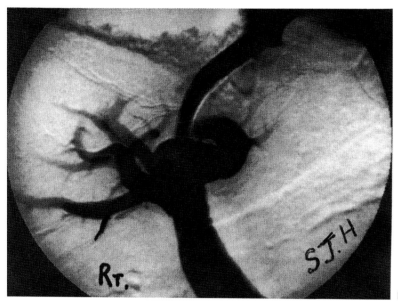

Fig. 19.**4   a Advanced alcohol cirrhosis in a 46-year-old man.** Arterial portography shows a small liver and patent portal vein and numerous lower abdominal collaterals. Sclerotherapy had failed to control hemorrhage **b** TIPSS inserted from the right hepatic vein. Bleeding did not recur

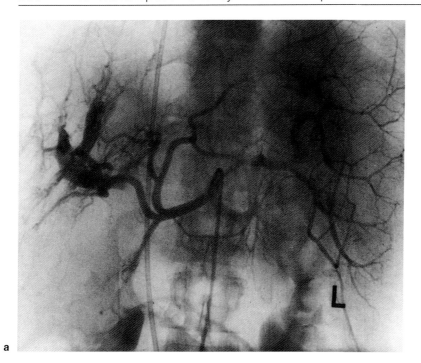

a

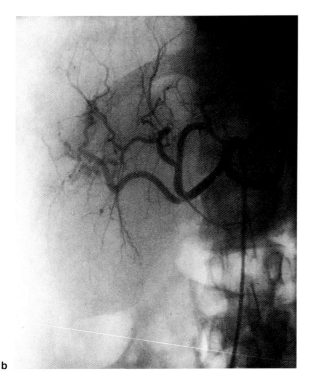

b

Fig. 19.**5   a A 52-year-old woman with a known case of Crohn disease developed portal hypertension after liver biopsy.** Arterial portography showed splenomegaly and an intrahepatic artery–portal vein fistula
b The right hepatic artery was embolized with Gelfoam strips and a repeat arteriogram at 1 week shows closure of the A/V fistula

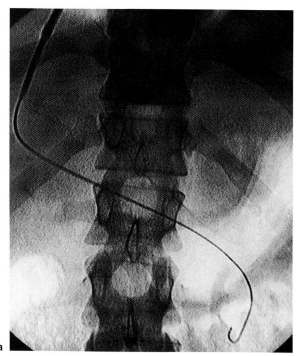

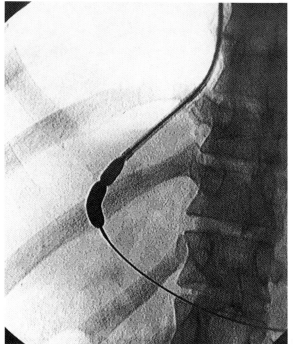

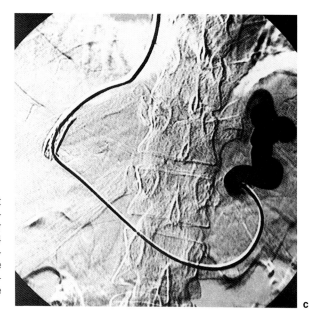

Fig. 19.**6** **a** Catheterization of the portal vein via the right hepatic vein. **b** Hepatic–portal liver track dilatation by balloon catheter. **c** Palmaz stent inserted across the liver track shunt. **d** Transjugular portal hepatic venogram at 4 weeks showing shunt patency. The patient was a 45-year-old alcoholic man with portal hypertension and massive gastric varices. Sclerotherapy had failed to control hemorrhage. The latter has not recurred up to 6 months after the TIPSS procedure

(Continued on p. 202)

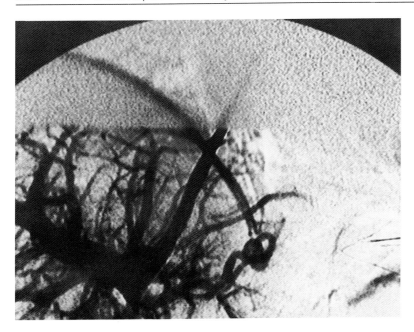

Fig. 19.**6d**

References

1. Becker CD, Cooperberg PL. Sonography of the hepatic vascular system. AJR 1988; 150:999–1005.
2. Chambers N, Readhead DN, Simpkin KJ, Hayes PC. Transjugular intrahepatic portosystemic stent shunts: Early clinical experience. Clin Radiol 1992; 46:166–169.
3. Dick R, Mc Cormick PA, Burroughs AK. Transjugular intrahepatic portosystemic stent shunt: which metal stent. Clin Radiol 1993; 47:143–144.
4. Grant EG, Tessler FN, Gomes AS, et al. Color Doppler imaging of portosystemic shunts AJR 1990; 154:393–397.
5. Hederstrom E, Forsberg L, Ivanek K, et al. Ultrasonography and Doppler duplex compared with angiography in the follow up of mesocaval shunt patency. Acta Radiol 1990; 31:341–345.
6. Laberge JM, Ferrell LD, Ring EJ, et al. Histopathological study of transjugular intrahepatic portosystemic stent shunts. JVIR 1991; 2:549–556.
7. Longo JM, Bilbao JI, Rousseau HP, et al. Transjugula intrahepatic portosystemic shunt: Evaluation with Doppler sonography. Radiology 1993; 186:529–534.
8. Pugh RN, Murray-Lyon IM, Dawson JL, et al. Transection of the oesophagus for bleeding oesophageal varices. Br J Surg 1973; 560:646–649.

9. Radosevich PM, Ring EJ, LaBerge JM, et al. Transjugular intrahepatic portosystemic shunts in patients with portal vein occlusion. Radiology 1993; 186:523–527.
10. Ralls PW. Color Doppler sonography of the hepatic artery and portal venous system. AJR 1990; 155:517–522.
11. Richter GM, Noeldge G, Palmaz JC, Roessle M. The transjugular intrahepatic portosystemic stent shunt. Results of a pilot study. Cardiovasc Intervent Radiol 1990; 13:200–207.
12. Ring EJ. Interventions in portal hypertension, In: Mueller PR, VanSonnenberg E, Becker GJ, eds. Syllabus: a diagnostic categorial course in interventional radiology. RSNA Chicago: 1991; 219–227.
13. Ring EJ, Lake JR, Roberts JP, et al. Using transjugular intrahepatic portosystemic shunts to control variceal hemorrhage before liver transplantation. Ann Intern Med 1992; 116:304–309.
14. Rosch J, Hanafee WN, Snow H. Transjugular portal venography and radiological portal caval shunt: an experimental study. Radiology 1969; 92:1112–1114.
15. Zemel G, Ketzen BT, Becker GJ, et al. Percutaneous transjugular porto-systemic shunt. JAMA 1991; 266:390–393.

Index